D1469291

PRAISE FOR
BILL KATOVSKY:

"A great, funny page-turner that you simply don't expect . . . It's packed with excellent advice on training, diet, and injury prevention . . . [and] the anecdotes and biographies are so enjoyable and well-told that I came away both enriched by newfound fitness knowledge and by the people I 'met' in the book and the examples they set."

—Michael Frank, Deputy Editor, *Bicycling and Mountain Bike*

"*Bike for Life* could be the most important book in your life. This informative and entertaining read gives solid advice and soaring inspiration for riders of all abilities."

—Sal Ruibal, *USA Today* cycling writer

"What a great book! . . . The concept of using cycling to stay young is being proven by the stars and regular folk interviewed in *Bike for Life* and many thousands more every day. To ride a century when you turn 100 can and should be everyone's goal after reading this book."

—Steve Boehmke, Mountain Bike Hall of Fame inductee

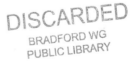

RETURN TO
FITNESS

RETURN TO
FITNESS

Getting Back in Shape after Injury,
Illness, or Prolonged Inactivity

BILL KATOVSKY

Da Capo
LIFE
LONG

A MEMBER OF THE PERSEUS BOOKS GROUP

Designed by Pauline Brown
Set in 10.5 point Utopia Std by the Perseus Books Group

Library of Congress Cataloging-in-Publication Data

Katovsky, Bill.
   Return to fitness : getting back in shape after injury, illness, or prolonged inactivity / Bill Katovsky.
      p. cm.
   Includes bibliographical references and index.
   ISBN 978-0-7382-1231-9 (alk. paper)
1. Physical fitness. 2. Sports injuries. 3. Health I. Title.
   GV481.K37 2010
   613.7—dc22

                                                2010023405

First Da Capo Press edition 2010

Published by Da Capo Press
A Member of the Perseus Books Group
www.dacapopress.com

Da Capo Press books are available at special discounts for bulk purchases in the United States by corporations, institutions, and other organizations. For more information, please contact the Special Markets Department at the Perseus Books Group, 2300 Chestnut Street, Suite 200, Philadelphia, PA 19103, or call (800) 255-1514, or e-mail special.markets@perseusbooks.com.

10 9 8 7 6 5 4 3 2 1

To Phil Maffetone
who showed me the way back

CONTENTS

CONTENTS

INTRODUCTION

I looked up at Mount Tam, its East Peak poking out of the clouds and mist, and then reflexively turned away. Instead I stared down at the muddy ground, feeling deep shame and embarrassment. Yes, I had been to the top of this revered San Francisco Bay Area mountain. Many times, in fact—running, biking, hiking. That was all in the past, but memories mocked the present. I now existed near Tam's bottom—emotionally and physically. I had betrayed more than just the mountain; I had been disloyal to my body. As I walked the few hundred yards back home, I asked myself, "Will I ever make it to the summit again?"

I was not the same young buck who could run for several hours on the mountain or who twice finished the Hawaii Ironman or who biked solo across America in his early twenties. In the space of several years right after I turned forty, I'd look in the mirror and be shocked to see this middle-aged stranger staring back. I felt like a victim of identity theft. Who was that imposter with a receding hairline, protruding gut, and mini–man boobs? Whatever happened to the hard-bodied college grad who successfully auditioned to become a nude model for a drawing class at Lake Tahoe Community College because the female art instructor needed a "muscular-looking male?"

I had once been a multisport athlete regularly drawn to the addictive rush of endorphins—trail running, swimming from Alcatraz, snowshoeing, adventure racing, kayaking, backpacking, mountain biking, road cycling. Then my athletic world collapsed. The decline didn't happen all at once, but was the direct consequence of a steady erosion of motivation that ended in my losing all interest in exercise. Apart from taking one- or two-mile walks every now and then, I saw little point in working out. It was much easier to remain slothful and indolent.

I didn't break a sweat for nearly a decade. Muscles dissolved. My body went softer than Silly Putty. I started wearing baggy clothes to cloak an increasingly pear-shaped physique. Being sedentary worsened my depression. Even though I didn't smoke or drink, and I was only about twenty pounds overweight, it was soul-shattering to discover how unfit I had become. One Christmas morning, as a grim yet perverse experiment to see how far I had fallen, I decided to go jogging. Gasping, lurching, and rubbery-legged, I went one hundred yards before stopping. There was no more gas in my tank. I was forty-nine years old.

Throughout this inactive period, a pesky inner voice kept insisting, "Stop making excuses *and* start exercising!" But the plea went unheeded because I first had to liberate myself from all the jostling inner demons intent on snuffing out resolve and desire. Only when I finally made a conscious decision to get back in shape—and then put that thought into action—was I able to reverse the physical meltdown.

Return to Fitness is a memoir of my struggle to reclaim a semblance of my expired athleticism. It is also a guide to help others learn how to recapture their former fitness, or become fit for the first time. These complementary aspects are braided together with the hope that my journey and the knowledge I've picked up along the way will serve to inspire and educate. Because fitness is a moving target, defined by natural ability, age, temperament, and self-discipline, the information found in these pages can apply to anyone who once abandoned exercise, whether it was a precipitous freefall or a more lackadaisical slide.

The precise reason for your layoff is immaterial. As is how many years you've been idle. You might have played high school and college sports, but then work and family responsibilities took over your life. Instead of being able to play hoops or soccer, you get winded climbing stairs or taking out the trash. Or you might have once been a recreational or competitive runner, but an injury caused you to leave the sport.

Yet you'd love to return to that earlier more vital and athletic phase of your prime—only you don't know how or think it's too difficult to achieve. Trust me, it isn't. I've been there.

As pitiful as my own fitness decline was, it was *not* irreversible. The entire healing or rebirthing process to get back in shape took nearly two years— punctuated early on by various extended periods of illness and injury. Once I was healthy enough for consistent, unimpeded training, it required six months before I began to feel like a jock. Of course I wanted speedier results— but you have to be more tortoise than hare if you want to succeed once middle age arrives.

The fitness gains were dramatic. I lost weight. Muscles resurfaced. I had greater energy. Mornings were brighter. Nights felt calmer. I even physically reconnected with Mount Tam, our estrangement a thing of the past.

As part of my long, slow climb back to an active lifestyle, I interviewed fitness experts and coaches whose instructive insights about diet and exercise were valuable. I spoke with a *New York Times* health and fitness reporter; a senior exercise researcher at the Mayo Clinic who participated in a deconditioning study; an astronaut who spent five months in space and returned to earth feeling like an old, bedridden man despite running on a treadmill on the space station; a nutritional and wellness guru who trained world-class runners and endurance athletes; and a top sports scientist who tested Lance Armstrong in his Texas exercise lab in the nineties before and after the cycling great had cancer. Each interview opened a valuable window into critical areas of fitness and health.

I also talked with several accomplished athletes whose illness, injury, or change in lifestyle had temporarily forced them to stop working out—but then they successfully bounced back. Represented here are a former Wall Street trader who lost seventy-five pounds and became Hawaii's Fittest CEO; a retired two-time world-champion Hawaii Ironman triathlete with a bum hip that required a bionic partial replacement so he could run pain-free; a Yosemite park employee who broke her spine in a hiking accident and is now back on the trails; and a sixty-seven-year-old business educator who's had six heart bypasses but still backpacks and goes to the gym.

With *Return to Fitness*, you won't find any quick-fix formulas that guarantee overnight results. Getting back in shape requires that you make a long-term commitment to diet and regular exercise. Having specific goals helps. We all need our own Mount Tam because it provides additional motivation and facilitates self-empowerment. Pointing yourself toward a lofty, admirable challenge—whether it's a 10K, marathon, triathlon, or bike trip—allows you to weather the occasional bad days, while making the good days richer and more meaningful.

Along the way, as you gradually become fitter, you will find yourself enjoying that confident feeling that comes with taking charge of your own health. But I want to emphasize that there is no one-size-fits-all return to fitness. Each individual will respond differently to this task. And always remember that well-burnished truism: The journey is more important than the destination. Yes, I wanted to return to the top of Tam, but not without first making fundamental lifestyle changes that would stick around long after I reached its summit.

Bill Katovsky
Northern California

$$\textbf{\large \textcircled{1}}$$

WHEN I WAS REALLY FIT . . .

Becoming an Ironman and
How This Race Changed My Life

was in the best shape of my life in the fall of 1982. I had been training for the Hawaii Ironman Triathlon since late spring. I was chiseled and ripped, weighed 170 pounds, sported low body fat, and looked great in a pair of jeans. I had rock-hard quads and calves forged from cycling, a wide trapezoidal back developed through swimming, and flat, serrated abs created by running.

This newly sculpted body belonged to me, the welcomed byproduct of working out between ten and fifteen hours per week for nearly half a year. Yet it also felt like I was inhabiting someone else's physique. It's not that I missed having a slightly protruding carbo-belly hang around like a houseguest who refuses to leave. It just seemed unusual to be this fit. Walking past mirrors, instead of sucking in my gut, I'd silently nod in approval. I liked wearing shorts or going without a shirt in the sun.

Strange, then, that the journey taking me to the Big Island for the Ironman almost never happened in the first place. Fate, luck, timing, perseverance, and desire all played their respective roles.

One lazy Sunday afternoon in February 1982, I happened to watch ABC's *Wide World of Sports* coverage of the Ironman, which featured one of the most remarkable finishes of any race, any sport, any time. Julie Moss was leading the women's race but collapsed from fatigue and leg cramps only yards from the finish line. As she crawled along the ground, second-place woman Kathleen McCartney ran right past her and won.

Julie's finish was nearly as epic and unforgettable as the Greek warrior Phidippedes crossing the plains of Marathon and dying after delivering his battlefield message to the Athenians. But in Julie's case, television cameras were right there in her face, broadcasting her courageous plight to millions.

I turned off the television and said to my girlfriend Terri, "Wow! I'm gonna do the Ironman."

She replied, "But Bill, you don't know how to swim."

"Yeah, you're right. What am I thinking?"

Terri was two years younger and a senior at the University of California at Berkeley, where I was a graduate student in political science. We had met six months earlier in a rooming house near campus. She was the practical and levelheaded one in our relationship.

I was first drawn to the Ironman after America's foremost cyclist, John Howard, won in 1980. I idolized Howard and yet he was a lousy swimmer. Someday, I used to fantasize, there might come a time when I would overcome my fear of ocean-water swimming and compete in the Ironman. With my cycling background, the 112-mile bike portion seemed doable. And the third event, the 26.2-mile run, would require adequate preparation. But the swim distance—2.4 miles—was too daunting, way beyond anything I could imagine completing. I would most likely drown. So I mentally scratched off the Ironman from my Adventure To Do List, and began thinking about alternate physical challenges because I wanted to take an extended break from academic studies. I was in my second year of the PhD program and, certainly not looking forward to an endless grind of at least a half-dozen years before possibly getting a doctorate, I contemplated going on another long-distance bike trip—starting in Alaska and traveling down the coast to Mexico. It would be an arduous trip, with winds, logging trucks, rain, snow, mosquitoes, bears, moose, and gravel roads, but I believed in pushing myself beyond the everyday comfort zone.

One evening as I was grocery shopping at the Safeway in Oakland, I stopped at the magazine newsstand rack. *Bicycling*'s cover caught my eye. I thumbed through its pages and saw a small race entry ad for the Ironman that fall. Was this a sign, an omen to follow? Naughtily, I ripped out the ad, stuffed it in my jacket pocket, and went off to pay for my groceries.

When I got home, I taped that ad to the refrigerator door. Alaska would have to wait. Hawaii, only six months away, marked my new destiny. Heat replaced cold. I needed to learn how to swim.

TRAINING BEGINS

I signed up for a swimming class at a nearby recreation pool in Oakland. The swim instructor assigned me the slowest lane, which I shared with two elderly women in swim caps. He asked me to swim two lengths of the twenty-five-yard pool using the freestyle stroke. I thrashed, splashed, and gasped those fifty yards. I had no idea what I was doing—how to breathe, how to stroke, how to kick. How was I ever going to swim two hundred laps—the landlocked equivalent of 2.4 miles at sea? When I told the instructor that I was planning to do the Ironman, he shook his head and snickered. I never went back to that pool or class. I would endure humiliation on my own private terms.

I went to a bookstore and purchased legendary swim coach Doc Counsilman's guide to swimming. Standing in front of our bathroom mirror, I practiced the freestyle's S-stroke, looking like a tone-deaf, rhythmless music conductor.

I put my new stroke to the test at one of the outdoor pools on the Berkeley campus. I went two lengths of the twenty-five-yard pool. It felt easier. I wasn't floundering like someone about to drown. I got my breathing down, though only from the left side. Relieved, I hopped out, and treated myself to a slice of pizza for dinner. The following day, I returned to the pool, and swam four laps. Then, once again, I got out and had another pizza slice. This was my routine for several weeks, increasing the distance by fifty yards each time. I was soon swimming a half-mile or thirty-six laps.

Yet my form was rather laughable. Instead of my body hydroplaning near the water surface to reduce drag, my stocky frame plowed through the water like a tugboat, with my head and torso horizontal, while my legs dragged behind like anchors because I had trouble kicking. (Apart from generating propulsion, kicking's main purpose is to stabilize your body's flat-plane position.) There were other significant stroke defects: limited arm and shoulder flexibility, poor hand entry into the water, and weak follow-through at the end of each stroke. I was losing a significant amount of energy and efficiency, maybe more than 50 percent. I didn't dare try doing flip turns.

Despite this chronic inability to move gracefully through the water, I continued adding laps almost every time I went to the pool. Eventually, I reached one mile, grinding out seventy-two laps. When my hand touched the final wall, I didn't exactly feel like Mark Spitz or Johnny Weissmuller, since it had taken fifty-five minutes. Elite Ironman triathletes swam the same distance in under twenty minutes. Because there was a two hour and fifteen minute mandatory Ironman swim cutoff, my big concern was time. Could I swim fast enough to not become disqualified? But first I needed to know whether I could even go that far without the assistance of black lines painted on the sea floor or a cement wall to push off with my legs every seventy-five feet.

I probably spent more time fretting about the Ironman swim than accumulating mileage in the pool. Biking and running, however, produced far less anxiety. But what did take some time getting used to was making the transition from biking to running. After an hour or two of riding, the last thing your legs want to do is hit the pavement and begin running. For the first mile or two, the quads and calves feel like someone smacked them with a baseball bat. But after several weeks, I grew accustomed to the lead-legs syndrome, and it became easier to jog through the temporary unpleasantness as the muscles warmed up.

Of the three triathlon disciplines, biking was my strongest and the most enjoyable. I usually averaged between 100 and 150 miles per week. Where I fell behind was running. I never seemed to have a week that went beyond 20 or 25 miles, because I was fearful of adding too many miles and risking a running injury that would then derail my Ironman dreams altogether. I wasn't aiming to finish in the top half of the field—I just wanted to get through the race. Be a survivor. Hopefully finish in thirteen hours, which would theoretically mean a 2:00 swim, 6:30 bike, 4:30 marathon. Those idealized splits were based upon a laborious analysis of competitors' times from the February 1982 race. In order to break eleven hours, one's weekly training average should optimally be 250 miles on the bike, 50 miles running, and 10 to 15 miles swimming. To go sub-ten hours like the elites, you have to continue adding more miles and higher intensity workouts and be blessed with terrific athletic genes. Pros now go eight hours and spare change in the Ironman.

Then why wasn't I working out harder and putting in more miles? I had the time and opportunity to train. I had the summer off from classes. There was no job holding me back. Yet my Ironman regimen lacked any real consistency or sustained self-discipline. My training was haphazard and sporadic, apathetically undermined by too many rest or easy days, as if I were deliberately rebelling against the Ironman despite being obsessed by the race. Terri once said, "Bill, all you ever talk about *is* the Ironman."

WHY I BIKED AND TRAINED THE WAY I DID: A BRIEF AUTOBIOGRAPHICAL DETOUR OFFERS SEVERAL CLUES

I was a conflicted athlete. During long bike rides, for example, I'd sometimes bring along a literary magazine (usually *The New Republic* or *The New Yorker*) and read it at the turnaround point over a lingering lunch, followed perhaps by a nap in the sun. I felt like a man of leisure, not someone who was training his body to race 112 miles.

I biked in a pack of one. I didn't belong to a cycling club. Nor did I have a riding partner. I rode upright, not in an aerodynamic tuck, while tooling along at a comfortable pace.

I felt perfectly at ease training in my own idiosyncratic and unconventional manner. Such unrepentant individualism was a natural extension to a lifelong aversion to coaches and authority figures. I took a judo class at age twelve, but the instructor insisted that we shout, "Kill!" every time we tried to throw an opponent. I never went back after that first class. During tennis lessons, I often found myself daydreaming rather than focusing on smacking smooth forehands and backhands. With swim lessons at Beechmont Country Club, I preferred to float on my stomach and gaze down at the pool bottom. My father gave up trying to improve my awkward batting swing, though he spent countless hours with my older brother Tommy who shined as a second baseman in Little League.

Only during loosely organized football games with my neighborhood chums or at summer camp did I truly excel. I was quick-footed, fast, tough, a real bruiser. I dreamed of playing professional football. Black-and-white glossies of Cleveland Browns players lined my bedroom walls. These gridiron gladiators, with their crew cuts and fierce, no-nonsense expressions, were my heroes. But to my future disappointment, a long-delayed puberty derailed this career ambition.

In seventh grade, I was the starting fullback on Byron Junior High's lightweight football team. I weighed ninety-five pounds and was about average size for my age. In our two intra-squad games, the coach insisted on calling the same play that forced me to run up the middle into a dense knot of bodies. Every time, whether it was 22 Right or 22 Left, I'd get tackled at the line of scrimmage. So on one play, I defied the call and took matters in my own hands, scampering around the right end without any blocking, and scored an eighty-yard touchdown. The coach offered congratulations, then berated me for disobeying him. In our next game, I pulled off the identical play, once again ignoring the coach's signal, and went untouched for forty-five yards, and another touchdown. Instead of chewing me out, the coach started calling me "Killer Katovsky" in practice.

In addition to getting top grades, I was also a Byron gym leader—a coveted position awarded to those who scored in the top percentile on a fitness and agility test that included the following: football pass, football punt, 6/10 of a mile cross-country run, pull-ups, sit-ups, basketball dribbling around cones, basketball layups in sixty seconds, shuffle test, standing broad jump, standing vertical jump, push-ups, and grip squeeze for hand strength.

In eighth and ninth grade, I went out for soccer because I had yet to reach puberty and the guys on the football team were suddenly much larger. In ninth grade, I weighed just 101 pounds and stood five-two.

That summer, our family moved to a new neighborhood—and different school district. Gym class turned scary. The fat, balding, gone-to-seed gym teacher indulged his sadism by having us play a variation of dodgeball known as scatterball with those in the eleventh grade who were bigger, stronger, hairier, meaner. Since I was still undersized, I started avoiding gym with the assistance of parental and doctor notes. I used a bad back as an excuse.

In eleventh grade, I decided to sit out gym for the entire year. Physically and psychologically, I was a puny, pint-sized outsider, wondering why God liked screwing with my growth hormones. I wanted to look normal, not like someone who could pass for a middle schooler. During the final week of classes, the new gym teacher—a young, wiry redneck from a small Ohio farm town—was going to flunk me unless I passed two phys-ed tests. The first was pull-ups. I did ten in my street clothes, one of the highest totals in the class. (I kept a set of barbells in my bedroom.) When I dropped to the floor, Coach snapped, "Katovsky, why have you been hiding this from me?" He then herded everyone outside to the football field for the fifty-yard dash.

When it was my turn to run, I took off my shoes and socks. I was wearing beige Levi cords. At the whistle's blow, I sprinted hard, but as I approached the finish line, I overextended my right leg and immediately felt a body part tear away near my hip. I crumpled to the grass, screaming in pain. Coach came over and shouted, "Stop faking, Katovsky, and get up!" I was seeing stars; the pain was intense. With my eyes squeezed shut, I tried lifting myself off the grass, but couldn't since my right side was now useless. I fell back to the ground, rocking back and forth in agony. Coach came closer. His voice suddenly became quieter and more concerned. "Maybe you *are* hurt." The other students gathered around me, whispering. Coach then decided to send someone to contact the school nurse, who called an ambulance. I was wheeled off the field on a stretcher. It was my first time in an ambulance. The driver kept the vehicle's siren silent.

I spent a week in traction at St. Luke's Hospital. At least I had a private room. What happened was that a large upper thigh muscle had ripped itself away from the hip. No surgery was required to repair the damage. Sufficient rest and time would heal the injury. The doctor recommended that I use crutches for the rest of the summer, but I tossed them aside after a week and started hobbling about unaided. The last six weeks of the summer, I got a job working for a tree service company where I was on my feet all day long. My leg and hip were pretty much healed when it was time to head back to school in the fall. In the end, Coach rewarded me with a passing grade.

Gym wasn't required in twelfth grade. That was fine with me. At our high school graduation, I was the smallest boy to walk onto the stage and receive a diploma. I would have gladly exchanged my 3.95 GPA for some height. Six, eight inches. I wouldn't have been fussy.

Apart from playing lackluster tennis and being the starting halfback on the soccer team in the fall of my senior year, I stayed clear of all sports and did little to stay in shape throughout those emotionally disorienting high school years. I watched a lot of television. I even stopped thinking of myself in jock terms. Those two touchdown runs in seventh grade comprised the entirety of an all-too-brief athletic highlight reel.

During my freshman year at the University of Michigan, the tardy growth spurt finally arrived. I shot up to five-nine and weighed 165 pounds. I began to bulk up in the weight room. I was drawn to fitness again. But the most I ever ran was a mile on the rickety indoor wooden track—eight laps to a mile. I hated running. A guy on my dorm floor ran seven miles every morning, even in the snow and rain. I never asked him why. I just assumed that his daily running ritual made him weirder than he already was. His sink-washed white tube socks were always drying on the radiator in his room.

On my first summer break from college, I took up cycling. My dorm friend David Farber had planted the two-wheel seed. He had spent several weeks bike-touring Michigan's Upper Peninsula. (He's now a highly accomplished scholar and history professor at Temple University.) I bought an English ten-speed made by Falcon for $270 with savings from a job in a lumberyard, and started biking throughout northeastern Ohio. The farthest I had previously biked on my heavy five-speed green Schwinn Varsity was a tiring eleven miles. But with my new lightweight British road bike, I was biking forty or fifty miles. The sport piqued my interest, not as a racer, but as a means to open-road freedom. I liked biking through the lushly forested Cuyahoga Valley and metro parks that girdled Cleveland. Two years later, I biked solo across America. And two summers after that adventure, I biked 1,500 miles from Berkeley to the Grand Canyon and back. David accompanied me on the first half of that tough, hot slog. He *was* competitive and enjoyed beating me to the top of long climbs, often by up to a half-hour. "What took you so long?" he'd usually ask when I reached the crest.

The bike I used for the Grand Canyon trip had been custom-built by an Oakland frame-builder named Bernie Mikkelsen whose cluttered live-work studio was located in a small building underneath a downtown freeway overpass. The mustachioed Bernie had a peculiar method of determining the size of my new bike frame. He jammed a steel pipe under my crotch, took out a tape measure, and checked its distance to the dirty concrete floor.

"Okay, I got what I need," he said.

"Is that it?" I asked.

"Yes."

This fitting took less time than getting measured for my bar mitzvah suit by a small, stoop-shouldered, Russian-accented tailor in Cleveland.

"Now what color do you want the frame?"

I chose pale blue. Bernie ended up painting it the wrong blue, the same color as the Trek that took me across America. The all-steel bike frame cost $750.

I trained for the Ironman on the Mikkelsen. But even with a custom bike, my riding form remained inefficient, clumsy, non-fluid, and bowlegged. I pedaled in squares rather than in circles, mashing down on the pedals in my Sidi cleats instead of smoothly applying force throughout the entire revolution. Then there was the question of cadence: Top cyclists spin at high RPMs; I probably motored in the 80s or lower. That is, when I wasn't coasting or looking at the scenery, contentedly letting my mind roam with stream-of-conscious thoughts.

This kind of riding was a poor way to prepare for Hawaii with its brutal heat.

BECOMING A RUNNER

When I was twenty-two, I took up running, in part to recuperate from thwarted love. A month after graduating college, I traveled out west with my girlfriend. We camped, hiked, and biked in the Canadian Rockies, and when we ran out of money, we crossed the border into Montana, where I got hired as a firefighter by the U.S. Forest Service and she worked in a deli in Kalispell. When summer ended, she returned to Ann Arbor for her senior year, and I went backpacking and biking in Yosemite for a month. Back in Ann Arbor, it took her about two weeks to decide that her next-door neighbor, a medical student, made better husband material. (They divorced after five years of marriage.) And that's how and why I started running. It was better than tending to a wounded heart. To my surprise, I discovered I liked running. I was hooked. To find out more about the sport, I bought one of the first books written on the topic by ultra-marathoner Tom Ostler, who raced in hundred-kilometer running events in the sixties. Inspired and fascinated by his endurance exploits, I got up to ten miles on my longest runs.

When I moved to Washington, D.C., to work as a political researcher at the Brookings Institution, I ran along the Potomac or canal towpath that started in Georgetown. On weekends, I went on fifty- or seventy-five-mile bike rides through the rolling Maryland countryside. I didn't know it at the time, but I was, in fact, cross-training, though the term—and exercise philosophy behind it—was still relatively new to athletes. Running and cycling lived in fenced-off athletic ghettos. But by combining biking and running, I seldom got injured. My knees held up fine, always a concern for runners.

In October 1981, I entered my first running race—a 13.1-mile hilly affair in Berkeley, where I now lived and toiled in the academic salt mines. I was running between ten and fifteen miles a week. I somehow can't remember what prompted me to show up on that cold fall morning near the majestic Claremont Hotel. About two hundred runners were already gathered on a side street, many hopping about in order to stay warm. I noticed several guys wearing running tights. I had never seen that before.

The first three miles went straight uphill, first along Ashby Avenue and then Tunnel Road, where all the homes would later burn to the ground in the devastating 1991 Oakland fire. I started out too fast and struggled in oxygen-debt, but I edged back and paced myself on the long climb. I must have been in the top half of the field at the 800-foot summit, feeling cocky, but on the flat and downhill sections that comprised the rest of the race, runner after runner zipped right past. Near the eight-mile mark, I finally asked a female runner, "How are you feeling? Tired?"

"No," she replied. "My legs feel fine."

Mine were weakening by the moment. "I'm curious, but can you tell me how much training you do?"

"About thirty or forty miles a week," she replied. She too pulled away. *Running is a number's game*, I thought. You need to put in the training mileage. Just like making bank deposits before making a withdrawal. I finished the half-marathon in a respectable 1:45, or just over eight minutes per mile. I received a small yellow fabric patch. Twenty-four hours later, I came down with the flu and spent three miserable days in bed because I had severely stressed my immune system. My body paid the penalty for being undertrained.

MY FIRST TRIATHLON

In the spring, I entered two more small, local running races—a five-miler and three-miler. That was it. The October Ironman was going to be my ultimate trial by fire. I was jumping right into the lava frying pan. Common sense dictated, however, that I should enter one triathlon beforehand. The Sierra Nevada half-Ironman, in the Sierra foothills of California east of Sacramento, was held a month before Hawaii, so I decided to make that race my Kona tune-up. The swim was two miles in cold Folsom Lake (wetsuits weren't used then in triathlon). I had never swum more than a mile in the pool.

About five hundred triathletes congregated on the beach as dawn broke. I seeded myself at the very back. When the starting gun sounded, swimmers charged into the water. I strolled into the lake like it was a Sunday outing. With the sun in my eyes, I had difficulty navigating in the choppy water. I kept swallowing water. Luckily it was fresh-tasting, not salty. When my arms grew tired from the crawl, I switched to the slower breaststroke. I was almost tempted to ask one fisherman if I could get in his boat because I didn't think that I could make it back to shore. I was one of the last swimmers to finish. It felt good when I reached the sandy beach and it was time for the fifty-six-mile bike ride.

But this is where I had made my second gross miscalculation. The day before I had gone on a forty-mile hilly bike ride, idiotically thinking that by doing so I was prepping my legs for the race. I had never heard of tapering.

Consequently, my legs felt sluggish and unresponsive on all three mountain passes. But I didn't get off and walk the steep sections (which some competitors were actually doing).

Famished and thirsty, I rolled into the bike transition area. Here's when I made the biggest mistake of the race: I wolfed down a peanut butter and jelly sandwich and quart of cold, delicious cherry fruit juice. My stomach immediately bloated from the sudden rush of food and liquid. Next up was the half-marathon.

Within the first few hundred yards, all that undigested sludge produced severe cramping. Gastric distress made it impossible to run. Clenching my sides with both hands, I walked hunched over. Two other stragglers soon joined me. We walked the entire half-marathon together. When we finally made it back to the beach, the race organizers were busy taking down the finish-line banner. I believe we were last.

I went over to the massage area and got my first-ever massage. Even though the white sheet was soiled with mineral oil, grime, and sweat from countless bodies, I appreciated the feel of a stranger's hands kneading out the stiffness in my legs and back.

My legs were sore for only two days. Then I was back to biking and running, but I realized that I had to ramp up my training, especially in the swimming department. I also had to come up with a better way to stay hydrated and fueled on the bike and run. At the time, sports nutrition was still in its infancy. You experimented with what you drank and ate. Energy bars hadn't yet been created.

Because the fall semester had already started at Berkeley—I was now a teaching assistant for an undergraduate class in American political theory—I had to squeeze my training around classes. When it was time to leave for Hawaii, I hoped that I was in decent enough condition to finish. But had I clocked sufficient quality miles? The final tally of six months of training was 75 miles swimming, 3,640 miles biking, and 505 miles running.

THE HAWAII IRONMAN

I arrived in Hawaii one week before race day. The sleepy, postcard-perfect town of Kailua-Kona resembled an Olympic training village set among palm and banyan trees. World-class athletes and multisport diehards strutted and flaunted their physical wares. For someone like myself, who was green as a papaya in this sports subculture, it was easy to feel intimidated. The intense hothouse atmosphere thrived on psyching-out and one-upsmanship. Ego-flexing was most visible during early morning swims in Kailua Bay or afternoon bike rides on the Queen K highway. Like a student cramming before the big exam, I logged my highest training mileage during pre-race week: two hundred miles biking, thirty miles running, six miles of swimming. Shouldn't I have been resting?

I swam the entire 2.4-mile course twice for practice. The only "buoy" was a single empty white bottle of bleach tethered to the seafloor 1.2 miles away. You had to aim toward a distant coastline knob for navigational bearing. I'd be all alone in the bay except for small schools of triathletes who motored right by like I was treading water (which I did a lot during those training swims). When I finally made it back to the small beach, my arms and shoulders were sore and rubbery, my throat raw from ingesting salt water. Both swims took well over two and a half hours. An early DQ on race day seemed imminent; I called my father in Cleveland and voiced my concerns about being so damn slow. He said that he believed in me and that I would finish the swim before the cutoff. He had faith in me, even if I didn't.

I spent many quiet hours alone in my hotel room, a sanctuary from the Kona scene that hummed and buzzed with triathlon testosterone, preferring instead to watch television and endlessly leaf through the Ironman race guide that featured short biographies of all 990 entrants. The magazine reminded me of a high school yearbook of super jocks. Many of the top-finishing returning Ironman veterans lived in southern California and listed "lifeguard" or "aquatics instructor" as their profession, but the majority of competitors were doctors, lawyers, engineers, pilots, bankers, realtors, housewives, and students living in all fifty states, Australia, Canada, and England.

The room lacked air conditioning. An overhead fan provided the only breeze, so I kept the windows open. The muggy sea air threw off a menacing, bullying presence. At night the rains came and the temperature would slightly drop. But in the mornings, the bright, happy tropic sun would reappear behind Mount Hualālai, and refresh the Hawaiian steam bath.

• • •

I woke up at four o'clock on race morning and prepared for the 7:00 A.M. start. It was still dark as I walked to the Kona pier, shuffling along in a semi-catatonic state of near-panic. A gathering storm of triathletes anxiously milled about under a bank of television lights, getting their limbs inked with race numbers, pumping air into bike tires, adjusting swim goggles. An ABC helicopter thumped overheard.

I seeded myself in the rear by the sea wall with the slow swimmers and waited for the cannon to go off. The water was waist-deep here. I kept an extra pair of Speedo swim goggles tucked inside my swimsuit.

The cannon blast sounded. The bay immediately turned into a wild, frothy maelstrom of numbered limbs and orange caps. Just fifty yards into the mass swimming frenzy, I felt my left calf pop. I don't exactly know how it happened. I would worry about the injury later.

I stayed clear of most swimmers and found a steady rhythm. *Hey, this isn't too bad*, I thought. Every now and then, I'd look up and keep close to the large inflatable orange buoys on my right to ensure I wasn't veering off course.

When I finally made it to the far side of the turnaround boat, known by locals as the Booze Cruise, I stopped swimming for several moments and asked a spectator on board for the time. He said, "7:45."

"You really mean it?" I yelled back.

"Yes," came his answer, which meant that I would make it back to the pier well before the cutoff time—I wasn't going to be DQ'd! I felt giddy, thrilled, in great (buoyant) spirits. Because of the current, it took longer to make it back to the pier, but most remarkably, I finished the 2.4-mile swim in 1:46. About seventy swimmers were still behind me. I wasn't in last place!

After quickly rinsing off the seawater with a hose in the transition area, I changed into my bike apparel—pink neon Italian bike shorts that I bought specifically for the race and a cotton tank top I picked up from a Kona gift shop for $5.95.

"Love your shorts!" I heard this often from spectators crowding the pier as I left the bike corral and climbed the short, steep hill out of town. Once on Queen K Highway, I felt like I was in my element. I began gobbling up other riders like a two-wheel Pac-Man, passing over two hundred cyclists within the first forty miles. I rode hard and strong along the rolling black lava fields, though my left calf ominously began to throb and tighten.

There were food and water aid stations every ten miles, and I loaded up each time with a new water bottle. I knew that I had to keep hydrated in the ninety-degree heat. I tried a banana, but it stuck in my throat and I gagged it out. I kept a stash of two Snickers bars in my fanny pack, which included a tool kit (rules stipulated that all mechanical repairs had to be made by competitors). I also carried several dollars just in case I felt like refueling at the small grocery store in Kawaihae, fifty miles away. (What would five minutes mean in the grand scheme of things?)

Long before I reached the base of the eleven-mile climb to Hawi, marking the bike turnaround point, the lead riders were already barreling down the other side of the highway. Drafting wasn't officially penalized, so the racers were arrayed in a dense, lengthy pack. I was amazed to see one guy on a mountain bike.

During the ascent to Hawi, the wind picked up and it started to rain. Howling gusts, up to 40 mph, forced riders to dismount and walk their bikes. Not me. I stood up on the pedals and grinded away into the unrelenting headwind, grateful that my bike training had been done in the hilly and windy Bay Area.

The descent from Hawi went by much too quickly. These were free miles to be savored. The ride back to Kona seemed endless. The winds were fickle, often changing from tailwind to crosswind. Outside of town, the early leaders were already running along the Queen K. When I turned onto Alii Drive, for the final six miles, a long line of grim-faced runners was now thundering my way. I did my very best to ignore this sun-baked herd who would finish hours before me, sternly reminding myself, "You are doing this race for yourself. Don't worry about the others."

One mile before the bike-to-run transition area at the Kona Surf Hotel, I got my first flat but decided to ignore it and kept riding, though at a slower pace. My bike split for 112 miles was 7:02. Entirely respectable. This was done without contemporary tri-gadgetry like clipless pedals, disk wheels, lightweight bike frames, and aero bars.

The bike-to-run-transition changing tent was a foul, wretched place, hot and smelly like a locker room from hell; you didn't want to dillydally here unless your body was entirely spent. I slipped off my bike shoes and laced up my Asics. Several competitors were seated in folding chairs, flushed from the heat, looking dazed and lifeless. They appeared uncertain about wanting to leave and run a marathon. Who could fault their reluctance? But I needed to get going. I hurried outside and charged up the steep one-quarter-mile Kona Surf driveway entrance on legs as wobbly and uncertain as a newborn colt's.

I had promised myself for months that I wouldn't walk during the marathon. I would gut it out, despite having never gone more than fourteen miles on a training run. That oath was broken before I even left the hotel grounds. My legs were shot. But along the more level Alii Drive, as vitality began to gradually seep back into exhausted muscle fibers, I began a slow, stilted jog, determined to walk only while passing through the aid stations positioned every mile. I tried not to pay too much attention to the dozens of runners flying past. These were the same folks I had passed on the bike.

The first six miles of the run followed coast-hugging Alii Drive. The spectacular views made for a pleasant distraction from an increasingly unpleasant sensation: The left calf pain was intensifying. While doing my damnedest to ignore it, I managed to make it out of town and back onto the murderously hot Queen K Highway. Up ahead: twenty miles of more suffering on the lava fields. Now, instead of walking through the aid stations, I was walking to them. My left leg had seized up. But as long as I continued to put one foot in front of the other, I was making headway.

Dusk comes rapidly in the tropics, illuminating the darkening sky with swirling bands of brilliant red, orange, and purple hues. Then an inky blackness descends like a velvet curtain. Back-of-the-packers like myself toiled alone in the pitch-dark torment, encased in a mobile cocoon of misery and fatigue. Aid stations offered us brief relief, small oases of light and comfort in an otherwise hostile, nocturnal kingdom.

I couldn't shed one constant thought: Why was I putting myself through such self-administered torture? The idea of quitting lured me like a wily, tempting seductress.

I decided to end things at the run turnaround near the airport, where I'd load up on snacks and drinks at the gift store and then take a taxi back into town. But once I had pivoted my aching, numb body around the turnaround's orange traffic cones, where a volunteer placed a checkmark by my race number (#501) on a sheet of paper, I experienced my own sudden turnaround. I was going to *finish* this race!

I was homeward bound. But the Ironman never lets you off easy. It indifferently finds ways to sap your spirit, upset your pre-race plans, erode your confidence. The calf pain worsened. I shifted my weight onto my right leg. That only worked to a limited degree, so I tried visualization. I recalled a passage from a Robert Stone novel called *Dog Soldiers* about the sixties gone sour. The plot involves a heroin drug-buy, with a crooked federal agent squared off against a Nietzsche-loving Merchant Marine named Ray Hicks, who was played by Nick Nolte in the film adaptation renamed *Who Will Stop the Rain?* Toward the end of the book, as a wounded Hicks bravely trudges along the train tracks in the New Mexican desert, his shoulder leaking blood from a gunshot wound, he triumphs over the pain by mentally isolating it as the letter *P* within a

Zen-like thought triangle. Mind over matter. I tried doing the same thing. The leg pain migrated inside the border of the triangle's three lines. The pain was geometrically locked away. I was its jailer. It would not escape or defeat me.

As Hicks's energy wanes in the desert heat, he starts chanting an off-color ditty favored by Marines during boot-camp marches: "I don't know, but I have been told that Eskimo pussy is mighty cold! Mmm, good! Feels good! Is good! Real good! Tastes good! Mighty good!" I began to recite those same crude lines nonstop. It got me through another two miles. Hicks never made it to safety. His two friends, whose lives he had earlier saved from several gunmen, found him dead by the train tracks, his body propped up by his M16 rifle. A warrior to the end. A dog soldier.

With less than ten miles to go, I realized that I would make it to the Kona pier finish line before the midnight cutoff but only if I continued moving. My top lava land speed was about fifteen minutes per mile. I tried hobbling faster. Another competitor joined me on this nocturnal death march for several miles. We chatted in the dark, bonded together by our common fate. He told me that he was a professional motocross racer. "Which sport is more difficult?" I asked.

"The Ironman," he said. "It's the hardest thing I have ever done."

Having company offered distraction from a weakening body. Kona was aglow in the distance, like a South Seas Oz. I began to jog. With my stiffening left leg, I felt like Ahab. Drawing nearer to Kona, I quickened my pace. An adrenaline surge masked the stabbing calf pain.

I descended into town and turned the corner onto Alii Drive, the Ironman's Via Dolorosa, where Julie Moss crumpled from exhaustion, as did six-time Hawaii Ironman champion Paula Newby-Fraser thirteen years later. Thousands of spectators lined both sides of the road. They were cheering and encouraging racers. The aloha atmosphere was democratic. It didn't matter if you had been out on the course four, five, or six hours after winner Californian Dave Scott broke the finish line tape. All Ironman triathletes who made it this far were true champions in their eyes.

Energized by the animated crowd, I sprinted the last four hundred yards. This got many spectators to yell even louder as I edged past fellow late-night travelers. I still had game.

On that full-moon night in October, I crossed the finish line in 15:02. I shot both arms upward in a victory salute. Race director Valerie Silk greeted me with a hug and fragrant lei, just like she had tirelessly done with each and every sweaty, smelly, and running-on-empty finisher. Two race officials escorted me to a guarded, roped-off area where I was handed a finisher's medallion and T-shirt; I was then directed to the massage area that had been set up next to the hospital tent. Both were doing brisk business. More than a hundred triathletes had withdrawn from the race due to heat, dehydration, or medical reasons, their hopes and dreams shattered by the unforgiving conditions. Many were getting IVs. I felt bad for them. Would they be stigmatized by failure, or try again next year?

There was one thing that I knew with absolute certainty. As I told the masseuse who attempted to revive my weary limbs with a sympathetic blend of tactile tenderness and *does this hurt?* prodding, "I will never do the Ironman a second time. Once is enough. That's it. Yup. You will never see me back here. This race is too tough, too hard."

She worked on my legs and shoulders for about thirty minutes before gingerly helping me off the table. I tried thanking her, but she interrupted, "You are the one who should be thanked for going through what you did." Her kind, appreciative words stayed with me as I limped off to a restaurant for a big plate of salty french fries and several ice-cold Cokes. Every few minutes, I would hear the crowd erupt in applause and cheers when another pre-midnight Ironman survivor made it down Alii. I called my father from a pay phone to let him know that I finished. I had never felt happier or more fulfilled in my life.

THE LAUNCH OF *TRI-ATHLETE* MAGAZINE

Three days later, I was back in Berkeley. Still limping from the calf injury, I wore my finisher's T-shirt on my first day back on campus because I wanted everyone to see those three-inch-high white letters printed on blue 100 percent heavy cotton: *1982 Hawaii Ironman Finisher.* The only ones who said anything about the shirt were some students in my political theory class. After listening to me ramble on about New England Puritans and the initial stirrings of representative democracy in the New World, they wanted to hear about Hawaii. I think I earned their respect for the first time that afternoon.

Then the inevitable happened. I stopped working out on a regular basis. My mileage began to decrease while my pre-Ironman appetite remained the same. I'd bike on the weekends and maybe run once or twice a week. Within a month I gained ten pounds. I also took a lot of afternoon naps. Around the Christmas holiday break, I found myself slipping into a restless, uneasy funk. What it came down to was this stark realization: I didn't know what I wanted to do with my life. I was twenty-five years old, indifferently marking time as a graduate student. I thought about moving to Israel, joining the Peace Corps, or opening up a bookstore/cafe in Santa Fe. I was looking for some kind of direction—meaning, a North Star, anything, in order to reorient an aimless, dithering life.

Then, on one sunny afternoon while sitting on the steps of the Student Union on the Berkeley campus, it came to me out of the ether: I would start a triathlon magazine. The Ironman had been such a life-altering experience, so why should it have to abruptly conclude at the Kona pier? The publication would become the voice of this new sport that changed lives.

When I got home, I told Terri about my latest brainstorm. She gave me her usual look that implied I was bonkers. If I had told her that I was planning to row solo across the Atlantic, it would have resulted in that same *oh, Bill* expression. How could I create a magazine when I had no prior journalism or business experience? In high school, I wrote a brief article on the men's cross-country team for the school paper, but the teacher rejected my short article, telling me that this was the worst story she had ever read. That juvenile attempt had been the first and last time I tried my hand at journalism. I knew zilch about the mechanics of publishing. Nor did I have any friends in triathlon to help me put together a publication. I had savings of only $16,000, and furthermore, I was busy taking and teaching classes at Berkeley.

I put the idea on hold for a few days, but I became more convinced than ever that my new purpose in life was to launch a triathlon magazine. Destiny by way of the Ironman beckoned.

I first needed a name for the magazine. I decided on *Tri-Athlete*. Yes, with a hyphen. Because back then, the term *triathlete* was seldom used. You were either an Ironman or a swimmer, cyclist, or runner who occasionally showed up at a triathlon. (In a short time, however, the hyphen seemed superfluous.)

I paid a local graphic artist seventy-five dollars for a logo; another one received fifty for making a subscription flyer. A local print shop then cranked out five hundred flyers, which I distributed in driving rain at the Oakland Marathon. I stood by the finish line chute shoving them into the hands of dazed, exhausted runners as they funneled past. Rethinking this strategy, I slipped the flyers under windshield wipers of nearby parked cars.

Over the next week, ten-dollar checks for subscriptions began to trickle in through the mail, accompanying water-damaged tear-off portions from the flyers. I also placed two small subscription ads in *VeloNews* and *Bicycling*. This netted around three hundred subscribers. The next step was sending out notices to race directors all across the country announcing the new magazine.

For postage, I made liberal use of a Pitney Bowes machine at a friend's office during weeknights. Terri expertly managed all the administrative matters. The office was the living room of our duplex. Our golden retriever Rockee was staff receptionist; he got paid in beef jerky and Bonz.

We produced the first issue within four work-crazed months. The pages were filled with race results, commentary, photos, interviews, and a race calendar. I ended up writing half the issue using an IBM Selectric typewriter. I found freelance contributors. Twenty thousand copies of *Tri-Athlete* were printed on high-quality newsprint. It was thirty-two pages, which included eight pages of color. We distributed our first issue at the season's first major race, the Ricoh Ironman in Los Angeles. We then handed out the remaining copies at races and bike and running stores throughout California. These copies were free. The three of us—Rockee, Terri, and me—logged thousands of miles in my Toyota pickup truck weighed down with the copies.

By late summer, *Tri-Athlete* became "the little magazine that could" by building a national reputation with pungent writing, incisive race commentary, and timely news coverage. Each monthly issue averaged about $10,000 in advertising revenue, which covered almost all our expenses except for printing. By fall, we had over 1,000 subscribers. I dreaded licking and affixing postage stamps on mail-bound copies. For California store distribution, I hired two part-time delivery employees. The rest of the copies filled the living room, giving Rockee a new place to climb and nap. The magazine had taken over our lives.

Tri-Athlete's main competition was Los Angeles–based *Triathlon*, which was being bankrolled, in part, by the J. David investment firm, and which later unraveled after the San Diego founder was arrested for orchestrating an $80 million Ponzi scheme. *Tri-Athlete* was the scrappy underdog. As the triathlon off-season approached, I believed that it made economic sense to join forces with a more established, well-capitalized publishing company. As a result, I sold a majority interest of *Tri-Athlete* to a Belgian sports magazine company that had recently launched *Winning: Bicycle Racing Illustrated*. Six things soon happened: One, the magazine became a slick color glossy; two, I was flying to Brussels every seventeen days to oversee the magazine's layout and production; three, *Tri-Athlete* became the international voice of the fledgling sport; four, Terri left me and enrolled in law school; five, I paid off my printing debt; and six, I officially withdrew from the PhD program in political science.

Triathlon's early years were a gold rush of frenzied participatory action and get-rich-quick event promoters, while media naysayers considered the sport a semi-legitimate "flash in the pan" athletic novelty. The notion of triathlon one day becoming an Olympic sport was far-fetched, an illusory dream. The sport was relatively unknown in Europe and Asia. About the only constant in the sport was triathlon's very own Mount Rushmore, better known as the Big Four: Scott Tinley, Dave Scott, Scott Molina, and Mark Allen. These four Californians ruled the triathlon planet. While each of them saw plenty of ink in *Tri-Athlete,* the magazine profiled new emerging stars, showcased events in tropical locales, tweaked sunburned noses of the triathlon establishment, and highlighted multisport lifestyles. Journalistic gaffes, too, were made along the way, such as dressing up Julie Moss as Madonna and putting her on the cover with the tagline "Material Girl." That became the worst-selling newsstand issue in *Tri-Athlete*'s history.

As I flew back and forth between the Bay Area and Brussels, I became so jetlagged that I allowed my overall fitness to decline. But I tried my best to run several times a week while in Brussels or bike when I returned to the States. The only time I went swimming was during a triathlon; each summer I'd choose one with short distances—1.5K swim, 40K bike, 10K run. I did the 1985 Dallas triathlon on my mountain bike—the only fat-tire bike in a field of 1,000 participants.

By the spring of 1986, I was burned out from triathlon and the accumulated strain of meeting monthly publishing deadlines. I decided to sell my remaining interest in *Tri-Athlete* and resign from the publication. I then quietly celebrated with a friend in Death Valley, where we spent a week hiking and mountain biking. The desert's stillness and quiet were relaxing, therapeutic, awe inspiring. Afterward, I biked two hundred miles up the California coast, traveling from Los Angeles to San Luis Obispo.

THE TRANSITION PERIOD

For the next seven years, I distanced myself from any conceivable interaction with triathlon and triathletes, even though I still biked and ran three to five hours per week. Exercise remained a much-needed outlet for stress. It also kept my weight from edging upward. But gone was a journalistic fascination with sweat and sport. Instead I launched a national literary magazine called *Arrival* with my *Tri-Athlete* earnings, but after three issues, it was too hard to sustain financially, so I closed it down. As a follow-up, I created a slick Bay Area lifestyle magazine irreverently named *Frisko*, in a city where only sailors, bikers, tourists, and relatives from the Midwest call the city by that name, albeit with a *c*. I found some investors, built up a staff, and this period in my life, known as the "*Frisko* Years," was a short-lived, wonderfully creative and productive era, stretching from 1989 through 1992.

Frisko had humble beginnings in a small two-hundred-square-foot office in the historic Flood Building. The rental manager informed me that Dashiell Hammett wrote *The Maltese Falcon* in this very same office. Looking back at these years running a magazine in a town not yet taken over by the dot-commers and Internet entrepreneurs, many memories tumble forth, triggering for the most part pleasant thoughts and associations. It was an exciting time for me, bracketed as it were by the quake of '89 and the advent of the digital age with the birth of *Wired* magazine that reshaped the San Francisco media landscape.

Frisko's pages were filled with articles and photos of celebrities, sports stars, authors, newsmakers, famous chefs, designers, fashionistas, actors, and politicians. International fashion model Carre Otis graced the cover of the first issue in full décolletage, followed by a morose-looking Nicholas Cage wearing an inside-out black T-shirt for the second issue. I remember the Cage issue as the "quake" issue. While I was talking to the printer on the phone, I felt the room shake, and then the entire Flood Building twisted about as if someone were wringing out a wet towel. Across the street, the huge plate glass window of the Emporium Capwell department store began popping and shattering onto the sidewalk. My staff fled for the stairs. Yet I remained on the phone, surprisingly calm, alone in the office. After all, the sturdy, nine-story Flood Building had survived the 1906 earthquake. It made it through the 1989 temblor intact.

As publisher and editor, I was invited to many lunches, dinners, and art gallery openings—and consequently, I made sure to keep working out at least three or four hours a week (mainly running or cycling) so I could enjoy the active social life and keep in moderately good shape. But even with an infusion of capital from several new investors, *Frisko* ran out of money in early 1993. With a heavy heart, I told my staff of twenty in our new North Beach digs that I had to close down the magazine. Hell's Angel founder and former Oakland resident Sonny Barger had been slated to appear on the next cover.

As I was wrapping up *Frisko*'s business affairs, I got a call from an old friend, Felix Magowan, who was the publisher of Boulder-based *VeloNews*. He said he was buying a triathlon magazine and wanted my editorial and creative advice. "But Felix," I said, "I have been out of the sport for seven years. Can't you find anyone else?" Felix persisted, and so I relented and flew to

Boulder for two days. He later offered me the job as editor-in-chief of *Inside Triathlon*. Two months later, I packed up all my books and belongings, hired a moving van, and relocated with Rockee to Boulder. I had returned to the triathlon fold.

BACK TO THE FUTURE WITH TRIATHLON

The sport had significantly changed while I was away during those seven jubilee years. It was now a global sport. There were triathlon wetsuits, steep-angle triathlon bikes, aero bars, disc wheels, energy bars, space-age bike helmets, and clipless pedals. *Tri-Athlete* had also dropped the hyphen in its name after merging with *Triathlon* to become *Triathlete*.

One of my first phone calls was to the new Hawaii Ironman race director to introduce myself and request an entry in the October race—four months away. He agreed. Getting in shape for the race would be an ideal way to get quickly up to speed on the sport's new dynamics.

Boulder, home to many top triathletes, was a splendid, high-altitude multisport playground. I'd go on short runs or bike rides before work. On weekends, I explored new running trails in the foothills with Rockee, or biked on the windswept prairies or up the few canyons that rose to meet Peak to Peak Highway. I joined a health club for swimming.

In late August, I did a sprint triathlon in Fort Collins. The swim was held in an indoor pool. It took me eleven minutes to go just a quarter-mile. October's Ironman was just eight weeks away, and so I began to focus more intently on training. When October arrived and the first heavy snow blanketed the ground, I was in decent enough condition though ten pounds over my 1982 Ironman weight. Compared with my Ironman prep work eleven years earlier, I had done half the mileage. A betting pool had formed at *Inside Triathlon* regarding the odds of my finishing the race. Almost all my colleagues wagered against me.

I felt much more relaxed in Kona the second time. The swim went fine, and I even trimmed five minutes from the 1982 split. Matters went differently, however, on the bike. Either I got much slower or everyone else biked much faster. Several dozen riders passed me, yet I only passed several in return. The bike ride took me 7:30. I still had plenty of time and energy left for the marathon, and despite stabbing pain above my left knee that forced me to walk nearly half the lava course, I managed to cross the finish line in 15:04, only two minutes slower than in 1982. Consistency must count for something. Though for the next two days I had to walk down stairs backward because of the leg pain, this seemed a small price to pay for being able to relive the experience of running down Alii Drive, while soaking up the crowd's energy and loud cheers.

. . .

Determined to stay in shape after this second Ironman, I continued working out between seven and ten hours every week. Keeping a training diary helped cement the motivation. But after a year of living in Boulder, I grew homesick for the Bay Area, and decided to move back and become the new editor of *Triathlete*. My multisport fitness followed me to the West coast, and the first triathlon I did there was Escape from Alcatraz.

Here's my journal entry from July 9, 1994, on swimming from the Rock:

Early Saturday morning in Frisco. T-shirt tourist shops in Fisherman's Wharf haven't yet opened. Crabs had a few more hours of limited freedom before the final indignity of being dropped into vats of boiling water. Also missing in action was the sweet aroma of sourdough bread. The only smell in the air was fear as five hundred triathletes solemnly boarded the Red & White Ferry for the 1.5-mile boat trip across the San Francisco Bay to Alcatraz Island. In order to escape from the Rock, you first have to get there. I was part of the reverse jailbreak.

We were Birdbrains of Alcatraz.

Almost everyone was encased in full-sleeved wetsuits. Dressed for chill. The only exception was a handful of beefy men and women. Body-fat would function as their natural insulation. As the ferry chugged across the slate-gray water, a raucous gang of sea lions lounging near Pier 39 began their cacophonous barking. The pinnipeds were all very resplendent in their shiny black wetsuits. No race numbers marked their flippers.

Before we disembarked from the ferry and tentatively walked onto the wooden-platform gangway leading to the island, some swimmers dipped their fingers into jumbo jars of Vaseline. Absolution for past sins of missed swim workouts? The petroleum jelly was smeared on the back of necks to prevent chafing from the wetsuit's collar. Two enterprising fellows wrapped duct tape around their necks. Surely this was a case of ducts taking to the water.

Alcatraz means "pelican" in Spanish, but swimmers stiffly milled about like emperor penguins. Nobody wanted to leave the joint. The water looked cold. In the high fifties. Borderline hypothermic conditions for slowpokes.

The race start approached. Faster swimmers dropped into the water near the rocky beach and stroked out toward the lead kayak. These wily front-of-the-packers weren't wet behind their ears; they jumped the start gun, which, in this case, was the boat's air blast, and sounded like an angry belch.

The water near Alcatraz turned angry as panicked swimmers scrambled into the water. Two thousand limbs into the sea.

The most vexing problem was navigation. Without orange DayGlo swim buoys lining the course, you had to focus on distant landmarks such as tall buildings in the background. These high-rises might serve as terrific backdrops for San Francisco–based films but were difficult to locate when your goggles were fogging up and waves rudely slapped seawater into your mouth.

But once you settle into a groove, a relaxed rhythm, swimming from Alcatraz can become an enjoyable experience—as long as the tide is behaving, wind chop is slight, and container ships the length of two football fields aren't motoring past.

The lesson of this swim was simple: Because of a fast-moving ebb tide, those who attempted to make a straight shot to the finish at Aquatic Park got swept out toward the Golden Gate Bridge. Those who aimed left, aimed right. Think of a golfer lining up a putt and correctly reading the green. The entrance to Aquatic Park is narrow. Miss it and you get a bogey or worse. Talk about a water hazard!

I made it to the small beach in fifty-five minutes. A bike ride across the Golden Gate Bridge was next, followed by an eleven-mile trail run in the hilly Marin Headlands. I didn't see any sharks during the swim. I read somewhere that the more "docile" leopard sharks patrol these urban waters. The great white shark, the true man-eaters, feed just outside the bay. So I was personally told by race director Dave Horning, who had swum from Alcatraz fifty times.

My next triathlon was an off-road affair near Lake Tahoe, where my main concern was to avoid crashing on the tricky, narrow technical bike course and smashing my head open on the rocks. Out of fifty triathletes in the race, I came in second-to-last. The winner, Scott Tinley, had already taken a nap and showered when he greeted the late arrivals. A race photo of me biking shows a muscular fellow with taut upper body—and no gut!

Despite this penchant for being a back-of-the-packer, I continued sampling a smorgasbord of multisport events for the next several years. These included an eight-mile adventure run along the Santa Barbara shoreline called the "Scramble"; three more off-road triathlons; the San Francisco half-marathon, where I surprised myself by finishing 500 in a field of 1,500 with a time of 1:44; a twenty-four-hour mountain bike race; the 129-mile Death Ride of Markleeville in the High Sierras with five mountain passes and 15,000 feet of climbing (I made three of the passes); a three-day mountain bike race in Coast Rica; a twenty-four-hour adventure race in the Golden Gate National Recreational Area; Bay to Breakers (I ran to the start from home—a distance of 11 miles—and then joined the costumed herd for the 7.2-mile run); and two additional swims from Alcatraz.

The last escape from the Rock seemed like a scene from *Waterworld*. When a strong ebb tide began sweeping swimmers out toward the Golden Gate Bridge, a flotilla of jet skis, kayaks, and support boats was on standby to assist wayward and weaker swimmers. Like myself. The current was too strong to fight. About one-tenth of the field were harpooned onto these rescue vessels. Though it was the height of the salmon fishing season, triathletes were the catch of the day.

. . .

While many endurance athletes trained to race, I preferred the experience of training—but without having scheduled events marked on the calendar. I liked nothing better than going on one- or two-hour trail runs with Rockee on the many trails that crisscrossed Mount Tam in Marin County. When I wanted to go for a bike ride, I always felt guilty about leaving Rockee behind, so I would scatter dog biscuits in different rooms. While he diligently hunted for his treats, I'd make a quick exit with either my road or mountain bike.

Whenever I traveled, I made every effort to challenge myself on long solo runs. Once, after watching a pro mountain bike race in Monterrey, California, I drove to nearby 17 Mile Drive, parked my jeep by the entrance, and then ran the entire coastal route. I brought along no water or food, so I was nearly delirious when I finished in Carmel. Shivering and chilled in my sweat-soaked T-shirt, I went over to a gift store, but the only shirts it had in stock were monogrammed purple golf shirts with pink collars. I bought one anyway. After lunch and nap in the sun, I walked up Ocean Avenue to Highway 1 and hitchhiked back to my vehicle.

Two other do-it-myself memorable runs: a twenty-mile Saturday run from the Santa Monica pier to the top of Topanga Canyon, where I loaded up on food at the small well-stocked market before heading back down the narrow canyon, which had no shoulder. Cars rushed by only inches from my left side. The descent was scary.

The other run was an 11.5-mile uphill affair along the highway shoulder from Lee Vining, a town on the eastern side of the Sierras, all the way to the 9,945-foot Tioga Pass entrance station to Yosemite, an elevation gain of about two-thirds of a mile. The slow, steady climb was exhilarating, but about a mile from the snow-covered pass—it was August—I began to bonk since I'd failed to bring along any food. I stopped running and tried to hitchhike back to Lee Vining. But traffic was scarce, just a few vacationers who sped right by. One driver heading to Yosemite did pull over to see if everything was okay. He handed me a piece of hard candy. That's all he had. I sucked on it, hoping for a miracle burst of energy. I then ran the entire way to Lee Vining—11.5 additional miles. My first destination was a café where I downed two pitchers of ice water and ordered two plates of French toast and hash browns. (Years later, I discovered that there's an annual Tioga Pass running race held each September.)

On the publishing front, I eventually left *Triathlete* after seven months to start my own magazine called *Multisport*. I raised funds for it and produced two issues, but it was difficult to convince advertisers of my vision of an emerging athletic trend—that the overlapping sports of cycling, running, swimming, triathlon, adventure racing, and hiking were successfully feeding off one another, while attracting many new participants. It could be argued that *Multisport* was ahead of its time. Lance had yet to win his first Tour de France. Charity bike rides were only just forming, The Ironman hadn't rolled out its massive event expansion to cities all over the globe. Big-city marathons were just beginning to regain their lost momentum from an earlier slowdown.

I might have clearly seen the future of participatory sports, but where my clairvoyance ultimately failed was with my own life as a multisport athlete. I never saw the fall coming. And it was some fall—a sorry, unplanned plunge into the zero-fitness abyss, which lasted ten years.

②

THE LOST YEARS

My Health and Fitness
Spiraled Downward for a Decade

My training diaries from 1993 through 1998 offered no hint that one day I would stop working out altogether—and that my hiatus from exercise would eventually telescope into a desultory decade.

How did this ever happen? And why?

First, my dog Rockee, a golden retriever, died at age fourteen. We had run together for practically his entire life. We romped through the parks in the Berkeley and Oakland hills, we explored Marin County fire roads and trails, and we had a grand time in the Boulder foothills. But with his passing, I lost almost all interest in running. Occasionally, I would go on a half-hour or hour run, but it never seemed the same without him at my side. Sometimes I'd imagine seeing Rockee's spectral presence—a beaming, curious, tail-wagging hologram—checking out his favorite creeks or bushes. Morosely tethered to this memory, I would stop running and sit on a moss-covered rock, hoping to ward off the enveloping sadness. I missed him so much that my heart ached.

Friends often asked, "Why not get another dog?" But I remained in mourning.

Right after Rockee's death, my father began to show early signs of Alzheimer's. The cruel disease progressively wipes away memory, identity, and self. My father, who had been a confident, assertive, kind, and generous man, soon became childlike and helpless. He had once run a successful food and candy brokerage in northern Ohio with over fifty employees. His vibrant, larger-than-life personality was replaced by a timid, forgetful individual who no longer remembered his own phone number or how to boil water on the stove. He had difficulty finishing sentences. He liked watching *Teletubbies*. This was a man who had built an indoor tennis club in Cleveland with seventeen courts. My mother now had to keep a strict eye on him. She said, "It's like having a child always around." Witnessing his mental decline burdened me with sorrow. At times, working out seemed meaningless—but I somehow managed to push through the gloom and go bike riding.

This period also marked my involvement with La Ruta de Los Conquistadores, a three-day mountain bike race in Costa Rica that proudly calls itself "the toughest mountain bike race on the planet." There's a 50 percent dropout rate among competitors. Little surprise—La Ruta boasts 26,000 feet of climbing over 250 miles of varying terrain. It starts at the Pacific and ends at the Atlantic. Between both coasts is a series of harsh riding conditions: tropical heat and humidity, mountains, poorly maintained dirt roads, tire-sucking mud, stream crossings, banana plantations, and intermittent rain.

In late fall 1997, I flew down to Costa Rica with my friend Roy Wallack, an endurance cyclist and magazine colleague. The event was small and virtually unknown, attracting one hundred Costa Ricans and a dozen Americans. I was in adequate multisport shape and didn't specifically train for the race, which I realized was a lapse in judgment several hours into the first day of riding. The climbs were endless and often steep. I began to walk the uphill grades with my bike, then began using my bike as a *walker* to get up them. I was in last place, but it had its benefits: I had my own private police motorcycle escort. I felt sorry for these two *policias* following me on their Kawasakis. Since they had no food, I shared some of my cookies with them. I covered fifty miles that day—which was thirty miles short of the day's finish line—before finally getting scooped up by the sag or broom wagon—a battered African safari jeep. Other whipped competitors soon joined me in the rattling vehicle. We were a glum-looking bunch huddled inside the cargo area as we bounced along the dirt roads, sweeping up several more slow cyclists.

The next day at La Ruta was even worse—it began with a twenty-mile body-buster up the flanks of the dormant 11,000-foot Irazu volcano. The elite riders passed me near Irazu's base as if I were riding in the opposite direction. My sore, aching quads were shot midway up the climb, so I asked a support Jeep to take my bike. I then began jogging and walking up the mountain for several miles. At the summit, I got back my bike and rode down the other side—a harrowing seventeen-mile, brake-pad melting descent—to the small town of Turriabla.

Day three was difficult just trying to get out of bed. My legs were numb, battered, weak. We had another seventy miles of mountainous riding. I managed to bike for about three hours before surrendering and climbing inside the empty support jeep. But the vehicle broke its axle on a rocky descent, and I had to wait by a coffee farm for five hours in the hot sun for another jeep to retrieve me. I had no water or food; I plucked a few unripe coffee berries from a tree but they were inedible. By the time I arrived at the finish line in Limon, on the Atlantic Coast, all the riders were busy getting on the bus for a return trip back to the capital San Jose.

I didn't finish a single La Ruta stage. "Okay," I promised myself, "You will do better next year. You *will* train."

That spring, I entered a twenty-four-hour solo mountain bike race in Monterey, California. It was fun for about twelve hours until complete exhaustion forced me to quit.

I trained hard for La Ruta by logging numerous six-hour mountain bike rides in Marin, though I belatedly discovered that I should have been doing at least two or three consecutive days of these long rides for several months. In any case, I was determined to finish each day of La Ruta, come jungle hell or high water.

The field had doubled in size when I returned to Costa Rica. Word was getting out to hard-core mountain bike riders that La Ruta was *the* race you wanted to have on your racing resumé. La Ruta organizer Roman Urbina told everyone that *policias* were once again assigned the thankless task of shadowing slowpokes. I recognized one of the motorcycle cops from last year. When he saw me, he told Roman, "Oh, no, not *him* again!" All this took place in Spanish, so I was spared the initial embarrassment. Roman, who became a close friend, told me all this afterward.

Once again I failed to finish any of the three stages. It was a miserable and humiliating experience, I was simply too slow of a rider. Or rather, the other cyclists were much faster and better prepared.

I returned to the Bay Area demoralized by what had happened in Costa Rica. I gradually began losing interest in cycling. This attitudinal change took several months to solidify into something obdurate. Three rides per week dissolved into a single-hour ride, if that. As my motivation to bike continued to wane, I became more apathetic about riding. *Not* biking developed into a vicious cycle of disinterest. My once-muscular calves and quads turned spongy. And before I knew it, I stopped cycling altogether—for the first time in two decades. I had mentally flatted.

ILLNESS ARRIVED

A year went by, then two years, and I still wasn't riding. The longer I stayed away from cycling, the more powerful became this separation, as if I didn't deserve to get back on the bike. Whenever I walked past my three bikes parked right outside the front door, collecting dust, leaves, and cobwebs, I did my best to look away—a coward's reaction to his own failing.

Meanwhile, my father's health deteriorated. The neural-choking disease took seven years to completely ravage his brain. On January 2, 2004, he died in a nursing home—mute, immobile, unresponsive, unable to recognize his wife of nearly five decades. It was as if he had died twice when his heart stopped and he took his last breath.

Several months after my father's funeral, I developed dermatitis in both legs. Was this condition stress-related? My legs became stiff, swollen, and terribly inflamed, the affliction spreading from feet to butt. I wrapped them in gauze or cloth three or four times a day. Hot showers provided momentary relief. But the legs remained a weepy, gooey mess. Bending down or walking even a few steps became painful. It was difficult taking out the trash, going to the bathroom, or trudging up the driveway to the mailbox—a distance of seventy-five yards one way. I once remarked to a friend that the driveway seemed like an eternity, as physically agonizing as the last half of the 26.2-mile marathon at the Hawaii Ironman. That might sound like an exaggeration—but it wasn't. Not with this around-the-clock misery.

The dermatitis led to edema. As a result of fluid retention beneath the skin, each leg ballooned to twice its size. My feet looked unrecognizable, as if they had been inflated with a bike pump. I couldn't wear shoes. I looked freakish, and was alarmed over what was happening to my body. Had the edema been caused by the topical anti-itch hydrocortisone Cortaid cream that I had applied to my legs? Or were the dermatitis and edema caused by an addiction to Advil?

For several years, to help cope with insomnia, I had been gulping down handfuls of Advil, popping them in my mouth like M&Ms. The pills seemed to having a calming effect, whereas sleep aids like Omnicom or Tylenol PM left me too groggy the next day. I tried Ambien, but it instigated too many disturbing nightmares. I was soon swallowing twenty, thirty Advil pills every day. In the mornings and afternoons, I balanced the brown pills with a two-liter bottle of Coke. Taken in large quantities, Advil's main ingredient, ibuprofen, can damage the liver and, in turn, this can cause skin problems and buildup of excess fluid. My blood was being polluted. By my own choosing! All that caffeine and sugar from Coke didn't help matters.

There was one incredibly bad period—lasting about three months—when the dermatitis spread to both my hands and arms. They too needed to be swaddled in gauze. I looked and felt like the Mummy. The affliction made it impossible to work on my current project: an oral history book focusing on political dissent in post-9/11 America. I couldn't hold a book or magazine to read, a pen to write, or knife to spread peanut butter and jelly on bread. I would lie in bed and call old friends from the past who were always surprised to hear from me, especially after ten or twenty years. I spent most of my time in the horizontal position, in bed, cut off from all physical activity. I was exiled from normal life, an invalid locked away in his own mattress prison. The cruel and ironic joke was that the year before, I had written my first book with a colleague and friend Timothy Carlson on Iraq War correspondents. The title of this oral history was *Embedded: The Media at War in Iraq.* The book received positive reviews in places like the *New York Times, Washington Post,* and *Michigan Law Review* and won a national book prize from Harvard. I had gone from *Embedded* to being trapped in bed.

Through continued bed rest, the edema eventually subsided. I tried walking for exercise. Even though my ravaged legs still hurt from the dermatitis, I refused to give in to the pain and discomfort. I'd walk several times a week, getting up to two miles, but for some inexplicable reason (most likely triggered by emotional or mental stress from simultaneously working on additional book projects as editor or author), the dermatitis, aggravated by intense itching and scratching, would flare up, and it was back to lying in bed, feeling sorry for myself and wondering what the hell was going on.

I finally stopped taking Advil and altered my diet. I had been a vegetarian since my early twenties. My diet lacked sufficient protein and healthy fat, which is good for the skin. I began to eat salmon, eggs, and vegetables like broccoli and spinach to help cleanse my liver. It took several months before these nutritional changes started paying off. After two and a half years of suffering, my legs were noticeably improving.

Just after my fiftieth birthday, my legs were almost completely healed. I decided that it was time to fight my way back to health and fitness. I was determined to climb out of the deep hole I had dug for myself. I had waited far too long. Plus I wasn't getting any younger.

STARTING OUT

We've all heard the saying, "A journey of a thousand miles begins with a single step." Here's what happened on that first day: I trotted up the driveway to the mailbox. Seventy-five yards. That was it. I was winded. My legs ached. I did this several days in a row. I then progressed to super-slow running—more like a fast walk—for about two hundred yards along the dead-end street to a splintering wooden guardrail that marked my finish line. The road has a gradual incline. That meager distance represented my absolute physical limit. My quads and calves seemed like they were on fire. Every breath felt forced and labored. The exertion drained me. I would walk home.

I was amazed at how unnatural running had become; it felt foreign to put one foot in front of the other and *not* think about the effort expended. I was aware of every plodding, earth-bound foot-strike. The exaggerated awkwardness of my gait and slowness of leg speed would have been laughable—only if it were happening to someone else. A disconnect existed between the upper and lower halves of my body, like it was constructed from mismatched parts.

I continued with the jogging-and-walking routine for about a month. I got up to one mile. My typical pace was twelve to fourteen minutes per mile. By contrast, at the 1996 San Francisco half-marathon, I had averaged 7:50 per mile—that's nearly twice as fast! But most importantly, my health and fitness were moving forward—not backward. The highlight of my day was going out for an evening run. Fancy that!

IRONY MAN

No one said it was going to be easy. My first setback occurred just after reaching the two-mile mark in my runs. I had recently finished editing a book on former Vice President Al Gore's speeches and interviews, and was anxiously awaiting the book's release in early October 2007. I dealt with the anxiety, stress, and insomnia the wrong way. I started taking Aleve, which is the brand name for a non-steroid compound called naproxen. Sleep came like a precious gift for several wonderful weeks. But I should have learned the lesson from my earlier Advil addiction. Aleve can also seriously affect the liver, disrupting the manufacture of blood-cleansing and healthy cellular enzymes. My skin went haywire again—hives, welts, intense itching, dermatitis. I was miserable and in perpetual discomfort, and stopped running altogether. I had screwed up my body with Aleve and my body now screwed me. It was lose-lose.

I eventually did the smart thing. I flushed the tiny blue Aleve pills down the toilet and began consuming more broccoli, spinach, brussels sprouts, onions, garlic, salmon, fish oil pills, and eggs. Relief came slowly over the following weeks. The hives disappeared, but my skin remained dry, inflamed, and itchy—a toxic epidermal legacy of unregulated over-the-counter medication that wreaked havoc on my body's metabolism. Two months went by before I started to jog again. I got winded after only going a quarter-mile. The dermatitis made my skin feel like construction paper being ripped whenever I moved about.

One Saturday afternoon, I happened to watch the delayed telecast of the 2007 Hawaii Ironman. NBC Sports did a masterful job following competitors—the winners, age-group triathletes, and those who deserve a special category all their own, such as a guy with two titanium prosthetic legs, a blind man, a sixty-five-year-old grandmother, and a college student who survived a near-fatal auto accident that left him in a coma. Each of these "triathlon success stories" would finish the race.

It was inspiring to witness their undiminished courage and personal heroism in one of the world's toughest endurance events. Seeing them push their bodies in the Hawaiian heat, I couldn't help but nostalgically reflect upon my own two Ironman experiences, that is, until a flashing neon mental billboard of my current unfit status interrupted the pleasant reverie.

Instead of thinking of myself as a former Ironman, I felt more like Irony Man—someone whose athletic identity had been forged by the race but who later allowed that identification to disintegrate. When the hour-long triathlon broadcast ended, I turned off the television and considered two options: I could abandon my fitness quest once and for all; or I could go for a short run, and simply learn to take one day at a time.

I decided to go running—sorry, I meant jogging—for several minutes. Afterward, I could almost sense my body thanking me for not giving up.

③

THE JOY OF RUNNING (AND WALKING)—

But Don't Overdo It at First!

Journal Entry—January 6, 2008

Our neighborhood has been without power for forty-eight hours, courtesy of the first of three fierce winter storms barreling out of the Gulf of Alaska that have lashed the Northern California coast. I live inland by about eight miles, but during the height of the storm, winds reached up to seventy-five miles per hour, knocking down trees and utility poles. Pacific Gas and Electric's toll-free outage hotline won't say when electricity will be restored. It feels like camping indoors, but I am low on food and candles, and the novelty of shivering under several blankets while listening to the radio for news and weather alerts grows dull and repetitive with each passing hour. Over one million Bay Area households are still off the power grid. I can't fall back asleep. At 3:30 A.M., I do something un-expected. I grab a flashlight, slip on my running shoes, and decide to run two miles to the 7-Eleven to buy some supplies. This will be my longest run in months. Fortunately, the first half of this nocturnal errand is all downhill.

The rain had stopped as I snaked down steep Summit Avenue in the dark, using a two-cell Maglite to navigate past the fallen branches littering the road.

Almost all the homes were dark, except a few that have loud, throaty portable gas-powered generators pumping electrical juice into their warm, cozy warrens. These homes also have recycling bins and pricy hybrids parked in their driveways.

I barely made it to the store on weakening legs. I had to push myself the final four hundred yards, almost like I were in a race, and the finish line was the 7-Eleven parking lot. Except when I get there, the store was closed. An employee was busy pumping out water from the flooded store with a generator. I asked him if I could go inside and buy some juice. He told me no. "The power is out and the cash register is closed."

I was thirsty so I walked another half-mile to a closed gas station, and bought an orange Fanta from the vending machine, and contemplated my trek back home—2.5 miles away. I was not looking forward to going up Summit Avenue whose average grade ranges between 5 and 10 percent. There was a time when I could run this one-mile uphill stretch without resting, but these were memories best left quiet, undisturbed, and out of sight.

Earlier in the week, I had read The Courage To Start, *a collection of essays by* Runner's World's *popular columnist John Bingham, who is widely known as the Pied Piper of recreational runners. His down-to-earth wisdom about getting into running shape is based on his own experience as a former coach potato and smoker who took up running for the very first time in his early forties. On his first day, he could only manage thirty lung-bursting seconds. I could relate. That too was all I could go before redlining. But he stuck with running and walking over several months, and with steely, admirable determination, he built up his cardio, stamina, and endurance. He eventually became hooked on competing in 5Ks, 10Ks, and marathons, where his presence was always welcomed by everyman and everywoman runners.* The *New York* Times *called him one of the most influential people in the sport of running because he inspires tens of thousands who flock to the big-city running events and have little expectation beyond obtaining a finisher's medallion.*

Bingham preaches the importance of setting achievable goals and living day-by-day as a way to overcome frustration and futility, because there will be both good and bad days. Tonight, my goal was to make it back home on foot. An hour later, as I reached my driveway, the rain began to fall again. I went inside and immediately warmed up beneath a layer of blankets. Drifting off to sleep, I watched the yellow flame of the vanilla-scented candle dance in the dark.

• • •

I never took physics in high school or college, but I was familiar with Sir Isaac Newton's first law of motion, which states that "an object at rest tends to stay at rest and an object in motion tends to stay in motion." Simply put, it's hard to get going when you have given up exercising for a long time, but once you get with the program, you will want to continue working out. Inactivity begets inactivity. Activity spurs activity. A body at rest in an Ikea recliner stays at rest and muscles atrophy. A body in motion on the trails or roads will continue burning calories even when you get home. Then there are the psychological benefits—the runner's high, which is addictive and will inspire you to continue training.

Scientists employ another term to describe the physical process of action and inaction; it's called inertia. We all resist change, but once we begin moving, we don't want to stop. This represents a personal choice between "Just Do It" or Just Screw It.

Walking is a simple and effective way to break free from inertia's Krazy Glue–hold on doing little or nothing. Running is the other. But in order to properly arrive at the running phase, fitness experts recommend that you first do a lot of walking. Don't expect to run a 5K or 10K at the end of week one, or even month one. Maybe not even in the initial three months, depending on how out of shape you have been. Don't be alarmed if you are unable to jog a mile those introductory weeks. Walk instead.

The American College of Sports Medicine and the American Heart Association urge walking as the ideal workout, and in terms of tempo, suggest reaching an elevated heart rate and breathing rate that will still enable you to carry on a conversation. In 2007, both organizations updated their physical activity guidelines and came to the following conclusion: All healthy adults need endurance exercise, which noticeably accelerates their heart rate for at least ten minutes at a time. This requires a minimum of thirty minutes a day five days a week, though the thirty minutes can be broken up into ten-minute increments.

Of course, you don't need to restrict your cardio activity solely to walking, since the elliptical trainer, bike riding, or swimming are ideal substitutes. Yet walking is the easiest to do. You don't need to join a gym, hire a trainer, buy a pedometer, GPS, walking poles, or expensive "walking shoes." You might, however, want to keep a walking diary, and there are plenty of online walking sites that provide all sorts of fitness and weight-loss calculators. The iPod, iPhone, and Blackberry have walking calculators that help measure distance and pace.

A recent study by the Duke University Medical Center found that mild exercise such as walking briskly for a total of twelve miles a week, or a total of two to three and a half hours a week, improved aerobic fitness and decreased risk of cardiovascular disease. The study examined 133 subjects who were divided into the following categories: sedentary, overweight, aged forty to sixty-five, with too much fat in their blood. All exercise groups significantly improved their absolute and relative peak oxygen consumption and lost an average of 2.87 pounds. "You don't have to be gasping for breath to get good aerobic benefits from walking," concluded the study. "People find exercise 'hard' and few people want to exercise at an intensity higher than they have to. Walking briskly for twelve miles a week per week is realistic and does not require anyone to incorporate a hardcore training regimen. Increasing your mileage or intensity will give you even greater health benefits."

TWENTY WALKING TIPS

You can get in admirable shape simply by walking. The well-respected multi-sport author and trainer Phil Maffetone, who pioneered the use of heart-rate monitors and was named coach of the year by *Triathlete* magazine, believes that walking is the cornerstone of building an aerobic base for health and fitness. "Most people will succeed with walking, which can provide people with the most difficult part of getting back into shape," he says. "Many will not need or want more exercise, while other people can use this base as an essential platform to build more fitness for running, competition, or just higher levels of working out."

I asked Phil to put together a list of twenty walking pointers for *Return to Fitness.* Here are his foolproof recommendations:

1. Have a regular routine. People who fit a regular workout into their daily schedule usually stick with it.
2. Work out near home rather than driving somewhere. A treadmill at the gym can be intimidating, especially if you're even a bit overweight or out of shape. There are lots of mirrors and sweaty jocks with enlarged muscles. Personal trainers can be okay, but often have their own agenda that may not fit your specific needs.
3. Don't buy special workout attire. Cheap shoes, simple gym shorts, and T-shirts work great.

4. Wear the flattest and most comfortable shoes you can get. The flattest, most inexpensive shoes are best because they won't increase your risk of getting injured (as studies have shown).

5. I strongly advise using a heart-rate monitor so you don't work out too hard. Your workout should be so easy that when you're done, it feels like you haven't done much of anything. The "no pain, no gain" attitude causes injury and is a common reason why people don't remain in a routine. You want to train your body to burn fat. This is accomplished at moderate levels of training intensity, not high levels. A heart monitor serves as a biofeedback device (like a coach), informing you that your level of intensity is too high or low (as indicated by your heart rate).

6. Don't count calories. You want to burn fat, not just calories. Diet (not dieting) and exercise must go together.

7. Keep your walking simple. There's no need to add more stress to your life. There's no special way to walk (some people look like zombies when they walk as a workout). Just walk.

8. Work out in a pleasant environment—a park, quiet streets. Don't walk along a busy road.

9. Schedule your workout in the morning if possible, before you start the day. Those who do this generally stay on course. As the day progresses, if you've not done your workout, you keep adding more things to do. Now your workout is in jeopardy because you're too busy. Get it done early in the day, and it's done.

10. Don't eat sweets before working out. Actually, don't eat sweets at all, but if you eat them before working out, they can reduce fat-burning. Sweets can raise the hormone insulin, which could impair metabolism to turn down fat-burning, so the calories you burn from your workout (and for some time afterward) are sugar calories not fat calories. This could result in more fat storage.

11. Drink a small glass of water before working out. No need to carry water with you as you can have some immediately upon completion.

12. Make your walking workouts a time of peace and relaxation. That means not chatting on the cell phone or to others around you. It's a time to meditate on your life and dream of getting more fit and healthy (and anything else you want to dream about).

13. Don't work out if you have an elevated temperature, even a half-degree. The body raises the temperature when it has to work very hard

(to fight an infection, for example). Exercise can interfere with that process. You could stress your immune system even more if you work out when you're getting sick. Your body requires rest at that time.

14. Don't work out in extremes of weather, especially severe cold or heat. Have an alternative when those days arrive: an indoor workout, a mall (better than not working out), or it may be time to buy that treadmill.

15. Don't worry about how far you go. Base your workout on time. Start with twenty minutes, if that feels physically easy. Build from there, as you are consistent, to thirty, then forty-five minutes. No need to exceed an hour unless you love it so much that longer weekend walks are fun.

16. Slowly start your workout with a warm-up. After about ten to twelve minutes, maintain a good comfortable pace. End the same way: by slowing down again.

17. Work out at least five or six days a week. Choose your busiest days, such as Monday or Friday, for an off-day from exercise. The body needs recovery, and this will help guarantee that.

18. Don't overtrain: Working out with too high a heart rate (which gauges the kind of workout you're having) increases stress hormones, and is not unlike other stress reactions. This is an unhealthy condition. Easy, low-heart–rate workouts don't trigger stress responses and are examples of healthy fitness.

19. The most difficult part in getting started is making room in one's schedule. Changing habits is always perceived as difficult; it's really just a matter of deciding to do it. Once you do that, the rest is relatively easy.

20. Occasionally, a particular disability might restrict you from doing certain activities (most people complain of things they believe limit them from working out, yet most of these are not valid excuses). Heart conditions, previous surgery, certain medications, and other things may require an adjustment in workout schedule. Ask your doctor if anything could be a problem.

DO RUNNING SHOES CAUSE INJURIES?

If you haven't been running for years but suspect that your feet will need extra pampering, do you buy a new pair of costly, shock-absorbing running shoes? Or go cheap and minimalist? Which option is best and will lead to many miles of injury-free running? Despite the universal availability of tricked-out running shoes, with amply cushioned soles, rigid foot boxes, and inch-thick heels, the injury rates among runners have virtually stayed the same since the 1970s. How can this be?

In a widely publicized 1999 study, Dr. Steven Robbins, a biomechanics expert at the McGill University Centre for Studies in Aging at Montreal, discovered that expensive running shoes aren't worth the money and may even increase your risk of injury. Dr. Robbins found that overly thick soles cause a loss of balance. "It's a myth that thick soles offer the most protection," he told reporters.

Subsequent studies by other researchers confirmed Robbins's findings. Runners in thick-soled shoes were more than twice as likely to suffer injuries as runners in thin soles. Robbins even went on to suggest that athletic shoes should be classified as "safety hazards" rather than "protective devices." His red-alert warning was certainly not the message footwear giants like Nike, New Balance, or Reebok wanted the public to hear.

The main problem with most running shoes is that the human foot was anatomically designed to provide a flexible yet durable platform to allow the lower body to move along the ground. (Our closest living relatives, the orangutans and chimpanzees, use their feet primarily for grasping and climbing; they seldom walk very far.) For eons, man walked, trotted, loped, and ran barefoot. Even the Egyptian pharaohs went barefoot. Because the foot is not dainty or fragile, it doesn't require a stiff, unyielding container to protect it from repetitive-motion impact. But when encased in a protective sheath like an excessively built-up running shoe, the muscles, tendons, and ligaments in the lower extremities begin to atrophy, leading to what one exercise researcher called "wimpy feet." Another critic called running shoes "little foot coffins." Instead of the foot and lower leg acting as shock absorbers, it's the shoe doing the work—which in turn causes a weakening of foot muscles, nerves, and tendons. Artificially supporting the foot contributes to its structural and biomechanical deterioration. Yet people who go around barefoot, observed Robbins, don't suffer from chronic foot, ankle, or knee problems.

"The problem is, the fancy running shoes have allowed us to develop lazy feet," Dr. Nicholas Romanov, a sports physiologist in Naples, Florida, told the *New York Times* in 2005. Romanov, an émigré from Russia, is best known for having created the "pose running method," which retrains your body to run more efficiently by making you land on the forefoot in what he calls

(continues)

"controlled falling." The forward-leaning, soft-landing action, coupled with a short stride and partially bent legs, allows gravity to propel you right along. Also known by some practitioners as "soft-running," the Romanov approach has become increasingly popular among injury-averse, high-mileage triathletes.

Bermuda orthopedic surgeon Dr. Joseph Froncioni wondered why he saw so many runners limping into his office. He blamed the flashy, built-up modern running shoe for their injuries. He recommends racing flats with minimal cushioning and arch support instead. On his blog, Quickswood, he wrote, "Don't listen to the store clerk who will try to dissuade you from buying a racing flat and may even go as far as telling you that they are for elite runners and are meant to be used for one marathon only. Don't believe him. I keep my flats for at least 400 to 500 miles with no problem."

Optimally, you want to run on the ball or forefront of your foot, not the heel. But the thick soles used in today's running shoes force you to land on your heels. Running on the heel is unnatural and will cause excessive stress throughout your foot and lower leg. Try running barefoot; no matter how slow or fast you go, it's nearly impossible to land on your heel. Yet we often hear that heel-to-toe striking is the proper way to run. Wrong. Chase your dog or kid around the home with your shoes off, and you will notice that your heels barely touch the ground.

Footwear companies have finally begun to address the paradox behind the sky-high frequency of running injuries and large number of new high-tech shoe models that arrive in stores each year. Nike, for example, introduced in 2004 a thin-soled minimalist shoe called the Free that partially mimics barefoot running. It performs more like a lightweight slipper or moccasin. Newton Shoes, of Boulder, Colorado, recently developed a revolutionary lightweight shoe with a thin sole and a spongy midsection that provides a push-off, touchy-feely rapport with the ground. It's virtually impossible to initially land on your heel. Then there's the truly bizarre-looking Vibram FiveFingers, which one running magazine reviewer likened to "a kind of below-the-ankle nudism that simulates not wearing shoes." The FiveFingers' upper section is made with a thin, abrasion-resistant stretch polyamide fabric; the sole is lightweight rubber Vibram; and here's the real kicker: Small green rubber sleeves individually encase the toes. Each of your little piggies has its own home. The shoe literally fits like a glove—for your foot. Sales of this distinctive footwear have reached $10 million annually.

Sensing that minimalism is here to stay, Nike now sells a lightweight shoe called the LunarGlide+, while New Balance has come out with its 1225 (it weighs just twelve ounces). Asics has its simple Gel-Plus, Brooks debuted the Ghost 2, and Avia's Avi-Stoltz is a stripped-down shoe for trail running. Who knows if the back-to-basics movement will eventually radicalize the multi-billion-dollar running shoe industry?

At the extreme end of the anti-shoe movement is barefoot running. Numerous websites and blogs are passionately devoted to the subject. Even *Runner's World* suggested that runners might consider incorporating brief sessions of barefoot running into their training: "Running barefoot a couple of times per week can decrease your risk of injury and boost your 'push-off' power."

If you do decide to go barefoot, it's recommended that you start with small distances since your biomechanics behave much differently. Think of these short training sessions as rehab or physical therapy since they will gradually strengthen underutilized tendons, ligaments, joints, and muscles in your feet and lower legs. After a while, you should discover additional barefoot benefits for your entire body, such as better balance and improved posture.

Running barefoot, however, is nothing new. Most Kenyan children and teenagers run without shoes, and the African nation perpetually produces the greatest long-distance runners in the world. Even Olympians go barefoot. At the 1960 Rome games, Ethiopia's Abebe Bikila won his first Olympic marathon and broke the world record while running barefoot. (One of the most amazing things I ever saw at the Hawaii Ironman was a barefoot, bearded competitor in 1985 wearing only a loincloth adorned with a marijuana leaf; he went sub-four hours in the marathon on the scorching hot asphalt to finish the triathlon in just under twelve hours.)

And what about me? What shoes did I use during my fitness comeback? At first, I went with an expensive pair of New Balance 801 all-terrain trail running shoes. The 801's product literature boasted "lightweight compression molded EVA midsole for cushioning and flexibility" and an "aggressive solid rubber lugged outsole" that could easily pound nails into sheetrock if I happened to misplace a hammer. But these shoes deprived my feet of any real kinesthetic awareness of the ground; they could barely feel any of the roots, ruts, and rocks along the trail. Was this cushy desensitization helping or hurting my feet? I traded these New Balance shoes for a pair of $39

(continues)

flat-soled Jack Purcell sneakers with hardly any cushioning support. Then I upgraded to the Nike Frees and even removed their insoles. After several months of running unimpeded in my Frees, I had zero complaints, except for pebbles occasionally getting wedged inside the shoe bottom's narrow channels. I'm a true believer in pared-down, thin-soled running shoes, no matter the terrain.

Certainly the last word about footwear should go to the Tarahumara Indians who live in small isolated villages scattered throughout northern Mexico's Sierra Madre. The impoverished Tarahumara depend on subsistence farming, make colorful crafts, enjoy drinking fermented maize beer, and are known for running long distances. *Tarahumara* comes from the native word *Raramuri*, which means "foot runner." From a young age, these reclusive people run as their primary mode of transportation and for social bonding, often covering between seventy and a hundred miles per day on foot while kicking a small wooden ball. In 1992, Rick Fisher, a Tucson-based wilderness guide and photographer, invited several Tarahumarans to compete in the Leadville Trail 100 Ultramarathon held in the Colorado Rockies. Most of the course's elevation is over 10,000 feet. The first time out, the Indians didn't fare too well in the hundred-mile contest, not because they were under-trained but due to culture shock.

"The problem, it turned out, was an unfamiliarity with the trail and the strange ways of the North," wrote Don Kardong of *Runner's World*. "The Indians stood shyly at aid stations, waiting to be offered food. They held their flashlights pointed skyward, unaware that these 'torches' needed to be aimed forward to illuminate the treacherous trail. And so on. All five Tarahumara dropped out before the halfway point."

But the following year, the first-, second-, and fifth-place finishers were Tarahumarans. Victoriano Churro, fifty-five, won the race in 20:02:33. All three men ran eighty-seven miles in open-toed sandals that were made from leather straps and discarded tires they had found at the Leadville landfill. At the first aid station, thirteen miles into the race, the Indian trio removed their running shoes, provided by Rockport, one of the sponsors. They then laced up their homemade *huaraches*, and continued running on the rock-strewn trail.

In 2009, the Tarahumara received a fresh new jolt of American recognition with the publication of the nonfiction bestseller *Born to Run: A Hidden Tribe,*

Superathletes, and the Greatest Race the World Has Never Seen, by Christopher McDougall, a formerly injured runner who now runs barefoot or in FiveFingers and other minimalist shoes. Waging a kind of jock jihad against thick-soled, heel-striking running shoes, McDougall cites additional scientific studies to conclude that "running shoes may be the most destructive force to ever hit the human foot."

So when footwear companies make bold, extravagant claims regarding their newest, priciest, and overdesigned shoe models, you should ignore the marketing hype, and instead buy a cheap pair of thin-soled shoes. You will save money. You will lessen the risk of foot or leg injury. Because isn't that the real purpose of running shoes—to keep you running?

TAKE IT SLOW AND EASY AS YOU START TO RUN REGULARLY

Walking might not seem like it will achieve much in terms of building fitness. You might even get through an entire hour barely breaking a sweat. This is perfectly normal. Think long term. Your body needs to gradually readjust to the new (and healthy) physical strain that it's now experiencing. Still, you must fight the temptation to run on under-trained legs. This is a recipe for disaster. And guess what: It's how I initially messed up my own return. Frisky and impatient to start running, I got ahead of myself despite the fact that my heart, lungs, and leg muscles had not been on speaking terms for years. I went too far on a mountain run one weekend. Within days of that two-hour alpine spree, my body rebelled from overexertion. (See the following chapter for an in-depth discussion on overtraining.) There was barely any zip in my legs to even walk a quarter-mile. Running was out of the question. This general tiredness lasted for nearly two months. When I felt healthy enough to start training again, I could barely jog a hundred yards. Not to get overly philosophical here, but this setback sucked.

For the next three months, as I once again jogged my way back to fitness, I never felt like a real runner. Certainly not like I used to be. My mileage hovered just shy of ten miles per week. This amount sounds small, but the majority of my running was on hills. I was either going up or down. My pal Timothy Carlson, a triathlon journalist who once ran 3:28 at the Boston Marathon, frequently reprimanded me for not running flats and increasing mileage to build up leg strength. I would always counter, "But I love hills, especially gradual one- and two-mile inclines. It symbolizes the ordeal I am enduring by trying to get back in shape. You know, like Sisyphus."

Tim wasn't buying what I was selling. "Run longer on the flats," he'd respond. I never told him that one day I wanted to run up Mount Tam—just over six uphill miles to the 2,500-foot summit.

Because I lived on the mountain's southern, forested flanks in Mill Valley, California, with my cottage located on a ridge about 500 feet above sea level, you can see where I am coming from. A run right out the door is either downhill or uphill. There is not much middle ground or flat stretches. Of course, I could drive to somewhere flat, like to the bike path that connected Mill Valley to Sausalito, but running along the tidal waterfront never excited me, and it often smelled at low tide.

. . .

When I was fit in my thirties, I had run on Tam countless times. But the sad, unforgiving truth is that despite living on the mountain, I hadn't run on its trails for ages. During those lost years when my fitness hollowed out, when I felt ashamed by my lack of interest, motivation, and ability to exercise, it was problematic to live on the mountain yet not feel associated with it. Instead of looking longingly at its peak during the natural cycles of gorgeous sunsets or late summer afternoons when thick fog encircled its sprawling midsection like giant pearls made from cotton candy, I viewed the mountain as a symbol of my personal failure to connect with nature. I lived in exile from the mountain and its numerous trails and streams. But somewhere in the back of my mind, I felt that our former relationship would someday be rekindled. That desire was kept alive through memory—by fondly remembering past runs as if they were ex-lovers.

Thankfully, a love of running doesn't have to remain unrequited.

After watching *Dancing with the Stars* one evening, I felt the overwhelming urge to prance under the stars. I put on my running shoes and headed outside into the cool nighttime air. The moon was full, an orange disc. Equipped with a small flashlight, I started running uphill, taking small grandfatherly strides, refusing to rest until I reached the half-mile mark where the road switchbacked onto another road. I could see the lights of San Francisco off in the distance. But my attention soon moved away from the city's gauzy amber glow to the immediate task at hand: tackling Tam's darkened hulk. After waiting for my heart rate to ratchet down, I continued slowly jogging uphill. I went another mile and then took another brief rest on a fallen redwood log. Since my calves and quads were tired, I debated whether to continue ascending or return home. On a whim, I impulsively left my wooden perch and lumbered upward and onward, carefully dodging ruts and rocks. As I chugged along, I felt like I was in pursuit of the shadow of my youth who was always running just ahead, making fun of my glacial pace. After going another mile, I reached Railroad Grade's intersection with the Hoo-kee-hoo-kee Trail. It was a fantastic place to stop and review what I had just accomplished. I didn't have any water, so I sat down on some wooden steps and drank in the mountain's silent splendor.

I had not been to this spot on the mountain in ten years. But here I was, feeling reborn, and though the summit was another 3.5 miles and 1,000 feet in elevation, I was not yet in the kind of shape to make it there on this triumphant night. I had already run over an hour—straight uphill. As I headed downhill, it seemed like I was gliding above the dirt path, as if wings instead of feet were doing all the work.

It would take another year before I reached a level of conditioning that would allow an attempt to run to Tam's summit. Why the long delay? I kept colliding into additional health setbacks, including a lengthy bout with vertigo from an inner ear ailment that left me unable to walk more than several yards.

With vertigo, the ground seemed to move with every step. It not only affected my balance and equilibrium, but kept me bedridden for four months. Just standing left me dizzy and wanting to hold onto a wall for support. I likened the sensation to standing in a rowboat in heavy seas while sauced to the gills. One time, after a five-minute hot shower, I was reaching for a towel to dry off when my legs buckled and I suddenly blacked out and struck the floor with the back of my head. As I lay sprawled naked on the wet floor, I stared at the ceiling for about a half hour, not moving, hoping that I didn't have a concussion. The fall did leave a nasty bruise on my head for about a week.

The vertigo eventually went away after all that bed rest. I was then finally able to start walking, before being able to jog short distances. I was determined to get in decent running shape. In a deep and profound way, I felt like Tam's distant peak was invisibly holding me up, like a giant puppeteer with his string. It was awaiting my return.

A BRIEF HISTORY OF TAM

Because this popular Bay Area landmark loomed magnificently large as both playground and battleground in my struggle to get back in shape, I thought it might be relevant to take a short break from fitness matters and briefly discuss Mount Tam's natural history and colorful past. Many locals call the mountain Marin's Everest, and despite its being only 2,574 feet high at the East Peak summit, one can understand why: It dominates both the geography and imagination.

First officially recorded on maps in 1845 as Mount Tamalpais (pronounced *tam-el-pi-ess*), the name is thought to have derived from what its original inhabitants, the Coast Miwoks, called "coast mountain" (*tamal pais*). Many want to believe that Tamalpais is the Miwok word for "sleeping maiden," but this is simply untrue. Yet this myth perseveres because, seen from afar, the mountain's outline does resemble a snoozing lass.

Because the Miwoks believed that their god, Coyote, who created man, resided at its peak, they refused to visit the sacred summit; to do so meant instant death. A local trader named Jacob Leese made the first recorded ascent of Tamalpais in the 1830s. When he returned alive, Miwok's Chief Marin, after whom the county is named, climbed to the top and solidified his reputation among his villagers as the bravest man in the world.

Tam's sleeping maiden silhouette is what drivers often first notice on non-foggy days after crossing the Golden Gate Bridge and emerging from the Waldo Grade tunnel heading north on Highway 101. Tam is part of the Northern California Coast Range. Its heft, height, and girth are a direct result of geological tectonic forces pushing and folding the North American plate, which slides along the Pacific Plate near the San Andreas Fault zone.

While the towns of Mill Valley, Corte Madera, Greensbrae, Larkspur, Ross, Kentfield, San Anselmo, and Fairfax form a crescent around the lower elevation along the southern and eastern sides, most of the mountain lies within protected public lands. Almost all the original redwood trees were logged between 1840 and 1870. Second-growth redwoods now cover the lower slopes. Only one virgin stand of redwoods was spared the saw—Sequoia Canyon's federally protected grove of towering redwoods, which is part of tourist-friendly Muir Woods National Monument.

Tam used to be home to black and grizzly bears. The last recorded bear was killed in Muir Woods in 1880. Mountain lions are still sometimes sighted, but the most common four-legged inhabitants are deer. (Once, at dusk, I saw a bobcat.) Over seven hundred types of plants and trees are found here, including oak, bay, madrone, manzanita, and chaparral, in exposed areas with thin, rocky soil and scant moisture.

On weekends, Tam's nearly two hundred miles of trails are clotted with mountain bikers, hikers, and runners, who are definitely in the minority and can usually be identified by their lean muscular torsos, water-bottle waist-belts, and nylon shorts no matter the weather or season.

Yes, the weather. Tam is a meteorological wonderland with several distinctive microclimates. Since its steep slopes wring out moisture from incoming Pacific storms and thick coastal fog, the mountain supports several year-round streams. In the summer, it can be cool and foggy at lower elevations, hot and dry on the higher manzanita-covered slopes, cold and windy at the summit, and mild and shady on the heavily Douglas-fir-forested north slopes. The cold, wet winter storms occasionally bring snow, but it's usually the hurricane-force winds that make this region prone to frequent power outages due to trees toppling onto power lines.

In 1896, a railway track was built from downtown Mill Valley to the summit. Known as "The Crookedest Railroad in the World," the Mount Tamalpais Scenic Railroad, with its 281 turns and curves, carried 23,000 passengers up its eight-mile track during its inaugural year of operation. A luxury hotel was erected at the summit. But by 1930, the steam-powered railroad proved no match for the automobile, and it was shut down and the hotel demolished in the 1950s. The former track is now a popular hiking and biking trail known as Railroad Grade, and was the one on which I frequently ran and mountain biked in the past. When I became fit enough to run to the summit, I would take this grade. There are other peak-bound trails, but they are Sherpa-steep; my goal was to run, *not* walk to the top.

West Point Inn is the only surviving structure from the storied railway days. Located near the 5.5-mile mark on the upper southern slope, the inn is still open to the public and accepts overnight reservations three months in advance. Rustic is an understatement. Heat, light, and refrigeration are generated by propane. Candles are not allowed because of the fire hazard. Guests are asked to bring flashlights and sleeping bags or linens and towels. The "honeymoon cabin" does have its own toilet with a sink.

As the birthplace of mountain biking, it's ironic that virtually all of Tam's single-track trails are off limits to off-road riding. If park rangers catch you riding these illegal trails, the fine is hefty—several hundred dollars—which

(continues)

is why many local "outlaw" riders prefer biking these trails at night with their high-powered, helmet-mounted and handlebar LED lights.

One of the darkest chapters in Tam's history occurred between 1979 and 1981 when a serial killer stalked, raped, and murdered at least five women who were either hiking or running alone. The press came up with a chilling moniker for this unknown predator: "The Trailside Killer." A terrified public began avoiding Tam while the heinous crimes went unsolved. David Carpenter, an ex-convict and San Francisco print shop employee, was eventually arrested. A jury found him guilty of the murders and sentenced him to death. He remains on death row at San Quentin State Prison.

During the Second World War, a radar station was established on West Peak to detect Japanese aircraft. During the early days of the Cold War, an Air Force station sprouted up at this location. The base was like a small city with sixty-two buildings and two hundred airmen, many with families. It was also the tactical command center for twelve Nike missile-launching sites located throughout the Bay Area. When the last Nike missile site was dismantled in 1979, the Tam station was deactivated; the buildings were torn down in 2005. The FAA currently keeps a radar station there for air traffic control.

Throughout its contemporary history, Tam has inspired legions of artists, photographers, writers, conservationists, outdoor enthusiasts, and Bay Area businesses like Tam Bikes and Cowgirl Creamery, which named its top-selling creamy organic cheese "Mt. Tam." The tasty, aromatic cheese took second place at the California State Fair in 2009.

The late Lew Welch, an American poet associated with the Beat Generation, briefly lived in Marin in the early sixties. He penned a well-loved tribute to the mountain entitled "The Song Mt. Tamalpais Sings." The first two lines are:

This is the last place.

There is nowhere else to go.

MORE ON AVOIDANCE OF
DOING TOO MUCH, TOO SOON

One of America's most popular running coaches, Jeff Galloway, champions a relaxed training program—one that involves walking. He suggests using a heart-rate monitor to prevent overtraining, which, he maintains, is one of the primary causes of fatigue, burnout, and injury. "When you're running below 70 percent of your maximum heart rate," writes Galloway in *Marathon: You Can Do It!*, "you are unlikely to overtrain in intensity." This percentage will vary from person to person, but the cardinal rule is this: "When you push beyond 80 percent of your maximum heart rate, you increase the recovery time for that workout." Going too far is also a factor that affects overtraining.

Aging is also an issue. "When you are past the age of 35," continues Galloway, "fatigue sets in more quickly but is usually masked by stressed hormones. It's easier to push yourself into overtraining without seeing any warning signs. Then, the worse the overtraining, the longer the recovery."

To reduce the chance of injury over the age of thirty-five, Galloway also recommends these guidelines:

1. Add an extra day off, though keep to a minimum of three running days per week.
2. Restrict your long runs to a pace of three minutes per mile slower than you could run that day.
3. Insert walking breaks during your runs.
4. Keep tabs on your heart rate.

If you don't have a heart-rate monitor, don't despair. I didn't start using one at first. *Runner's World*'s long-time columnist Joe Henderson, who teaches a class for beginning runners at the University of Oregon, says "Listen to your breathing. If you aren't gasping for air, and you can talk while you're running, your pace is just right."

Dr. Kenneth Cooper, whose 1968 bestselling book *Aerobics* turbo-charged the fitness revolution and running boom, once believed in high, strenuous levels of exertion to achieve maximum aerobic fitness. Not only did he encourage people to walk or run at least four times a week, but he believed that the harder you physically pushed yourself, the healthier you'd become. But over the years, Cooper came to rethink his position. "Overtraining might not only be unnecessary, but might even be harmful," he told the *New York Times* in 1995. More exercise isn't better; in fact, too much of it can lead to injury, chronic inflammation, hormonal imbalance, sickness, and possibly death.

His reversal about sweaty, blood-pumping exercise resulted from ongoing research that had been conducted with volunteers at the Cooper Institute for Aerobics Research in Dallas. After his friend Jim Fixx, the popular author and runner, died from a massive heart attack at the age of fifty-two following his daily run, Cooper recognized that moderation should be the primary objective for most athletes. To exercise for health, Cooper insisted that one should walk two miles in thirty minutes, three times a week, or walk two miles in forty minutes, five times a week.

Now in his late seventies, Cooper continues to practice what he preaches. Standing six-feet-one, he weighs 170 pounds. In 1960, after graduating from the University of Oklahoma Medical School, Cooper became sedentary for eight years and watched his weight balloon from 165 pounds to 204. He then took up running, lost the weight, and has not gained any pounds since then. Following a ski accident that fractured his leg, he abandoned running—which he had been doing for forty-four years and 38,000 miles—and became a speed walker, averaging two to three miles a day, five days a week. He also follows a low-fat diet that substitutes fish and chicken for red meat, and takes a daily "antioxidant cocktail" of vitamins E and C and beta carotene to fight an excess of free radicals, which are unstable oxygen molecules that can cause permanent cellular damage.

Cooper explained his philosophical turnabout in a fascinating interview in *Run for Life*. "I'm smart enough to realize I've made a mistake. Over the years, we found that more is not better, more may cause more harm than good. You can get detrimental effects from exercising too much. From 1968 to 1982, I used to say, if you can run enough, forget about cigarette smoking, your diet, your body weight; if you exercise enough, it's a panacea. Don't worry about anything else. Well, then I had too many times during that fourteen-year period telephone calls from distraught widows. They told me that their husbands followed my recommendations for running exactly but ignored their diet, ignored their weight, their smoking, and had a heart attack at fifty-five years of age. That shocked me into reality."

Cooper went on to say that for all athletes, whether they are world-class runners or weekend warriors, there "may be a point of diminishing return" when it comes to training. "I tell my runners, if you listen to your body, the most important thing you can do is to watch out for overtraining. I tell my patients that they are 'straining, not training.' You aren't conditioning your body; you're deconditioning your body." And because your immune system is weakened, it opens the door to illness or injury.

RUNNER'S DILEMMA:
TO STRETCH OR NOT TO STRETCH?

If overtraining should be guarded against, then what about stretching? And why is the running community so divided on this topic? I certainly didn't stretch. And though in theory, stretching seemed like the smart thing to do, the more I read about the topic, the less convinced I became of its usefulness.

Your junior high gym teacher probably required you to do a series of stretches at the beginning of each class. These exercises might have included toe touches and hamstring stretches. Proper form was usually neglected. But did these exercises actually warm up your muscles and joints? Well, science now suggests that your whistle-blowing phys-ed instructor was ill-advised. In 2008, the *New York Times* reported that "researchers now believe that some of the more entrenched elements of many athletes' warm-up regimens are not only a waste of time but actually bad for you. The old presumption that holding a stretch for 20 to 30 seconds—known as static stretching—primes muscles for a workout is dead wrong. It actually weakens them."

So runners, take heed. Don't stretch before running. You can risk injury.

"There is a neuromuscular inhibitory response to static stretching," Malachy McHugh, the director of research at the Nicholas Institute of Sports Medicine and Athletic Trauma at Lenox Hill Hospital in New York City, told the *Times*. "The straining muscle becomes less responsive and stays weakened for up to 30 minutes after stretching, which is not how an athlete wants to begin a workout."

Here's Galloway's anti-stretching view: "Stretching is the third leading cause of injury among runners. You can injure yourself while doing a stretch that seems perfectly safe." Ouch! "Stretching *does not* warm you up for a run," he continues. "The best warm-up for running is walking or very slow jogging."

"The right way to warm-up should do two things: loosen muscles and tendons to increase the range of motion of various joints, and literally warm up the body," Duane Knudson, professor of kinesiology at California State University, Chico, also told the *Times*. "When you're at rest, there's less blood flow to muscles and tendons, and they stiffen. You need to make tissues and tendons compliant before beginning exercise."

"Warming up is the first step of exercise," emphasizes Phil Maffetone. "It's the slow shifting of blood into the working muscles. The key word is slow. Shifting the blood into the muscles too quickly can be a significant stress on the rest of the body. Specifically, the blood going into the muscles comes from other important areas of the body including the nervous system, adrenal glands and intestines. Diverting the blood out of these areas and circulating it into the muscles too quickly can be much like going into shock. When a warm-up is done slowly, the organs and glands can properly compensate for this normal activity. Warming up provides several important benefits: It increases the blood flow, bringing oxygen and nutrients into the muscles, and removing waste products. It increases the fats in the blood that are used for muscle energy. It increases flexibility in all the joints by gently lengthening the muscles."

You should spend at least five or ten minutes warming up with a brisk walk to prime your legs. Ease into your run. Don't start out sprinting. Cooling off is just as important following a run. Once again, five or ten minutes of walking will help restore your body's equilibrium, and, according to Maffetone, "will establish nearly normal circulation without pooling blood in the muscles."

Does this mean that stretching should be avoided at all costs? It all depends on your sport. "For those who require a wider range of motion, stretching may be necessary," adds Maffetone. "These include dancers, sprinters and gymnasts, but usually not most people doing aerobic exercise." He does caution that "even people who don't work out sometimes think stretching is a good way to get rid of body aches and pains and so-called tight muscles, but there's very little, if any, scientific information demonstrating that static stretching is beneficial, especially the way most people do it. You see this in health clubs, people stretching when they shouldn't. One of many examples given is the hamstring muscles. It is both the most frequently injured muscle group and the most stretched."

However, there is beneficial stretching—using slow, deliberate, unhurried movements, without bouncing, that will lightly stretch a muscle without tearing fibers. Yoga and other "whole-body" flexibility activities are very different from stretching. "When properly done in a slow easy motion," says Maffetone, "they are healthy, safe, and effective. They're also recommended as a source of relaxation and meditation."

FORM FOLLOWS FUNCTION: RUN LIKE A KENYAN!

After several months of consistent running, with longer runs averaging forty-five minutes, I noticed several things happening. First, my form was smoother and more relaxed. I wasn't erratically moving my arms like an over-caffeinated Bangkok traffic cop. I felt more in control of stride length, body posture, foot strike, and breathing. But I was only running at a ten- to twelve-minute clip. Imagine if I suddenly tried running seven-and-a-half- or eight-minute miles like I used to do in my thirties. In all likelihood, I'd turn into a herky-jerky comical figure, with flailing arms and feet slapping the pavement like a really pissed-off beaver.

The beauty of running is learning how to allow your body to transcend the physical act itself: to run but not feel like you are running; to decouple the conscious from the unconscious, to have thoughts travel elsewhere and miles disappear inside an invisible whoosh of free association. Zen indeed! During this heightened mental and physical state, you magically enter a different world in which you are often aware of everything but putting one foot in front of the other. It's like when you drive somewhere in your car and your mind goes on autopilot. You obey all the traffic laws and stoplights but afterward you don't even remember driving. It can be the same with running. This might be hard on short runs or when going nowhere on the treadmill. Yet on runs over thirty minutes, especially on trails or quiet country lanes, you will be surprised at how enjoyable and liberating running can be.

Perfect running technique is a different story. When you look at the long-distance running champions, such as the Kenyans, Moroccans, and Ethiopians, and even the well-trained Americans, you see little upper body movement and shoes that barely kiss the pavement. The very best even manage to click off sub five-minute miles during a marathon. Ever try running just *one* sub five-minute mile? At the Berkeley track after classes, I would sometimes run two miles at all-out speed. My first mile would average seven minutes, and the second one about six and a half. I was twenty-three years old, and it took every scintilla of heart-pounding, lungs-burning, legs-aching effort to break 13:30. When I finished, I'd lay sprawled on the infield grass, sucking down oxygen as if through a straw.

So how do world-class runners make it look like so easy? It's a question that mocks and defies probably 99 percent of all runners. Is it genetics? Weight? Training? The laws of gravity seemingly don't apply to top runners. These athletically gifted sprites must have secret jetpacks.

Surely there's a right way and wrong way to run, just like there is a correct way to hit a golf or tennis ball. The running books and magazines pretty much all say the same thing about proper running form. It's not all that complicated.

Ten Basic Techniques for Good Running Form:

1. Take short strides with quick cadence or leg turnover.
2. Land lightly on the middle portion of your foot—*not* the heels, or toes like a sprinter.
3. Quickly lift your foot off the ground instead of scraping it along the ground or pushing off with excessive force.
4. Don't overstride to go faster; this will wreck your knees and awkwardly stretch leg muscles.
5. Keep arms close to your side with the elbows tucked in.
6. Don't swing your arms back and forth like you are a drum major in a marching band.
7. Hands should not be squeezed tight or balled in a fist, but relaxed and loosely cupped, thumbs gently grazing a finger or two.
8. Don't look at the ground right in front of your feet; keep your head up instead while trying to maintain relaxed facial muscles.
9. Don't run leaning too far forward.
10. Run upright, but not with your shoulders pulled back like a soldier at attention on the parade grounds.

There are plenty of proper running form videos on YouTube. Or you can bribe someone in your family to film you running, so you can review your technique. But don't get discouraged if you fail to resemble an Olympic distance runner. They have put in tens of thousands of miles. Who cares if you look like you are bobbing for apples and the neighborhood kids snicker as you run past. The fact is that you *are* running.

Still, if you really, really want to run like a Kenyan, you will need to do several things differently.

- Try to do all your running on dirt trails; avoid asphalt if you can. Your knees, ankles, and feet will appreciate the consideration and care, because it's less jarring on your joints to run on soft surfaces.
- Find hills and run them regularly. By doing so, your leg strength will improve. Another benefit of hill work is that it helps promote a smoother, faster, and shorter stride.
- Vary the tempo of your runs: start slow at an easy jog, rev up the metabolic engine for quick intervals, and then blast to the finish. Just don't neglect the cool down afterward.

- Run early in the morning and preferably as part of a group. You seldom see Kenyans train alone. They like pushing and challenging one another. But above all, they look like they are having fun.
- You need to be lottery-lucky when it comes to physiology and genetics. In 2000, the Danish Sports Science Institute conducted a study of young Kenyan runners and theorized that their remarkable ability might be a result of their "birdlike legs." What the study failed to address is that Kenyans have a fierce work ethic when it comes to running. Early in the season, they will run three times a day. The elite marathoners will often run 150 miles per week in training. That kind of mileage is insane and ill-suited for anyone simply hoping to return to fitness. But the Kenyans' commitment and love of running serve as a vivid and inspiring example of what the human body is truly capable of achieving.
- Finally, and this is obviously impractical for many, move to a high-altitude region where the air is thinner. Consider running meccas like Boulder or Flagstaff, which, respectively, are 5,400 and 7,000 feet above sea level. Living and running at a higher elevation increases lung capacity and produces more red blood cells for enhanced muscle function.

CONCLUSION

Stripped to its essence, there is something pure and beautiful about running. Watch little kids run around in the playground. They are uninhibited. They live in the moment. That's what running can and should be. As you increase the time or distance spent running, your mind and body will undergo all sorts of wonderful changes. Push yourself too far or too fast, however, and those changes can reverse course and make for an unpleasant experience. The goal then is to find a happy balance between too much and too little. Pursue moderation with your running, and your time on the trails and roads will become the highlight of your day. Homo sapiens were born to run. Several million years of natural-selection tinkering and evolutionary trial and error have provided us with a marvelous physiological gift. Use that inheritance wisely.

As you become a better runner, you will probably want to challenge yourself in local races. But don't feel that you must enter a marathon to become a "real runner." Going 26.2 miles on untrained legs marks an open invitation to injury—and just might set back your fitness for months. Why take that unnecessary risk? Instead, gradually work your way up to a marathon, if that's what you ultimately want to complete, beginning with 5Ks or 10Ks, and followed up with half-marathons.

It might take you a year or longer to get in marathon shape. There's no ticking clock demanding urgency. Some coaches recommend training for two years before running a marathon.

Each year, several hundred thousand Americans will participate in a marathon. That number goes even higher for 10Ks and half-marathons. Being part of a growing movement like this will make a return to fitness all the more meaningful on a personal level.

ASK THE EXPERT

WHAT I LOST IN SPACE: INTERVIEW WITH NASA ASTRONAUT JERRY LINENGER, WHO RETURNED TO EARTH FEELING LIKE AN OLD MAN

What happens to the human body in outer space? What is the severity of physical deterioration and muscle loss? And what does this physical breakdown mean for those of us living right here on earth who have shunned exercise or were forced to spend months in bed? Since both scenarios applied to me, it was with great interest that I tracked down U.S. Navy flight surgeon and NASA astronaut Jerry Linenger, who had endured five months on the Russian space station Mir.

When he touched down on Russian soil on May 24, 1997, Linenger discovered that he was ill-prepared for the shock awaiting him. "Imagine going to bed in January and getting out of bed, for the first time, at the end of May," he wrote in his memoir Off the Planet. "That was how inactive my body had become in space. As I had found during my first restless night at the crew quarters, bed rest on earth is actually strenuous since it takes effort to roll over. My post-flight bone scan showed that I had lost a disturbing 13 percent of my bone density in the weight-bearing areas of the hip and lower spine."

Linenger, a highly competitive cyclist, runner, and age-group triathlete, had run on a treadmill every day aboard Mir—a dank, dangerous, cluttered place that he likened to "six school buses all hooked together." But even the treadmill was insufficient to arrest the atrophy. Obviously anxious to get back in shape after his 132-day sojourn in space, he encountered several unexpected obstacles. He explained in his memoir:

On the advice of experts in sports medicine, the first month I would train exclusively in the water. With my bones now weakened to a level similar to the bone loss experienced by an older woman with osteoporosis, I was prone to fracture. Furthermore, my muscles had atrophied somewhat and would not be able to protect my bones from repeated low-level impact [from running].

So, I plunged into the pool bright and early each day. Upon entering the water for the first time, I thought I was going to drown. The water felt as thick as mud, like quicksand trying to pull me under. I slugged my way through the dense medium for a couple of laps, breathing heavily. By the beginning of the second week, the water felt more like mercury, by the third week it felt like water should.

In addition to swimming laps, I would exercise in the water. Strapping on a restrained harness attached to a line to the side of the pool, I would run in place. In the shallow end, I would squat and explosively lunge from the bottom of the pool, first with both feet planted, then alternating on each leg. I also used Styrofoam dumbbells to re-strengthen my upper body.

Linenger ended each workout with a deep body massage, because his paraspinal muscles—the muscles running along both sides of the spine—had significantly weakened since they had not been used to maintain an erect posture in space. Most importantly, given the extent to which his muscles and bones had deteriorated, Linenger felt vulnerable to injury. "So strong was this feeling of vulnerability that if someone had offered me a thousand dollars to stand on a three-foot platform and jump to the floor, I would have staunchly refused."

By the end of the first month, Linenger had regained about 70 percent of his full strength. He continued working out regularly in the pool for three more months before graduating to jogging and weight training. It took an entire year of rehab before he felt confident about going on long bike rides and runs. "I did an occasional hundred-miler [bike ride] and ran a half-marathon just to convince myself that I was, indeed, back to normal."

Eleven years after his Mir mission, the fifty-four-year-old retired astronaut now

lives with his family in a small town in northern Michigan. He keeps busy doing corporate motivational speaking. I was eager to learn how his time in space affected his general attitude toward exercise, what lessons he had for those wanting to break free from the surly bonds of inactivity, and how in the world he'd kept from going bonkers on the treadmill. So the next time you hit the treadmill at the gym, even for only ten minutes, think of Linenger's daily mind-bending workouts in deep space.

Question: What was it like to work out in space, and then back on earth?

Jerry Linenger: My case is a unique thing because it wasn't a voluntary deconditioning by any means. It was an imposed deconditioning for five months beyond my control. No matter what you do up there on Mir, I found that you do get deconditioned. When I came back, for the first time in my life, I lost my testosterone or something. I would lift weights, for example, do a bench press and at five, I'd say, "That's enough," whereas in the past I'd say, "Push, push, push" to get stronger. The other aspect of what I lost is that in space, for the first time in my life, it took effort to get up and actually get on that treadmill on Mir and strap myself down with bungee cords every day; it took determination. It was something I dreaded doing because, to be frank, it was pretty painful strapping myself down. Sometimes the soles of my feet lost sensation; it felt like I had pins shooting into them. Or the strap would wear on my shoulder. It was just the first time in my life that a lightbulb went on and I said, "Wow, this is what a lot of people that I'm always trying to motivate to get out and get active must feel like." It's absolutely unbelievable how hard it was to motivate myself to get on that treadmill twice a day. And then again, during my first half a year back on earth, it was the same difficult thing to try to get moving again.

Q: What about using a stationary bicycle on Mir?

JL: In space, I found that with the bicycle, you basically got no exercise. Most people resorted to going on the bicycle because it met the space agency requirement; you got to check the box of "exercising," but it was not real exercise in my mind. For the treadmill, I'd get on it and I did it pretty religiously; I would try to do close to an hour a day, not just running, but also doing squats, using the hold-down plates along with bungee cords.

Q: Where would you put the weights? Affix them to your legs?

JL: No weights. In space nothing like that would work. What I would use is bungee cords; it kind of looks like a windsurfer harness and that would yank me down with a spring force, if you will. It was the equivalent of loading your body up. It felt like carrying a heavy pack on your back. So it wasn't a natural run. It was not comfortable;

plus you're just staring at walls inside of a cave. The only way I could get through those workouts was to close my eyes and literally visualize step-by-step a run that I would take on earth. In the park, I could see the kids playing. I'd just escape the reality of where I was and just go back and use my imagination to get through the workout, and by doing that sometimes I'd find myself twenty-five minutes later virtually in front of my house. I'd finish my run and then I'd open my eyes and realize, of course, I'm in this space station. That's the way I was able to do the workouts.

Q: What about your fellow astronauts? Did they run to this extent?

JL: Again, seeing people exercise in space, you can tell that they're basically looking for an excuse not to do it, which again goes back to my navy days: people are looking for an excuse not to stay in shape. But everyone has a ready excuse—in space or on earth. "I've got a lot of work to do; I'm busy on the computer; I have to get through this email." I used every ounce of self-discipline I had to make myself get on the treadmill.

Q: When you came back to earth, what was it like to run?

JL: At the beginning, I had what I felt was a sort of neuro-muscular disconnect that lasted for almost a year and a half after that flight. The best analogy I can give you is a baseball pitcher who is still able to throw the fast ball, but just can't locate it over the plate. My strength measurements were back to normal after probably six months, but in the back of my mind, I knew my own body wasn't right; it was just lack of coordination. I'd say in two years I was fully recovered.

Q: You're a doctor. Did you locate any causes for this disconnect?

JL: No. NASA had some good physiologists looking very hard at it. Another analogy is a high-speed, slow-motion film of a foot strike of a runner; it is a very complex thing the way that the heel strikes the ground, the way the foot then follows through with fine muscle control to dampen out the shock that would be going into your leg otherwise. And what I felt is that I did not have that fine muscle control. Basically, I could plop my foot down while I ran, but I did not have that muscle control that turned a foot strike from a plop to an absolutely incredible thing—a beautiful dampening of that strike force.

Q: What was the decline in your VO_2 max? And was the bone-loss temporary?

JL: I don't remember any substantial decline with the VO_2 max. They did all the lung function tests and it all kind of looked okay. Of course, at the beginning, you don't come back and try to do your max-out on the treadmill because everyone realizes that you are prone to injury at that point, and so you gradually work your way back up to it. But with the bone loss, I was at 12, 13 percent loss, then cut it down to

about 6 percent after one year; 2 percent at two years.

Q: In your memoir, you describe being in space for five months as like being in bed for that entire time.

JL: It's true, though. But it is worse than going to bed, because you would be fighting gravity in bed as you rolled over, where in space, there is effortlessness with everything you do. I don't think I've ever conveyed it properly to anyone because you've got to live it to know what it's like, but in space you can use a fingertip to push on something and then you go flying away. Everything is so effortless and underwhelming to your muscular-skeletal system that you basically are just going to keep getting weaker and weaker unless you do something to try to counter it with those two one-hour periods a day of exercise.

Q: During your first few months back, you did a lot of water walking and pool training. Do you still do these workouts?

JL: I still do water workouts. For example, a lunge off the bottom of a pool is a great way to get those fast-twitch muscle fibers developed because you're in a nice forgiving medium; it dampens out when you land. I play hockey now and I find doing these lunges off the bottom of a pool is a very good workout. If I'm traveling at a hotel, when no one's around, you'll see me jumping up and down in the pool. It's a great way to work out especially as you get older;

you're in cold water, which is good to keep inflammation down so the next day you feel fine after working out.

Q: During the past decade, have you been doing triathlons, century rides, marathons?

JL: I'm up here in a small 500-person town. So, no, I haven't, but I've done a half-marathon. I've done 10Ks and I bike hundred-mile stretches at a time, but not competitively. I've got four small children, and when I have time, I go out and I do my workouts. I'm pretty consistent in doing them still.

Q: I understand that you were a top age-group triathlete.

JL: I was a reasonable triathlete. I'd finish ten out of a hundred or something; and I'd finish ten out of a hundred on a bike; and probably ten out of a hundred on a run, and so you put those together in triathlons, I did okay. I did maybe fifteen years straight of triathlons, maybe two or three a year and that was mainly in San Diego. I was living with SEAL Team guys and it was just part of our lifestyle. I was competitive, but at this stage in life, I've mellowed out enough to know that I consider exercise kind of like brushing your teeth. It's something you do every day.

Q: Have you experienced any lingering effects from outer space?

JL: No, not really. If I run a slow 10K, it just goes on slowly.

Q: Anything else you want to add about your return to fitness, or tips for others seeking to get back in shape?

JL: What's relevant is that I was finally able to put myself in the shoes of someone who has a hard time going out to exercise. I learned a lot about empathy, whereas before, it was like, "Come on, this guy's being lazy; he's making excuses. Just get out and run. Get out and do something." In space, I had to use every ounce of self-discipline to get on that treadmill everyday or do my exercises. I finally could relate to what people on earth go through. In my own case back on earth, I found that you've just got to do it—exercise—for those first six weeks, and that it's critical to do things very lightly during this time. When you get past that six-week point, you just start incorporating it into your lifestyle, and it just feels so normal after a while that if you don't do something, you feel like you're missing something in your life. You don't think about it; it's just part of maintenance of the human body. You have to look at exercise that way if you have the sort of psychological makeup that says, "This is tough. It's not what I want to do." You've just got to tell yourself this is part of living and I'm going to do it. Probably just a half-hour walk would do well for 90 percent of the people. Let me give you my mellower, over-fifty advice: Grab your wife by the hand and take about a half-hour walk every day and it'll do wonders for communication. It does wonders for your health and you can sustain that forever; you're not sore, it's not painful, and I think if you start doing that, you don't have to start saying, "Do it three times a week or four times a week." You'll just do it because you enjoy doing it and you find out again it's just part of the way you live; it makes you feel good about yourself and it helps everything in life.

We often make things way too complicated in lots of aspects of our life. It's the same thing with exercise. With elite athletes, you've got to get that last half percent if you're going to be the champ. But for 99 percent of us, you just need to move and don't make it complicated or sound like it's something that you have to study for a year. You don't have to worry about your VO_2 max; and you don't have to worry about your time in a race or anything else. You've just got to get out. It's as simple as moving, or walking, running, bicycling, going out and having fun and moving your body.

④

THE PHYSICAL INJURY

Successfully Addressing the
Athlete's Number-One Nemesis

"The healthy, slightly less trained athlete
beats the injured superstar every time!"

—Dr. David Goltz, of Mt. Tam Orthopedics,
official provider of the U.S. ski team

Given the duration of my sabbatical from exercise, one legitimate concern kept me worried during my fitness return: How would my aging body respond to renewed physical stress? Which body part would scheme against making an athletic comeback? Would too-tight hamstrings rebel in silent protest? Groin tendons groan and act up? Lower back issue an SOS? And could I blame them for possibly having to misbehave? My muscles had been out of work longer than a Flint, Michigan, autoworker.

Genetics handed me the body of a Russian peasant—stocky, thick in trunk and torso. A Boulder sports message therapist once told me that I had the most inflexible body she had ever worked on. Was her observation offered as praise or personal rebuke?

My body was like a Swiss Army Knife unable to fully open. Oh, to have a smidgen of Gumby-like limberness! There was a foot of daylight between my outstretched fingertips and feet when I leaned over. But I shied away from yoga's pretzel-bending demands and the somatic charms of downward facing dog or reverse warrior pose. It all seemed too unnatural, too difficult.

Then I came across an article on the *New York Times* Well Blog that reviewed the latest scientific findings on flexibility. Some of us will always remain inflexible—such hard, unyielding truth! All those hours of Pilates won't make much difference to the stiff set. "To a large degree, flexibility is genetic," Dr. Malachy McHugh, the sports medical expert on flexibility, told the *Times*. "You're born stretchy or not. Some small portion of [each person's flexibility] is adaptable, but it takes a long time and a lot of work to get even that small adaptation. It's a bit depressing, really."

Yet I still needed to be kinder and gentler toward my half-century-old body. That meant being extra cautious on running trails, especially when navigating narrow single-track with exposed tree roots waiting to snare a careless foot. Then there was the larger issue of training—just how much was enough, especially during the early phase? Too much, too soon—then the obvious most likely happens: injury.

I erred by upping the hilly mileage too quickly. One morning as I began running, I wondered why I was out of breath after only several hundred yards. My legs also felt soft, unresponsive, and weak. I had to take frequent rests. After only going a half-mile, I turned back home, thinking that this was just an off-day. The next morning, a similar thing occurred: A regular 2.5-mile hilly loop took two hours to complete, since I had to sit down and take a break every few hundred years. Something was wrong. But what exactly? Later in the week, it was even tiring to walk short distances. Running was entirely out of the question.

I was forced to stop running altogether for several months. My body had shut down due to overtraining and adrenal fatigue. This diagnosis came from my friend, multisport coach and author Dr. Phil Maffetone, who spent thirty years treating and coaching endurance athletes.

Overtraining isn't something that only happens to elite distance runners who average a hundred miles or more per week. Overtraining can happen to anyone, of any age or ability, and especially to those starting out. The body needs adequate time for recovery following arduous physical activity or it will run down like a broken clock. Getting fit rewinds that timepiece. Even elite endurance athletes must schedule sufficient recovery time to avoid injury and exhaustion. The body can't go hard every workout. For someone like myself, who had been inactive for a decade, it was foolish to assume that I could somehow coax my body into regular hour-long mountain runs without first establishing an adequate conditioning base. In the end, you can't outsmart the body. It holds all the cards.

OVERTRAINING: PAY ATTENTION TO ADRENAL BURNOUT AND FATIGUE

So what happens when you overtrain, when you continually push your body deep into the red zone? Maybe nothing will go wrong during the actual workout. Or even the next day. That's probably because your adrenal glands have produced a flood of stress hormones such as cortisol to make you feel peppy and strong by replenishing gone-to-exhaustion muscles with extra energy and strength. It can take up to forty-eight hours before the real trouble surfaces.

The adrenals are small glands that rest on top of each kidney. In addition to regulating production of other hormones, these glands are responsible for helping the body cope with physical and mental stress. Ever hear the expression "fight or flight"? The adrenals are responsible for the fight reaction, an evolutionary mechanism designed to deal with peril and unexpected danger. For early man, that chance encounter with a wolf, lion, or bear would send the adrenals into overdrive. The adrenals do much the same thing in today's world, but here the on-off switch can be something non-physical like getting cutoff in traffic, losing a job, or discovering that you were a victim of identity theft. Your heart rate increases, your mind races, and you feel prepared for battle. (See sidebar on stress in the following chapter.)

With physical exercise, the adrenals spring into action to help you adjust to intensity and duration. When all systems are working properly, physical conditioning improves. However, a common cause of excessive adrenal stress is over-exercising.

In the early 1900s, a medical student named Hans Selye discovered several conditions related to adrenal stress. Selye identified three distinct stages of adrenal response to stress, which later became known as the "General Adaptation Syndrome." The first, or alarm stage, is marked by increased adrenal hormone output. This is followed by the resistance stage, in which the adrenal glands actually enlarge in an attempt to cope with the added stress load. Ultimately, however, the adrenals can be overwhelmed, culminating in the third, or exhaustion, stage.

The further the progression of the General Adaptation Syndrome, the more difficult it is to return to normal adrenal function.

Warning signs of this syndrome leading to overtraining can include:

- Lack of energy
- Leg soreness, general aches and pains
- Pain in muscles and joints
- Decreased performance times
- Insomnia
- Headaches
- Decreased immunity (increased number of colds and sore throats)
- Moodiness and irritability
- Apathy
- Decreased appetite
- Increased incidence of injuries

If you experience just one of these symptoms, there's a strong likelihood that you may have some degree of adrenal stress. The likelihood increases significantly if you show more than two symptoms. Then, the best thing to do is to take a salivary adrenal hormone test to precisely determine the specific imbalance and what stage of adrenal stress you may be in. Depending on the results of this test, certain natural remedies may also be helpful in correcting hormone imbalances. In this case, a competent health-care professional should be consulted, as improper treatment can further worsen the problem. A poor diet also affects adrenal function. Avoid sugar, refined carbohydrates, and caffeine.

When I started running again, it was as if someone had pressed the reset button, just like in *Groundhog Day*. I could only jog about two hundred yards, but each week, I increased the distance by another hundred yards. I was taking it slow, gradual. It took three months to get up to three miles. I feared another recurrence of adrenal burnout.

Twenty years earlier, I had suffered through a running injury for over a year whose root cause was adrenal dysfunction—though I wasn't aware of the term or syndrome back then. While trail running, my left foot slipped into a small hole. I immediately felt a tendon just below my left knee twang, like a defective piano wire. The pain was sharp and intense, but I continued running, thinking that it was only a muscle pull that would work itself out. How wrong. The next few days, I could barely bend my leg. (At that point in my life, I had never taken Advil or any other pain medication.) I saw a sports massage therapist, hoping that his powerful fingers could alleviate the discomfort. He was able to pinpoint the trouble—an inflamed *gastrocnemius,* a fancy Latinate name for the calf. I visited him a half-dozen more times, but the pain continued to linger. I then went to see a Chinese acupuncturist who stuck needles up and down my left leg before attaching tiny electrodes to them. A low electric current was sent through the needles. It produced an odd, slight quivering sensation—nothing like being Tasered, I can assume. Each of these weekly acupuncture sessions lasted about forty-five minutes and cost sixty dollars. While the pain in my upper calf lessened after several months of this alternative-medicine treatment, I still had difficulty running more than two or three miles. Any longer, the calf would tighten and it felt like an ice pick was jammed into the top of my calf.

Stretching didn't work. I even stopped riding my bike because I thought that would only further aggravate the tender tendon. Growing ever more frustrated, I next saw a holistic sports doctor, who worked with elite triathletes and runners. He traced my problem to an adrenal gland deficiency. That was the first time I ever heard about the adrenals. I had no idea what they did. Nor did he explain their function. Instead, he sold me a thirty-dollar brown bottle of raw bovine adrenal gland extract pills to help strengthen my weakened adrenals. Since I was a vegetarian, I literally had trouble swallowing this unfamiliar type of meat-based medicine. Before I left his office, I asked him if I could begin biking. He said yes.

"What if the pain comes back?" I asked.

"Just deal with it," he responded.

I was miffed by his tart, callous reply. Nonetheless, later in the week, I went on a twenty-mile bike ride—the first time in months—and with about five miles to go, the *gastrocnemius* tendon stiffened, and the concentrated pain flared up just below my knee. But I kept cycling . . . through the pain. I made it home. And surprisingly, the next day, my leg felt fine. After a few more bike rides, I never felt pain in that region again. The *gastrocnemius* problem had disappeared, almost as mysteriously as it had arrived. The low-impact repetitive motion of pedaling must have healed the calf injury. I never did finish taking all those raw bovine adrenal pills.

"Motion is lotion," sports orthopedist, Dr. Nicholas Di Nubile, often says on his PBS-sponsored television health shows. He's right. Commit those three words to memory and you might possibly save yourself untold expense and months of frustration trying to rehab an ailing body part.

CROSS-TRAINING AND ACTIVE RECOVERY

One of literature's great opening lines is from Tolstoy's *Anna Karenina*: "All happy families are alike, but an unhappy family is unhappy in its own way." The human body is a lot like a family. When it's fit, healthy, and behaving well, there are no complaints. All the body parts seem to get along. But when injury or illness strikes, the body becomes incorrigible, disagreeable, indifferent to reason, pleading, and bribery. The symptoms and experience are different for each person, a function of pain threshold, severity of ailment, temperament, and meds.

Injury treatment also mirrors social and cultural priorities, including education, income, and health-care costs. In *The Healing of America,* journalist T. R. Reid examined the world's health systems. For purposes of global comparison, he used an old shoulder injury as a valid excuse to visit doctors in several countries. The results were fascinating. The American orthopedist was eager to suggest a major joint-replacement operation that would cost around $20,000. In France and Germany, with their socialized medicine, the doctors recommended a similar operation, either free or at minimal cost, but additionally pointed him toward regular physical therapy. In England, the doctor was unconcerned with his injury and wouldn't treat him. In Canada, home to national health insurance, he was told to wait up to a year before he could see a specialist. He fared best in India, where he was directed to an ayurvedic clinic, and after a treatment of herbs, massage, and meditation, his shoulder felt much better.

Runners, in particular, have been the proverbial golden goose to the healthcare industry. No other popular sport suffers from such a huge dropout in participants due to injuries. Yet enthusiasts keep on running, or trying to. The last time I checked, a quarter of all *Runner's World* marketplace ads showcased pain-reducing products for either the knee or foot.

Running doesn't have to lead to a broken-down body. Much to their detriment, many runners balk at the notion of cross-training, or at least fail to embrace it with the undiminished gusto of their triathlete brethren. Walking, cycling, and swimming place much less strain on joints, tendons, and ligaments, while ensuring the upkeep of the cardiovascular machinery.

I asked an old friend and retired world-champion adventure racer, Ian Adamson, about the injury-free benefits associated with cross-training. Now living in Boulder, the forty-six-year-old super athlete, race director, and motivational speaker emailed me the following:

It is well known and documented in the field of sports medicine that muscular balance is required to maintain optimal performance and prevent injury. A good example is runners who neglect their core strength. You see this especially at the elite level where runners lose abdominal tone, allowing their belly to protrude and their hips to rotate forward. This has the effect of shortening stride and causing excessive lower back curvature, ultimately leading to slower times, back and leg pain, and poor posture.

Cross-training done correctly provides balance between muscle groups. For example, cyclists develop big quadriceps and need to develop their leg adductors (muscles that pull a leg toward the body's central axis) to prevent chondromalacia, or anterior knee pain due to irritation of the cartilage on the undersurface of the kneecap, as well as iliotibial band syndrome, which is inflammation and pain on the outer side of the knee. Cross-training also allows you to recover and repair faster by maintaining cardiac output by using rested muscles. Swimming the day after a hard run or spinning on the bike after swimming hard intervals works well.

Developing core strength, balance, and non-propulsive muscles helps maintain posture and protects your joints by developing the connective tissue around them. Swimming and Nordic skiing (on snow and using dry-land trainers like in-line skates and poles) are two of the best cross-training sports since they demand high cardiac output, and use virtually all muscle groups, with minimal impact.

There is a strong argument that proper cross-training benefits performance in other sports when done correctly with a well-thought-out program. Runners may perform better if they mix swimming and weights into their training. In fact, injured runners regularly use pool training when recovering from injury, with water running and swimming.

Triathletes and adventure racers are incredibly robust endurance athletes and suffer far fewer injuries than athletes who only run. This is likely due to the cross-training effect and their ability and drive to simply switch their training focus from one sport to the others if injured.

I place a ton of credence in Ian's counsel. He dominated the adventure-racing scene for almost a decade, injury-free and achieving victories with his teammates in world champion events in Borneo, Fiji, Utah, Baja, New England, and Colorado. At five-seven and 160 pounds, the mild-mannered Ian possessed an amazing ability to race without sleep through treacherous wilderness. The Aussie-born stud is listed in *Guinness World Records* for setting the world record in marathon kayaking—217 miles in twenty-four hours along the Yukon River. Once on a trip to Costa Rica together, we had been kayaking for six straight hours, and both of my biceps went into spasm, so Ian towed me in his kayak for a mile, using bungee cords, while I leaned back and enjoyed the sunset as we zigged and zagged across the water. Consider this other piece of evidence regarding Ian's superhuman athletic prowess and pain management. During his last adventure race in 2006, the 420-mile Primal Quest, which was held in the Utah desert where daytime temperatures exceeded 110°F, his four-person team experienced an early equipment foul-up and Ian was forced to wear ill-fitting aquatic slippers for the sixty mile run. Race photos of him getting his wrecked feet wrapped with bandages at a medical aid station seemed like a scene out of a war zone. He still had to cover another 350 miles of desert via mountain biking, trekking, horseback riding, mountaineering, and white-water swimming.

Ian retired from competition not because of a chronic injury or because his body was beaten and battered from weeklong madcap marches through deserts, jungles, and mountains. "I retired because I had achieved everything I set out to and more in adventure racing," he says. "I was racing at the top of my game, and my retiring had nothing to do with my physical shape. I believe I could've raced at the top for another five years at least."

He currently engages in what he calls lifestyle training, which means biking to work a couple of times a week. "Since I live in the hills above Boulder, it takes me about thirty minutes to get to work and sixty minutes to ride back home. I also run two or three times during the week, do core strength a couple of times, and a long bike or run, averaging two to four hours, on weekends. So the difference between now and when I was in peak racing shape is that

I'm averaging between thirty minutes and an hour per day instead of one to four hours. I estimate that I'm probably at 70 percent of my fitness from my racing peak in 2006. And any time I miss a workout for a day or more I get grumpy. I definitely function better mentally and emotionally when I'm active and fit."

In 2010, Ian, who is a director of R&D and education at Newton Shoes, put on an all-day running demonstration at the San Diego Rock 'n' Roll Marathon Expo by going 47.3 miles on a treadmill. This running-in-place feat took him eight hours, which included brief bathroom and food breaks. Average speed was 10:15 per mile. "I was a little stiff the day after," he emailed me, "and so I went for a bike ride the following day, back to running two days later with no apparent aftereffects."

Cross-training also allows an injured athlete to keep working out. This is known as "active recovery" and helps maintain cardiovascular fitness. What you don't want to do is go to complete rest. Numerous research studies have shown that fitness rapidly declines after two or three weeks of no activity.

"There is nothing passive about recovery," says Robert Forster, a popular Santa Monica–based physical therapist who has treated Olympic athletes such as Jackie Joyner-Kersee and Gail Devers, and tennis legend Pete Sampras. "Recovery is an active process where light adaptation workouts stimulate recovery better than rest alone. Light workouts are akin to the self-cleaning oven where the heat is turned up but no roast is placed inside. Light workouts provide the body the same opportunity to do housecleaning functions without having to recover from the damaging effects of a new workout. The vascular system is stimulated to increase blood flow to the muscles delivering oxygen and nutrients to aid recovery. The muscle cells, stimulated by a release of hormones, step up the reparative functions and grow stronger. Similar occurrences improve connective tissue and bone repair as well."

THE DOMINO EFFECT—HOW AN INJURY EVOLVES

It can seemingly come out of nowhere, like a thief in the night. Or it might lie buried, like some ghoul in a horror film emerging from the crypt. No one welcomes the arrival of an injury. And when it shows up, life's priorities are immediately reshuffled, especially if you are an athlete or like working out. Your entire world narrows like a laser beam focusing on the ailing body part. Your sole desire is to return to that happier, pre-injury state. In many cases, that is not possible, even with the best medical care and treatment.

"An injury is, with some exceptions, simply an end result of a series of dominoes falling over," says Dr. Phil Maffetone. "One little, innocuous problem affects something else, and the dominoes start to fall. The end result is, sometimes after a half-dozen or so dominoes have fallen, a symptom—pain, dysfunction, loss of power, all depending on how the body adapts and compensates to the falling dominoes."

Phil used the example of a hamstring injury to show how these dominoes begin to fall.

One morning, the athlete bends over to tie his right running shoe and he feels a painful twinge in his right hamstring, but this is the end result of biomechanical inefficiencies piling up like falling dominos. Perhaps it was the left foot—on the opposite side—that underwent micro-trauma due to the running shoe not fitting properly. This placed stress on the foot and ankle. While this produced no overt symptoms, the body compensated by tilting the pelvis to lessen the weight bearing load on the left side, which in turn increased stress on the opposing right side, in particular the quadriceps. These muscles were forced to overcompensate due to the gait change resulting from the tilt in the pelvis. As a result, the quadriceps may become weaker or inhibited. And finally, the hamstrings compensate for the quad problem by tightening. So when the athlete bends forward to put on his right shoe, the too-tight hamstrings are being stretched. The pain he feels is from the micro-tearing.

Should the athlete ice it? Take anti-inflammatory drugs? Or find and correct the cause of the problem—which in this case was the shoes? "Generally, the body has a great natural ability to heal itself," says Phil. "When your body gives you a very obvious sign, such as a hamstring twinge, it's time to stop and assess what's going on. If you don't, it may soon be too late. Waiting until you're physically unable to train—the point at which your body forces you to stop—just results in more unnecessary damage and wasted time. And finally, consider that this whole process, from the time the first domino fell, may take weeks or months, or in some cases, years. And throughout this entire process, your performance is adversely affected."

During the summer of 1995 when I was mountain biking up to ten hours a week on fire roads and trails in hilly Marin County, I often experienced minor lower back pain. My back was stiff and aching after I woke up, but later in the day it would feel okay. One morning, as I bent down to pick up a magazine that had fallen on the floor, my back suddenly locked up. My upper body felt like it had been wedged inside a vise. I couldn't straighten up. There I was, ridiculously bent over at a ninety-degree angle, thinking "Now what?" For the rest of the day, I hobbled about like a hunched-over homeless guy looking for spare change on the sidewalk. I could only walk at a right angle—a carpenter's square with legs. When it became too painful to walk, I spent the next day at my girlfriend's apartment, curled up in bed, fetal and helpless.

It was obvious that I needed to see a chiropractor. My girlfriend drove me to one in Sausalito. After several quick tests, he identified the problem as subduction—the back muscles in the lumbar area had slipped under one another. This created further muscular-skeletal imbalance, making the left leg one inch shorter than the right.

I literally put myself in his hands as he carefully wrapped his arms around my body and tried to straighten my back. The loud crack of vertebrae shifting into place was both a startling and soothing sound. I felt instant relief in my lower back. He then placed me face down on a machine that gently rocked my entire body for thirty minutes. When the session was over, the back pain was gone, though I still couldn't stand full-mast. The following day, I wanted to celebrate my newfound freedom from subduction, so I went on a three-mile Quasimodo-like run with my dog Rockee.

That incident was my first real wake-up call that the body will eventually rebel from overuse or muscular-skeletal misalignment. Had I done warm-up exercises before I mountain biked and cool-down exercises after I finished riding, I might have avoided the back pain and seventy-five-dollar chiropractor sessions.

A sudden injury can occur even when you are not exercising, because the pressure has probably been building up over time—in gradual, almost infinitesimal increments. It's like the final dusting of snowflakes triggering an avalanche. It didn't take much to throw out my back that morning when I bent over.

THE NUMBERS DON'T LIE—WE'RE LIVING LONGER, WHICH MEANS MORE WEAR AND TEAR ON THE BODY

According to the London-based *Sports Injury Bulletin*, 60 to 65 percent of all runners are injured each year.

(continues)

Twenty million people a year visit a physician because of knee problems.

An artificial knee replacement that uses metal and plastic for joint reconstruction usually lasts for only ten to fifteen years.

According to a study presented at the American Academy of Orthopedic Surgeons' annual meeting in 2008, there will be an estimated 3.48 million knee replacements by 2030. This is approximately a 673 percent increase compared to today's procedures. Artificial hip replacements now averaging 200,000 per year are estimated to increase to 572,000 annually by 2030.

Hip replacement surgery is normally covered by health insurance, but for patients without coverage, the average cost of a total hip replacement is around $40,000.

For over-the-counter pain relief, 33 million Americans regularly use nonsteroidal anti-inflammatory drugs, also known as NSAIDs—aspirin, ibuprofen (Advil, Motrin), naproxen sodium (Aleve).

NSAIDs account for about 16,500 deaths annually; the culprit is usually ulcer-related complications associated with the drug's continued use.

One-quarter of the bones in the human body are located in the feet (twenty-six in each foot, excluding the *sesamoid* bones at the base of the big toe).

Each time a runner strikes the ground, the force of impact can be as high as eight times the body weight to the joints (feet, knees, hip).

BE PATIENT

When we are young, we want life to speed up. When we are older, we want life to slow down. It's a constant negotiation that requires balancing expectations with reality. Richard Kyle, MD, president of the American Academy of Orthopedic Surgeons, treats a broad range of sports-related injuries among fifty- and sixty-year-old patients. "We see a lot of people coming in who have decided they're going to get fit," he told *AARP* magazine. "So they start exercising the way they did in their 20s and 30s. All of a sudden they're in my office with pain in their knees, their hips, their shoulders. Don't start out by running five miles just because you could do it ten years ago. Be aware of how fit you are and how old you are."

To avoid injury during your return to fitness, you should start slowly and build up gradually. Never increase the amount or intensity of your workouts by more than 10 percent each week. Fitness doesn't occur overnight. It might have taken you years to get woefully out of shape, so don't expect magic-wand miracles that will suddenly transform your physique from blob to buff. "To make a change in how you look, you are talking about a significant period of training," William Kraemer, a kinesiology professor at the University of Connecticut, told the *New York Times* in 2009. "In our studies it takes six months to a year. That is what the reality is."

WHEN INJURY STRIKES: THREE STORIES OF SUCCESSFULLY REBOUNDING BACK

To learn more about how the body copes with an injury, I decided to speak with several athletes whose injury kept them temporarily sidelined. All three individuals eventually recovered and returned to fitness—but with an altered mental outlook. Their successful physical rehab was tempered by self-reflection, compromise, and appreciation for the body's remarkable ability to heal itself and bounce back from adversity. Here are their extraordinary stories, as told in their own words.

The Catastrophic Injury: Broken Back

Theresa Ho, thirty-eight, lives for the outdoors. She traded in her Berkeley doctoral degree in molecular and cell biology to become a full-time resident of Yosemite National Park, where she manages the website for the concessionaire of DNC Parks and Resort. In 2006, while hiking up a steep, unmarked section in the backcountry with her husband, Tom Lambert, a four-foot boulder came loose and crushed her body before skittering down the canyon. Tom rushed to her side, thinking she was dead.

I came to California from Wisconsin, originally, for a PhD program at Berkeley. I absolutely chose Berkeley for the outstanding research in molecular neuroscience, but I only applied to programs that I thought would put me within striking distance of the Sierras. While I was there, I spent as much time as I could in Yosemite rock climbing with Tom who has a PhD in European history from the University of Wisconsin.

We climbed the Salathe Wall together on El Capitan, and we did many of the classic moderate routes, including routes on Half Dome, Sentinel Rock, Middle and Higher Cathedrals, Washington Column, and Leaning Tower.

Once I graduated, we treated ourselves to a vacation that ended with a few months in Yosemite—a few months that turned into several years and a completely different life. I started out filling in at the front desk at the Yosemite Medical Clinic part-time, teaching skiing at the small local ski hill, Badger Pass, and after a summer of bean counting, became the Assistant Manager of the Mountaineering School and Guide Service, primarily managing the hiking and backpacking program there.

On October 22, 2006, Tom and I decided to go out hiking on my lunch break. The leaves in LeConte gully were a spectacular golden yellow, hiking uphill is always good exercise, and I had an idea that I'd like to check out the gully for a possible ski descent should the snow come into condition. Tom was a short distance ahead of me when I pulled on the loose rock— egg shaped and about four feet in diameter. At first it tipped so slowly that I tried to push it back into place; when that didn't work, I leapt backward, thinking that it would just fall over and come to a rest. Unfortunately, it kept rolling. I tried to get my feet on it, to push it away from me, but it was just too big. It felt like I got folded in two as the boulder rolled right over the top of me, blocking out the light. I remember thinking, "Please don't stop now." Fortunately, its momentum carried it over me and it bounced further down the gully.

My first thought was "I'm okay," but it quickly became clear that "okay" was relative. I could move a little, but had suffered many wounds on my legs and was not able to support my weight. My chest really hurt. Tom helped get me settled, and then ran to get help. As the sounds of his footsteps faded, I realized that it was going to get really lonely up there really fast.

Surprisingly, I heard sirens only twelve minutes later, and then in almost no time at all, Tom was back at my side, with a Yosemite Search and Rescue team close on his heels. There was John, the incident commander, Ernie, and Max, but I could hear in the background the large team of people supporting them, and working to set up a zip line in case it was needed. I was told later that, at that time of year, the park helicopter isn't active and the California Highway Patrol helicopter usually takes over an hour to scramble the team and fly into the park. This time, however, it was already in the air on some other business, and was able to re-route and responded in only twenty-two minutes. I felt amazingly lucky and grateful for the quality of care and the speed of response.

I was first flown to Doctor's Medical Hospital in Modesto where they did my initial imaging. The ER nurse reported that the doctor swore aloud when he first saw the images of my back, and ordered that I be transferred to a top-notch research hospital, and so I ended up at Stanford Hospital and Clinics.

In spite of horrific MRI images, with the exception of a bit of numbness on the insides of my knees (I also had broken ribs, a fractured fibula, and a punctured lung), I always had feeling and strength in my lower extremities. The surgery was postponed for a day while the doctors made sure that there were no other internal injuries that might complicate the surgery. That waiting period was the worst as I was transferred in and out of beds for more imaging. I was painfully aware of how exposed my spinal cord was, and terrified that some small mishap could mean paralysis.

Dr. Stephen Ryu, a neurosurgeon, then with Stanford Hospital, but currently working at Palo Alto Medical Foundation, fused my back from L1 to S1 using two eight-inch rods with a short connector bar between them, nine screws, and a piece of cadaver bone used to prop up the L4 vertebrae, which was shattered, and twisted ninety degrees. The surgery took about eight hours. Dr. Ryu was amazing, simply amazing.

When Tom (out of my hearing) asked Dr. Ryu for his prognosis, he only said that he had high hopes that I would be able to return to "normal" activity. He expressed some skepticism that I would ever climb again, but after seeing Tom's dismay, quickly added that I should just prove him wrong.

My team of doctors wanted me to get out of bed and move around as soon as possible, so I sat up and took my first steps the day after the surgery with the aid of a walker. My first walk was probably about fifty feet. My crushed legs and injured back hurt like crazy and I was exhausted afterward.

I continued with a number of therapists at Stanford. Some helped me with walking and climbing stairs and others had suggestions for making it easier for me to do simple tasks like putting on shoes and socks or leaning over a sink to brush my teeth.

Once home in Yosemite, I had little mobility at first. It was frustrating to be so helpless. I was home alone. I dropped the book I was reading on the floor. It was so close—yet completely inaccessible. I tried to pick it up a couple of different ways, all with no success, and then finally when it hurt too much to keep trying, I just lay back down in bed and cried.

Tom was incredibly busy during that time. He was finishing up one of his books for the University of Wisconsin, teaching downhill skiing at Badger Pass part-time, and working with our contractors to finish up construction on the house we were building in Yosemite West. He did a great job taking care of me, but it was hard.

In addition to walking, I also visited the physical therapist that works in Yosemite Valley. Prior to working there, she had experience working with major trauma rehabilitation in California's Central Valley. We worked on flexibility, scar tissue mobilization, and gentle core strengthening. Because of the severity of my back injury, we focused on isometric exercises that involved holding positions, such as planks, where you hold a push-up position with a straight back, or simply tightening the core muscles without moving at all.

During my slow rehab, the most amazing thing was the outpouring of support that I received from friends and family, and the Yosemite community in general. If there was an emotional high in all of that mess, that would have to be it. My husband was a source of strength, love, and good humor through everything. Also, I started to hear incredibly inspirational stories from friends about other people who had broken their backs and the amazing things that they were doing now. The wife of one of the climbing guides that I worked with, Eliza, had broken not only her back but also her pelvis. Unlike me, she spent a significant amount of time in a wheelchair before getting permission to start walking again. Now, not only is she incredibly active, she even teaches yoga at the local center.

My initial recovery took place during the winter in Yosemite, where slipping on the ice is always a possibility. I couldn't imagine how much it would have hurt to fall, because even the thought of throwing out my arms suddenly to catch myself and avoid that fall was horrifying. When I ventured outside, I clung to Tom's arm, or walked between two people when I could, and shuffled along painstakingly. Mostly, I was trapped indoors, in the shadow of the big Yosemite cliffs. I don't have a history of seasonal affective disorder, but the lack of sunshine along with all the other things that were going on made those dark days darker.

Whenever I was standing, the pressure from my leg injuries hurt the most. Whenever I was sitting, my back hurt the most. It left me in the strange situation of standing until my leg pain was too much, and then sitting until the back pain was too much. I would oscillate between the two positions in shorter and shorter intervals until I just had to find someplace to lie down.

I ended the official part of the rehab six to nine months after my injury, but my body has taken much longer than that to recover. At this point, most of the residual effects are secondary. Of course, my back is fused, so there is a certain amount of flexibility that I've lost, but the things I notice most are the lack of strength, especially core strength, that I used to have, and leg strength and hip flexibility. Fortunately, working on those things isn't a mystery. It will just take some time and effort. Some days I'm excited about how much progress I've made—hiking faster, lifting more weight in the gym, being less afraid of hurting myself. On other days, I shake my head about how far I still have to go. The other day I went to a friend's indoor bouldering wall, fell from the top-most holds, and didn't wince when I landed. I would never have described the sensation as painful before—but my back was fragile, tender. Now, it's more solid, and I'm less hesitant to try things. That is partly psychological too, but my mental state is also a reflection of how my body feels.

As I got stronger hiking, I thought that there'd be few, if any, psychological issues, that is, until I got out on a talus field two and a half years after the accident. Although the boulders were big, the angle of the slope was low, and the rocks were so stable that most of them were covered with lichen. The rational part of my mind knew that this was relatively safe terrain but there was another part that kept running disaster sequences through my head. What if this boulder were to roll? That one? The next one? These thoughts kept spiraling until I just sat down on one of those big, flat, stable rocks and cried. I shook my head when Tom came over to comfort me. "I'm sorry," I told him. "I know it isn't scary." But I was terrified.

Of course, the way to deal with fear is to embrace it. Since the talus field incident, I've hiked out on slopes that are considerably steeper and looser. I suppose at this point someone will point out that it would be safer to stay indoors, or on the trail, but there is also value in pushing your comfort zone a little bit, and the mountains are strong incentive.

In early August 2009, my husband and I hiked to the top of Mount Tyndall, just south of Yosemite. It was my first 14,000 ascent, and it was glorious. My legs were tired, of course. Tyndall involves thirteen miles and 8,000 feet of elevation gain, one way. We split the trip into three days, but it was still quite the challenge for me. I'm proud of the effort, the mountains are beautiful and wild, and I love seeing the high alpine flowers, and the tiny pikas which manage to put together a living in such a seemingly harsh alpine environment.

I'm sure I'll end up rock climbing again. It's just a matter of time. Plus, now that I don't wince at the idea of falling, and my fitness is increasing, I'm looking forward to the upcoming backcountry ski season as well.

I have always been inspired by stories of what people were able to overcome. But I'm a little more aware and those stories come into clearer focus. In the winter, a friend of mine is the hut keeper at a backcountry ski hut, the Glacier Point Ski Hut. He tells a story of going out to greet two skiers—a blind man pulling a paraplegic woman on a sit-ski—who had teamed up for the 10.5-mile ski-in.

I recently spoke with my surgeon, Dr. Stephen Ryu, who told me that he still uses me as a case study because, as he put it, I "should not be walking or going to the bathroom normally." He also mentioned that he hadn't seen that much damage without paralysis either before or since. That sure renews the sense of gratitude I have about my outcome.

The Overuse Injury: Faulty Hip

Scott Tinley, fifty-three, embodied the sculpted personification of triathlon for over two decades. The blond San Diegan multisport athlete was a two-time Hawaii Ironman champion, off-road racing pioneer, and consistent enough to bag nearly one hundred triathlon victories in his storied career. But his body eventually began to betray him—an unwanted occupational hazard for the self-styled Californian iconoclast. As he entered his early forties, all those weekly sessions of three hundred to four hundred miles on the bike, sixty miles running, and endless laps in the pool had exacted their physiological toll on his aging, weathered physique. The former superstar stud could now barely hold his own against top triathlete age-groupers. The more his race performances began to falter, the more his carefully constructed world began to collapse while he struggled to come to terms with the emotional and psychological fallout of slowing down. With great reluctance, he retired from the sport and started a new late-in-life career as a creative writing instructor and sports humanities professor at local San Diego colleges. He still stayed in shape, but his priority had transitioned to the heavy-lifting demands of literature, philosophy, and psychology.

I first met Scott in 1984 when I had flown down to San Diego to interview him for a Tri-Athlete *magazine cover story titled "Rebel With a Cause." Our interview took place in his kitchen. He was cocky, edgy, flippant, a surfer dude with an alpha male attitude. I was just as rude and helped myself to a can of Bud Light (an Ironman sponsor), which I plucked from the fridge without asking.*

Over time, our relationship mellowed after I asked him to write a monthly column for the magazine, which he continued doing until early 2010. His words, skillfully carved from a mountain of athletic experience, gave voice and direction to all triathletes. But even the sport's former demigod wasn't prepared for the ultimate physical injustice: He could no longer run because of a bum hip—a hip that had worn itself down from all that training and racing, a hip that seemed like it belonged to an eighty-year-old. So he did what had to be done:

He went under the knife and got the end part of the faulty hip resurfaced with a cuplike metallic gizmo that sets off airport security alarms but has allowed him to become physically active again.

When I first realized that I was no longer one of the best endurance athletes in the world, my life did not end at that precise moment in time. In fact, as that truism began to sink in, it could be said that my life was starting to look less stressful, more balanced, that I was healthier without the underlying need for constant training, and the oppressive guilt when that beast was not fed his daily mileage. I found some of my workouts were not as snappy and crisp as they had been twenty years ago. On others, I wondered why I was doing it at all. For me, that was the sign: when reason had no reason at all, when the obvious was obviously gone, when I would line up on the starting line and instead of being focused, I was distracted by deep thoughts of "Why?" and "Did I leave the burner on the stove?"

Since I'd been a professional athlete for over two decades, there had always been a sense of purpose and clarity to my life. It was a black-and-white world with all the emotional fuzziness cut off. I lived for the experience of being an athlete. No, that's not right, my entire being was an athlete. I was over-identified with the beast's icon and what it meant; I was the shiny cartoon superhero.

But all that was fading.

I had spent nearly twenty years immersed in thirty to forty hours per week at some form of endurance exercise: swimming, cycling, running, paddling—plus all the supplementary activities such as stretching, weight training, and miscellaneous body work. My body was addicted to the naturally occurring corticosteroids, to endorphin highs and constant Southern California sunshine, all further buoyed by a steadily increasing need for self medication—three or four cups of coffee in the morning to get me going, two or three glasses of wine at night to slow me down.

Someone once did the math of all my training miles before I was inducted into some hall of fame for triathletes. The journal said that I'd made it to the moon but not quite all the way back.

It was no wonder why my body had began to shut down. And so, I retired as a professional though kept in good shape. But then it got harder and harder to run. The pain in my hip started in the mid 1990s. I had trouble reaching down to tie my shoes on the starboard side. Gave up laces and wore beach slippers until 2006. My friends said I was walking like John Wayne on a hillside. It was time to seriously consider getting my hip surgically altered.

My once-dependable body that competed in the world of endurance sport will not and cannot ever be the same. I will have "parts."

The head of my femur, also buried near the core of something central, is the largest ball-and-socket joint in the human body. Mine looked more like a pumice stone than the shiny, well-lubed and smooth piston of my past. And the soft ligamental coating of the acetabulum that soaks up the pogoing had left the building with Elvis. So what were my options? Live with the grinding, painful issue of bone-on-bone or have the mechanic go in and replace the air conditioning unit even if it means having to cut through the intake manifold?

I ultimately decided to get a Birmingham Hip Replacement, also known as a BHR. If it sounds exotic, it's not. Unlike a total hip replacement, the BHR is just a very cool cobalt chrome alloy cap that is placed atop the worn-out head of the femur. You could drink Johnnie Walker Black from it. There's a hole to be drilled and a bit of fitting to be done. The reciprocating female side looks like a postmodern ashtray and the thing spins in there like a children's top. That part fits in the hip socket. First developed in England in 1997, the BHR has only been FDA-approved in America since 2006.

Hospitals normally scared me. They shouldn't. But other than watching my wife Virginia give birth to our two children and a few of the good days when I worked as a paramedic, nearly all of my experiences with hospitals have been related to something bad. Trauma, illness, death, the smell of Lysol and lime-green Jell-O. These are the things I conjure when considering hospitals. I also wasn't too keen about wearing a breezy white gingham gown that'd expose my lily-white ass. Or knowing that I would be lying in bed, a fifty-year-old ex-jock wondering why I was such a fool to think that eighty miles a week running on the concrete Mission Beach Boardwalk was as good as it gets.

The doctor who cut me open was a masterful surgeon by the name of Dr. John Rogerson. He's based in Madison, Wisconsin, and that's where I spent a week in early snowy December 2007 with Virginia. There are few great surgeons who have been doing it longer than Dr. Rogerson. I had spent two years searching for the very best surgeon on the planet to do this procedure. I almost went to India. I almost went to England. I'm glad I ended up at Meriter Hospital in Madison because my gut told me it was the right place. I love it when my gut is right.

The surgery went smoothly. Rogerson later checked up on me and told me that the BHR fit great and that I had plenty of bone spurs for him to shave and a few cysts to pack. When he left, I could urinate, and that made me happy. When you get cut, you resort to childhood pleasures. I liked the long thin cup with the cap that I could pee into without getting out of bed. I was feeling cavalier and decided that later in the evening I'd get out of bed and pee in the toilet. I nearly passed out and the kind nurse, Cherry, picked me up with one hand like a firefighter holding a buddy from falling off a fiery ledge. I asked her if she'd keep this between us—you know, that I couldn't walk to the bathroom after surgery. She said the secret was safe. She placed me back in bed and I peed in my little cup.

I began my rehab at a facility in Madison fittingly called the Hip Hab. It's a retirement facility replete with physical therapists, training rooms, warm-water exercise and lap pools, massage therapists, and the best damn group of octogenarian cheerleaders. It was the perfect place to rehab. Dr. Rogerson fashioned his post-op therapy on the European model: Find a place to land your patients after they come back from the hospital, teach them how to walk again, how to breathe, how to live without a computer. And teach their family and friends how to be involved with the entire process. Imagine if we took all of our returning combat vets and did the same thing. It's not the same but it has paradigmatic similarities—coming back from major surgery is like coming back from war.

During my first rehab appointment with a woman named Desiree, I walked nearly fifty yards, much of it with a cane. Then we did a series of standing exercises. She was gentle. I nearly fainted. She's worked with all but a few of Dr. Rogerson's patients. She's seen it all. Two days earlier, I was unable to will my legs to move. With great concentration I was now able to walk with a normal gait while putting all my weight on my operative leg. The human body is truly an amazing structure. And the technology available to fix it is nearly as awe-inspiring.

My rehab went quickly once I returned to San Diego. I was swimming at week two, paddling at three, jogging at four months, playing beach volleyball at six months.

So here I am one and one half years after Dr. Rogerson placed some new cobalt chromium parts inside me. My new BHR hip is bitchin'. That's the best way I can put it. Forget that I am running fifteen to twenty miles a week and could do thrice that if I could win the Super Lotto and give up my day job. Forget that the pain I feel is in other places from other activities and other poor choices. (Why do I think that I can play eight tough games of two-person beach volleyball just because I have blonde hair?) Forget that when I try to show someone the six-inch scar on my butt they don't believe me because they can't see it. Metal parts? What metal parts? Anyone want to hit some tennis balls? I now feel better than I have since eighth grade. I'm not as fit but I'm a hell of lot healthier, my liver notwithstanding.

The thing about working with the body in repair is that unlike the mind or the spirit, clichés work. When discussing rehabilitation from surgery, I can claim that a well-oiled and smartly driven machine rewards the driver. My ducks are in a row, and I shoot out of the blocks in the morning like a bullet and make a beeline for the stairs.

Here are a few final—and practical—thoughts on physical rehab.

Think about relearning many basic motor movement skills (for example, walking, standing up from a seated position) since you may have compensated for years of degeneration and need to rebalance your musculoskeletal alignment. You want to incorporate these basic techniques of proper movement along with gentle non-weight-bearing activities as you can tolerate them.

As soon as you feel ready (and even if you don't but are being well advised to), start moving that hip in the advised motions. Remember there are limitations on certain hip or leg angles for a few weeks post-op. Your surgeon and therapist should have advised you of this. But, the point is, you want to regenerate and reformat the soft tissue surrounding the operative joint. This begins by moving it—if only sliding your leg up and down on the bottom of your foot. Sitting on your ass for two weeks is the worst thing that you can do for a new hip. Old bodies and old cars need oil and fluids to run through their innards to keep them from rotting away.

Consider massage or an ART-styled (active-release therapy) session. Beginning three days post-op and continuing for five months, I had good hands-on body therapy to increase circulation to the area, break up scar tissue, and gradually increase ROM (range of motion). I think this was key to my successful rehab.

As soon as your suture site is healed, get in the pool and start moving. Even if you start with a pull-buoy, the simple act and idea of being physical and training again is a great benefit. Like Steinbeck said, "Good things love water. Bad things always been dry."

Get as much information about activity levels in rehab from as many good sources as you can and then come up with your own program. There is a wide disparity in the kinds of approaches. My surgeon, Dr. Rogerson, takes a moderate and mindful stance on rehab that considers a variety of factors surrounding the patient and the success of the surgery. Other surgeons can be more or less aggressive in what they suggest a patient do. Be your own best consultant.

Be cautious when considering weight-bearing activities. I waited four months before I ran a step and then worked my way up from a hundred yards to five miles over a one-year period. But, now I can run as long and as fast as I want; my BHR hip is not a limiting factor. I choose not to run more than fifteen to twenty miles a week and often only do half of that in considering that while the wear is likely minimal there's not yet enough empirical data to claim that excessive weight-bearing use will not increase metal-on-metal hip wear of the prosthesis.

Think like an athlete in training—you have a job to do and that's to get your physical life back. Make yourself a plan with regular goals and objectives and find the best "coaching" that you can out there. The resurfacing family is very supportive. It's quite amazing really: people coming out of nowhere to offer advice and support.

Eat well. Drink lots of fluids. Get good rest.

Think in terms of years and decades not weeks and months. Be patient with your body and your new hip, but also require it to serve its master. It's only a new body part.

Share what you learn with others.

The Near-Fatal Injury: Cardiac Arrest

On the morning of our interview, sixty-six-year-old Don Summers, of Seattle, had just returned from an arduous six-mile hike with 2,000 feet of climbing. Summers spends as much time as possible outdoors, a stark departure from his lengthy career in human resources, business consulting, and teaching MBA courses at Seattle Pacific University. Growing up in Michigan, he wasn't a high school jock, but he started running for relaxation in the late sixties. By the early seventies, he was averaging forty to fifty miles a week, six or seven days a week. He finished the Boston Marathon twice—in 1983 and 1996. He's also completed a number of triathlons on both coasts. When he moved to Seattle in 1985, he continued to run, but soon found his way to the mountains. He climbed the 14,410-foot Mount Rainier eight times, certainly not the easiest ascent since the final 4,500 feet is on glaciers. Climbers are roped up, wear crampons and use ice axes.

Summers is also passionate about cycling. One bike event he liked doing was Ride Around Mount Rainier in One Day (RAMROD), which covers 154 miles and 9,000 vertical feet of climbing. He was training for RAMROD on July 6, 2002, just another long, tiring day in the saddle, when something unexpected happened. His heart stopped.

I feel as if I won the lottery on that day. On that morning a group of cycling friends and I left from our homes first thing in the morning and met at our regular spot on Mercer Island, Washington. We headed east off the island, all of us in a good mood, on a warm, sunny day. Within a few minutes we were climbing up a steep hill with sparkling Lake Washington to our backs. My goal was simple: do a final hundred-mile training ride in preparation for the upcoming RAMROD. Of the four of us, I was the only one doing the RAMROD. The others were out to have a good time—and support me.

I was feeling great as we made our way up the hill, and could tell that my training was paying off. I was surprised that my pace kept me in stride with the group's fastest climber. I was right on his back tire. As I approached the crest, I looked down at my watch and noticed that my heart rate was registering a whopping 276. My resting heart rate is about 45. I dismissed it as a false reading. After all, I was feeling great. At the top, I stopped to wait for my remaining two colleagues, a bit puffed up because of my strong performance. Then bam, I passed out. My heart had stopped. I wasn't breathing.

But it was my good fortune that day, because as I was lying on the ground dying, the first driver who stopped, I later learned, was the wife of an EMT who had taught her CPR. Her name was Kristi Nipert, and as she was about to start working on me a second driver showed up. One lucky event after another kept happening. This person, Bridgett Jonas, was a critical-care nurse at a local hospital. So she took over from Kristi. Somebody had also called for 911 and before the first EMTs came, Bridgett had my heart pumping again. It hadn't been beating for several minutes. Any longer and I would have suffered brain damage, or worse.

At the hospital, I was awake and conscious by early afternoon. Meanwhile, the doctors were trying to figure out what caused the cardiac arrest. It was then determined that I had experienced ventricular fibrillation. A very high percentage of persons die from it. Some estimates are as high as 85 percent. Sudden cardiac death typically follows unless medical help is provided immediately. In my case, an unusual strong electrical impulse sent my heart into arrhythmia. My riding up that hill probably triggered arrhythmia. When you bring up your heart rate through intense exercise, you can send your heart into an arrhythmic state because the body creates too much adrenaline, and that in turn generates too strong or an irregular electric current in the heart.

Feeling better, I left the hospital after four days. I immediately started walking. The doctor told me to not allow my heart rate to get too high, no more than 120. I then went to my medical center for more testing, and they discovered how easily my heart goes into arrhythmia, both atrial and ventricular. So in August they implanted a defibrillator in my chest. If my heart goes over 220, the defibrillator activates and it shocks my heart back into rhythm. The gadget is smaller than a cigarette pack, and it was implanted in the left side of my chest.

After they implanted the defibrillator, I stayed overnight in the hospital for observation to make sure everything was working right. Then I went home and I was back up and running within a fairly short period of time and cycling and hiking and doing all the things that I love. But my cardiologist had also discovered during the examination that I had some blocked arteries. Now this had nothing to do with my cardiac arrest, but he figured that if this condition was left untreated, I would eventually have a heart attack, particularly because I was so active. With blocked arteries, you're not getting as much blood to your heart. So I waited until December when my teaching ended and my consulting load went down to get the six bypasses done.

The bypass surgery really slows you down because they crack your chest open. The recuperation took some time. After several days, I was back walking but at a slow pace. I did go to a business meeting a week after the operation, but the cardiologist warned me, "Take it easy, you've got stitches and your body's been through a lot. Ease yourself back into your normal level of activity." Within five weeks I was back snowshoeing. But at this point, everything had been tuned up. My arteries that were clogged were clear; I now had a backup with my defibrillator. I felt pretty confident that heart-wise nothing was going to happen.

It took a few months before I was running again but even then not at full speed. Not that I was a very fast runner to begin with. But I was weaker because of the surgery and because I was taking a beta blocker, which slows your heart down. The beta blocker's purpose is to put a ceiling on how high your heart will beat so there's less chance that it will go out of whack and into arrhythmia.

I remember when I was running for speed, I'd look at my heart rate and it'd be at 140 beats per minute. Now imagine you're trying to do that very same thing and your heart rate doesn't go over 100. It means that the heart is beating at a slower pace. You talk to anyone who's on a beta blocker and who has had an active life and they will say that it's frustrating because it just doesn't allow you to do things at the same level without putting a lot more effort into it. I'm usually the slowest one hiking with my friends and it's just frustrating, but I'm out there—I'm doing it. And I'm grateful that I can do these activities.

In 2004, I did an up-and-over backpacking trip of Mount Rainier with three friends. We climbed to the summit, stayed in the crater overnight, and descended via a different route. Climbers typically leave most of their equipment at the halfway point, so the second part allows you to carry a much lighter pack. The up-and-over meant that we had to carry everything, about fifty-five pounds each, up to the summit and down the other side.

My next big adventure was climbing Mount Kilimanjaro in Africa in 2006. The summit is 19,334 feet. Kilimanjaro is basically a long hike; it's not a technical climb. As you might imagine, I wondered how the elevation would affect my heart. Mount Rainier's 14,410 feet was fine. On Kilimanjaro you go slowly. This allows you to acclimate to the elevation gain. On the last day we had about 900 feet to do—very steep, slippery volcanic ash all the way to the top. While it was no walk in the park, I made it to the summit without a problem. It was a dream come true and as magnificent as I had expected.

I'm now doing much more hiking than in the past. Part of the reason is a renewed interest in photography and the need to provide my border collie Barclay with the massive amounts of exercise that he needs.

Once or twice a week, I lift weights even though I hate weight training, so about the only way I can do it is to work with my great trainer, Lisa Sabin. On other days, I do the Stairmaster or stationary bike because I can get a good workout, good sweat, and read at the same time.

Every few months, I download data from the defibrillator by holding a wand next to it. The data is sent through a machine in my home to Minneapolis where the company's server is and then the data gets sent back to my medical center in Seattle. And then they're able to see whether there've been any "incidents."

I have had only a few serious incidents since the implant. I did a strenuous hike into the Goat Rocks Wilderness. It was long and I ran out of beta-blocker medicine. My heart went into arrhythmia and left me very weak. Fortunately, I had a walkie-talkie and called a friend who was back at camp a mile away. He brought me the medicine. I sat for about twenty minutes and then I was back in the game. The two other incidents happened when I was running. My heart had gone over the magic number of 220 beats per minute. The shock from the defibrillator definitely gets your attention. In both cases, immediately after the shock, my heart returned to a more normal pace.

Since that day when my heart stopped, I have been often asked how my near-death experience affected me. Did it change my life? Did it send me on an entirely new trajectory? I wish that I could say that the drama surrounding it exploded into new possibilities. My sister, using her best gallows humor, asked me if I had seen Mom. The fact is I was here one moment and gone the next. No bright lights drawing me to the great beyond. The drama was with the other folks at the scene. It frightened the living daylights out of my three cycling friends. One of my good Samaritans, Bridgette, later told me that she spent the rest of the day worried that her CPR effort had not been successful. In the hospital where she works, she is part of a team and supported by an array of sophisticated equipment. Once she jumped in on the side of the road where I was lying, she was on her own.

As time has passed, I have become more and more aware of how much I appreciate my life, appreciate how fortunate I've been, and am concentrated more fully on using my time productively. I spend more of my time teaching. I've really enjoyed my life. I have been married for forty-four years and have two beautiful grown daughters. I love being active. I recently did a 5K with my younger daughter. She's twenty-seven and decided the day before the race that she'd better start getting in shape, so fortunately she didn't set a blistering pace.

I exercise almost every day, often walking, I love being outdoors. Being out in the middle of the wilderness really enriches your life. I'll do it for as long as I can.

SUDDEN CARDIAC ARREST IN RUNNING AND TRIATHLON—SHOULD YOU BE CONCERNED?

Whenever a runner or triathlete happens to die of heart failure in the middle of a race, the media often pounces on the unfortunate tragedy with a voyeuristic fascination, asking if it was "really worth it." The implication underlying this rhetorical query is that the individual probably should never have participated in the event in the first place. But this viewpoint comes up short in several regards.

(continues)

Exercise *is* healthy. It prolongs life and general well-being. The real question should be how *much* exercise is good for heart health, especially for high-risk individuals. "The well-established risk factors for heart disease," writes long-time *New York Times* health reporter Jane Brody, "remain intact: high cholesterol, high blood pressure, smoking, diabetes, abdominal obesity and sedentary living."

But when exercise enters the picture, matters significantly improve. As proof, Brody cites *The No Bull Book on Heart Disease* by Dr. Joel Okner, a cardiologist in Chicago, and Jeremy Clorfene, a cardiac psychologist. The authors point to a 1996 study that showed only fifteen minutes of exercise five days a week decreased the risk of cardiac death by 46 percent.

So why are people dying in triathlons, marathons, and half-marathons? Aren't these people fit? Nor do these deaths only occur in a race. They can even happen during training.

At the 2009 Detroit Half-Marathon, three male runners died within sixteen minutes of one another. Their ages were twenty-six, thirty-six, and sixty-five. The previous weekend, a twenty-three-year-old male competing in the Baltimore Marathon died.

A study published in the *British Medical Journal* examined twenty-six U.S. marathons between 1975 and 2004. Over this thirty-year period, there were twenty-six sudden cardiac deaths, statistically equivalent to 0.8 fatalities per 100,000 participants. The typical victim was a forty-one-year-old male; 19 percent were women. Five of these deaths occurred in individuals who had previously completed a marathon.

One fact from the study leapt out at me: Most of these deaths took place within one mile of the finish. Which meant that the individual was pushing too hard, far past his or her physical limits. These deaths were preventable.

Actuarially speaking, the risk of sudden cardiac death in a marathon is two deaths per million hours of exercise. (The odds of dying from a bee sting are one in 117,000; from lightning they're one in 79,000.)

Of the twenty-four marathon autopsy reports available in the *British Medical Journal* study, most of the cases were due to atherosclerosis, followed by electrolyte abnormalities (water intoxication coupled with severe salt loss) and heat stroke.

Sudden cardiac arrest is also the primary cause of death in triathlon, and unlike those fatalities in running races, triathlon deaths usually strike during the first few minutes of the swim. In the span of three weeks in 2008, three male triathletes suffered fatal heart attacks during the swim. Their ages were sixty, fifty-two, and thirty-two.

There have been nearly thirty deaths in triathlon since 2004, as recorded by the national governing body USA Triathlon. Close to 80 percent of these fatalities occurred during the swim. The average age was forty-three years.

Medical researchers have no definitive explanation for this phenomenon because in a few cases, autopsies revealed no blocked arteries; instead, they have several theories. "The combination of apparent good health and a negative autopsy suggests a fatality caused by abnormal heart rhythms," Dr. Pamela Douglas, a Duke University cardiologist who has studied triathletes, told the *New York Times*.

Another researcher, Dr. Michael Ackerman, a cardiologist and the director of the Windland Smith Rice Sudden Death Genomics Laboratory at the Mayo Clinic in Rochester, Minnesota, also told the *Times* that "swimming may trigger a certain type of cardiac arrhythmia caused by a genetic condition called long QT syndrome. About one in 2,000 people are born with a heart condition that causes a glitch in the heart's electrical system, and the most common of these is called long QT syndrome, after the telltale interval on an electrocardiogram. The long QT heart recharges itself sluggishly between beats, and that delay sets up the potential for a skipped beat."

That missing beat usually happens when the victim is still close to shore and in the first few minutes. Does the adrenaline rush of racing cause it? Inexperience in open water? An accidental kick to the torso from another swimmer? A wetsuit that fits too snugly and compresses the chest?

Dr. Kevin Harris, of the Minneapolis Heart Institute Foundation, and his colleagues presented a paper at the American College of Cardiology 2009 Scientific Sessions that reported that the risk of sudden death in triathlon was 1.5 out of 100,000 participants, a "not-inconsequential" risk that is nearly double the risk of sudden death in marathon runners.

Harris told the media there was *no* significant difference in the death rates for different triathlon distances. But he added something of particular note: "Maybe what's going on is that you're getting less well-conditioned athletes or more novice athletes, although what's interesting is that we know of only a couple of athletes where this was their first triathlon."

(continues)

By the time a triathlete suffers a heart attack in the mass frenzy of the swim start and drowns, it's often too late to save him or her, even with nearby lifeguards. So it's up to the individual to decide if there are pre-existing risk factors—poor diet, stressful lifestyle, family history of heart disease—that might trigger sudden cardiac arrest in a race. A medical checkup before entering a triathlon (no matter the distance) is recommended, especially if one had previously been inactive for a lengthy period. Electrocardiograms are simple and inexpensive tests that can help diagnose many potentially fatal heart problems. Italy, in fact, requires all participants in a marathon to complete a medical sports fitness test that includes an electrocardiogram.

Sadly, even the fittest people can be struck dead in a race. In 2007, Ryan Shay, twenty-eight, and one of the U.S.'s top long-distance runners, collapsed during the Olympic marathon trials. He had previously run seven marathons. His autopsy reported the cause of death to be cardiac arrhythmia and cardiac hypertrophy—abnormal beating due to an enlarged heart.

ASK THE EXPERT

THE EFFECTS OF "DETRAINING": INTERVIEW WITH DR. MICHAEL JOYNER OF THE MAYO CLINIC

Dr. Michael Joyner, fifty, wears several hats at the world-famous Mayo Clinic in Rochester, Minnesota. He's a clinical anesthesiologist and exercise researcher who studies how the human body adapts to physical and mental stress. When he's not in the lab or operating room, he is one of three senior scientists who administer the entire research program at Mayo Clinic, which has eighteen hundred physicians and scientists. "Our mission at Mayo," he says, "is that the needs of the patient come first through integrated practice of medicine, supported by research and education."

In college, Joyner ran track at the University of Arizona. Before entering medical school, he took part in an exercise physiology study at Washington University in St. Louis that measured the effects of detraining or deconditioning. For twelve weeks, Joyner completely stopped running. The following interview begins with Joyner discussing how even a short layoff impacted a highly conditioned athlete like himself.

Question: What was it like being a guinea pig in the deconditioning study

Michael Joyner: I was in my early twenties; I just finished my senior year in college at the University of Arizona, where I'd run 14:38 for 5,000 meters. I could run 2:25 for the marathon, just over thirty minutes for the 10,000 meters and a sixty-eight-minute half-marathon. I had known Eddie Coyle, who's now an outstanding exercise physiologist at the University of Texas. [See following Ask the Expert interview.] At the time, Eddie was at graduate school at the University of Arizona getting his PhD with a man called Jack Wilmorealbor, who is really one of the godfathers of exercise physiology, and when he finished his PhD he moved to St. Louis to work with Dr. John Holloszy another of the godfathers of exercise physiology. Eddie was looking for subjects to be "detrained." He knew a lot about how sedentary people adapted to training, but he and Dr. Holloszy wanted to pose the question in reverse to see if the rate of change is the same or different with athletes becoming sedentary. This was the first study that really looked at people who had trained for five, six, ten years, who'd really been doing prolonged endurance training. We were tested but we did not go to bed rest; NASA does a lot of studies where they put people at complete bed rest. We just did our normal activities and every so often we were tested regularly throughout the twelve-week study.

The study investigated the following questions: How did heart performance change? How did lung performance change? How did the ability to use fat versus carbohydrate change? How did muscle change—the ability of the muscle to use oxygen? And, did the number of capillaries change in quantity? And what Eddie found—and it was just actually important for me because I started helping in the lab and it was one of the things that really directed me to become a physician scientist—is that people lost about 20 percent of their VO_2 max, which is defined as how much oxygen you can use per minute when your heart rate is at its maximum. My VO_2 max was a little less than 70 and it went down to about 56, so I was still way above average, which is about 45, and this loss was mostly because my heart performance went down. The normal person has about five liters of blood volume, but with training you get extra blood volume that really helps the heart pump better. There are also more red cells floating around to deliver more oxygen and that extra volume facilitates performance of the heart. But the change in terms of the number of blood vessels in the muscle really did not change as much as we had expected, and the thought emerged from the study that

there may be some more permanent changes in the muscle that occur when you've been training for five or ten years. Previous studies had looked at people who only trained for a couple of months and they showed that the adaptations in the muscle went up and down very quickly. So we saw how consistently the muscle retained some of the characteristics of the highly trained person.

Q: After three months of detraining, what was it like to start running again?

MJ: I became tired fast, but it took a month to get back. I was tested later that fall, two months after I started training again. I started running some races and within two or three months, I was pretty much normal, but again, my skeletal muscle had retained many of its adaptations in spite of the detraining. My cardiac performance came back as soon as I started training again and got the blood volume up. I think I'd only gained a couple of pounds.

Q: Say that instead of three months of detraining, it was three years. How do you think your body would have responded?

MJ: If I'd gone to three years, some of those changes in the muscle probably would have gone away and, I think, my VO_2 max probably would have gone down to about 50, but it would always have been above average because when I started running in high school, I ran a 4:27 mile, so I had athletic potential.

Even if I'd taken three years off, I was still young. You really respond to training when you're young.

Q: Is there an optimal recovery period for an injured athlete?

MJ: There's tremendous individual variability in how people deal with injuries. The key thing to any kind of injury situation is, first, try to figure out what's wrong. Secondly, the one thing you don't want to ever do is tell the athlete to go to total rest. You have to find an alternative activity. If you're really committed to alternate conditioning and when you get back to running, you don't want to have the heart and lungs so out of shape that they put other parts of your body at risk. What can happen is you can get roving injuries, by which you injure one thing, and then you injure another thing because you're overcompensating. You risk getting hurt because you have an imbalance—one part of the body is stronger than the other. The important thing when a runner gets injured or a cyclist is injured or a swimmer is injured is to keep that base conditioning as much as you can by doing an alternate activity and then hopefully as you begin to feel better, phase back in your normal training. Again, this is common sense; this is what the coaches and athletic trainers have seen for years. So this is not rocket science; this is about routine daily physical activity. Don't go hog wild everyday. Use a hard-and-easy

approach. The point is, when you come back to running after an injury, to not start at zero. Do not start like you've been at bed rest, and you'll be able to recondition yourself relatively quickly.

If you look at the history of training, before World War II, athletes had really long off-seasons where they didn't do much and there was a lot of concern about staleness. Then, right before World War II but certainly after the war, people started training really hard and by the fifties, people were training a hundred miles a week in running. I don't know what they were doing in cycling, but I think they were spending a lot of time in the saddle. Swimming is a little different because they had to develop the goggles and get the pools in better shape, but anyway people were training as hard as possible and people really did become overtrained. The consensus now is that people need to base their training on some sort of hard-and-easy cycle. So do a hard day, do an easy day; do a hard week, do an easy week; do a hard month, do an easy month, but you never go to complete zero or complete rest. For multisport athletes, they're able to do the biking or running and then use the swimming to help the legs recover so they can balance things out by their various activities. The late great running coach Bill Bowerman's first rule of running was that it's better to be undertrained than overtrained because if you're undertrained, you have something in reserve; if you're overtrained, you're just spent. Some people train themselves into something similar to chronic fatigue syndrome—and it does take a while to recover from.

Q: Why does running have such a high incidence of injury? This creates a high attrition rate and runners leave the sport altogether. Is running fundamentally healthy?

MJ: One of the reasons that there are injuries is because obviously there's some pounding associated with it, whereas cycling and swimming are much more forgiving, where you don't have those foot strikes. It's also because people overtrain; they don't get into the hard-and-easy cycle. They really become a slave to their watch, a slave to their heart-rate monitors, a slave to their training diaries, and they're not able to manage their suffering. You have to learn to manage your suffering over time and dole it out, knowing when to go easy, when to take a day off, and when to do active rest, where you don't go out and run fifteen miles. In fact, I've been emailing a gal who's getting ready to run a hundred-mile race and she's tapering, but she wrote, "I should do ninety minutes of studio cycling a week before the race." My comment was: "Why?" A lot of endurance athletes are high achievers who believe that the amount that they put into something plays a key role with their return on investment of

their time and that's certainly true, but once people start training more than an hour or two a day, the return is really marginal, if it's there at all.

Q: Let's look at someone who was an athlete in college, but then got preoccupied with work and raising a family, and before you know it, he's forty-five years old and hasn't really worked out since his college days.

MJ: When you look at someone like that, they look an awful lot like their peers who've been sedentary up to that period in time. The question becomes, have they gotten fat, has there been some hidden physical activity? Maybe they take the stairs, but in general, those people would be more like starting at ground zero, except those individuals have a history and understand the process of training. So they understand what it takes to get in shape even though it was a long time ago, about what it's like to have your lungs burn and your legs hurt and so forth. But considering the case of a person starting out again, the first thing to do is look at any possible risk factors: Did the person start smoking? Did he develop hypertension? Does he have diabetes or pre-diabetes? Does he have high cholesterol? And does he need any kind of medical screening before he jumps right into exercise? The main thing is to recognize two things that happen: One is you've been detrained; and, two, you've gotten older, so you just need to slowly get yourself back into it. But again, the key to all of this is hard-and-easy training to avoid injury and be consistent. For example, I travel a lot now and I do competitive stuff with my swimming. Occasionally I miss a day, but I try never to miss more than two days in a row of swimming. I swim for an hour and then on the days I don't swim hard for an hour, I swim for maybe twenty minutes.

Q: Do you do any other physical activities?

MJ: I've been cycling or using the Stairmaster, but I have kind of a low-grade back and hamstring injury that needs to be resolved. In the summer, Rochester is a small city and a terrific place to ride your bike around when the snow melts. I live a mile from work so I ride my bike to work.

Q: What about your competitive running?

MJ: I've pretty much backed off of it, although I'm having these precognitive thoughts about doing some more. I'm a pretty good swimmer. I've been physically active. I gained a lot of weight from swimming. I put on a lot of muscle mass. I went from a 42 coat to a 48 coat! I'm six-five. I was probably too big to be a runner in the first place. I should have been a rower or a swimmer to begin with. I was like 170, 175 when I was running well, and now I am 205.

Q: How do you feel, athletically speaking, compared to your early twenties?

MJ: I would say that I'm probably much stronger than I was, because I was only doing distance running, and I had little upper-body strength. I probably only lost about 6 to 8 percent of my VO_2 max from my peak. People lose about 10 percent per decade. It's known that if people continue to train hard and keep their intensity up, they can reduce the VO_2 max rate of decline by about half, although if you look at cross-sectional studies of athletes over long periods of time, you find that they get hurt, they lose interest, they stop competing at the highest level.

Q: I have this buddy who is forty-five years old and a competitive triathlete. He had a weight problem before he did triathlons and running, but after he got sick with bronchitis, he gained fifteen pounds in one month. He says he's eating the same; is it fluid accumulation? Does the body's metabolism slow down with no exercise? What does the body do after two, three, four days versus seven days or a month?

MJ: What people need to realize is your body weight is calories in, calories out. That's 90 percent of it. There are some nuances, like changes in your basal metabolic rate, whether people fidget more or less, and changes in muscle mass. If you eat 3,500 calories more than you expend, in general, you're going to gain about a pound. Now again, that equation isn't perfect and some people are a little more resistant to weight gain than others, but the people that are resistant to weight gain start sleeping less, they start fidgeting more, so there are reasons they are resistant to weight gain.

Q: Fidgeting really creates weight loss? I heard about that.

MJ: In fact, my colleague, Dr. Jim Levine, at Mayo, did those studies along with Dr. Mike Jensen and they overfed people by about 1,000 calories a day. The individuals that had the weight gain were the people who fidgeted less.

Q: Fidgeting—is that different from Restless Leg Syndrome?

MJ: Restless Leg Syndrome's a medical condition, but fidgeting is very subtle, too. For example, let's say you're a secretary and the mailbox in your office is a hundred feet from where your desk is. Well, some people will wait to get a stack of things, and then go stick them in the outbox. People that stay lean are more likely that every time they complete a single task, they will go stick that one item in the outbox and come back. And over time, that little bit, those hundred feet here, hundred feet there, it adds up. Here's another example. Jim Levine measured the effect of the television remote control, and he thinks it's costing people ten or fifteen or twenty calories a day. If you look at how people get fat, people get fat ten calories a day just by using the remote control.

Q: Now ten calories a day, what does that compute to in five years?

MJ: It's five pounds in five years. The average person gains twenty to forty pounds between the ages of twenty and forty. So that's only a ten or

twenty calories per day mismatch. One of the reasons people are leaner in Manhattan than they are out in the suburbs is just the little extra walking that they do. And if you look at people who live in less mechanized cultures like the Amish who eat tremendous amounts of food, they aren't fat because they're doing manual labor all day. There's actually good data from around the early part of the twentieth century about what people were eating when working on non-mechanized farms. They were eating 4,000 or 5,000 calories a day but they were physically active all day long.

Q: Weight loss is a huge industry. Actually, it's a *growth* industry; 30 percent of Americans are obese. A lot of people only consider one aspect of weight loss. They diet, but they don't do exercise. Don't they go hand-in-hand?

MJ: There's a couple of things going on. One is you're going to get some health benefits from exercise, whether you lose weight or not. The interior lining of the blood vessels are going to get healthier, you're going to be much less likely to develop diabetes or if you do have mild diabetes, it's likely to get better. Your blood pressure is likely to be better. The other thing that people need to realize is that lean muscle mass burns more calories than fat does. And so by exercising, you tend to promote lean muscle mass, as opposed to loss of muscle mass. So when people lose weight, not only do they lose fat, they lose muscle mass; but when people lose weight with diet *and* exercise, studies tend to suggest that they retain a little bit more muscle mass. As the guidelines have emerged about physical activity, one of the reasons strength training has emerged as desirable is so that people do, in fact, keep their muscle mass up as protection against weight gain when they are not dieting. Strength training also has an anti-aging effect, which is an important element.

Q: It seems that people who do these diet programs like Jenny Craig or Weight Watchers tend to gain their weight back.

MJ: What the data show is no matter what diet plan people are on, there tends to be weight gain.

Q: Is that a result of psychological reasons or lifestyle choice?

MJ: What happens is that people enter into a program and there's an accountability element to it. But what's going to happen when the program is over? So I think what you have to do is have better programs that have some sort of maintenance element to them. People who are successful weight losers weigh themselves regularly, and as soon as their weight starts to drift back up several pounds, they do a little mini–weight loss program to get back on track. And a very high fraction of these people get one hour of physical activity per day. I think the other thing about big people is that many of them are afraid to come to the gym. We opened

a new Healthy Living Center at Mayo Clinic for employees to make sure that people had the opportunity to exercise, and we've really done everything we can to make it friendly for overweight people because we want those people being physically active whether they lose weight or not. We have a dress code so people aren't wearing tank tops in there and women aren't running with sports bras on. We don't want the hard bodies intimidating people that are a little bit leery of going into the gym. So when those individuals do show up, it's a relatively nurturing environment and you get a lot of positive feedback from the regulars who see somebody making progress toward their goals.

Q: I've read that the average person, just to stay healthy or keep the heart going a little bit better, should work out three times a week, twenty minutes each time. Is that a good benchmark?

MJ: That's a minimum. What's emerging now is about 150 minutes a week of moderate physical activity, either in smaller bites or five thirty-minute walking periods. It's really what's required to stave off type 2 diabetes. The studies show if you can get people walking thirty minutes a day at a brisk pace, five days a week, you reduce their chances of getting diabetes by about two-thirds.

Q: That's a high percentage.

MJ: If you take people who are prediabetic, it's much better than drugs.

Q: Those who are addicted to exercise get stressed-out if they don't work out every day. Or they miss a few days, which adds to the stress.

MJ: And then the mountain above you gets higher and higher. What people have to recognize is reality and not beat themselves up. I mean, most of us aren't going to the Olympics and most of us should be exercising for our health, to get some recreation, to spend time with people, family, and friends. To set goals. But once it gets too much into our achievement cycle, and once it activates "if some is good, more is better," you run the risk of getting into this internal dialogue: "I work out, so therefore I'm a good person; I didn't work out today, so I'm a slob." People really need to get out of that. It's one of the great problems of life. We're bombarded with stuff like "should be doing" versus giving ourselves some slack. What I would urge people to do is simultaneously be tough on themselves and set goals and do their best, but on the other hand, recognize we're all human. I'm always looking for quotes and I saw this one recently by the explorer Thor Hyerdahl. It's about setting boundaries. He said, "I've never seen any, but I hear they exist in most people's minds." So I think this is about getting past your boundaries, getting out of your comfort zone, pushing yourself a little bit,

but also having some compassion for yourself. That's really the trick in all this.

Q: So when I beat myself up thinking about the last decade when I didn't work out, I really do myself a disservice.

MJ: What can you do about it? You can't do a damn thing about it. You can't un-ring the bell. I was reading something in the *New York Times* about Crestone, Colorado, where all these unreconstructed hippies, Buddhist and Catholic monks, and Hindus live. And evidently, there's a guy who's a Zen Buddhist firefighter and he was asked, "What's the secret? What do you try to do with the fires?" And he said, "I try to greet the fire." That's what you have to do: You just have to greet it where you are in life.

Q: So you're telling former athletes wanting to get back in shape that they can't dwell on the past, that they just have to greet the present.

MJ: Greet the present and remind yourself, "I have some experience; I know how to get into shape. What I need to do is reactivate that skill-set I once had versus beating myself up for not doing it for ten years." But the larger question is: Are your workouts going to control you, or are you going to control the workouts? I became a much better runner after I decided to go to medical school because I had something else to focus on besides running.

⑤

MENTAL INJURY

Fighting Depression with Exercise

I have always had a shitty relationship with stress. Stress overwhelms my emotions, clouds my judgment, forces a retreat from the world, undermines the old self-confidence, and saps energy. I even get stressed-out reading magazine articles about how to reduce stress.

Stress was a major factor why I stopped working out for a decade. Stress also rode shotgun when I started working out again; I was perpetually concerned about failure.

To keep the S monster under control, I knew that by running, I'd have a way to eliminate stress, blow off steam, and not sink into a stupor or funk. Then why had I capitulated to stress and let it take dominion over my life during all those years of self-imposed inactivity and idleness? One answer: There was more than stress involved. Stress was only the forward scout for depression. By the time full-blown depression arrived, I was in its complete thrall.

Many don't always know when the big D looms overhead like a toxic cloud; I didn't recognize its harmful severity at first. One might exhibit several of its telltale symptoms, but doesn't necessarily connect all the dots. Denial makes one unwilling to confront the unvarnished truth about the affliction. "There is a terrible collusion in our society, a cultural cover-up about depression in men," writes Terrence Real, author of *I Don't Want to Talk about It* and family therapist in Massachusetts. "And part of the cultural influence involves the way men are taught from early childhood to be strong, silent, independent, and resistant to suffering." This cover-up is worse for men than women, who are three times more likely to seek outside counseling.

Denial exacerbates the underlying conditions of mental distress. Left untreated, depression is like any serious illness with life-threatening consequences. According to the Mayo Clinic, symptoms of depression include:

- Loss of interest in normal daily activities
- Feeling sad or down
- Feeling hopeless
- Crying spells for no apparent reason
- Problems sleeping
- Trouble focusing or concentrating
- Difficulty making decisions
- Unintentional weight gain or loss
- Irritability
- Restlessness
- Being easily annoyed
- Feeling fatigued or weak
- Feeling worthless
- Loss of interest in sex
- Thoughts of suicide or suicidal behavior
- Unexplained physical problems, such as back pain or headaches

Judging by this checklist, I qualified as your typical sad sack with 80 percent of these depressive symptoms. So what constructive actions did I take? Did I seek professional help? Gobble down antidepressants? Or even check myself into a psychiatric ward?

Stubbornness and pride kept me from seriously considering temporary hospitalization. Maybe because I envisioned the likely scenario of being in the company of zombified, pajama-clad patients playing checkers and chess with their therapists. It'd be like visiting another world without guaranteed reentry into the world you already know.

While depression can strip away your natural defenses, it also reinforces your inhibitions. The malady fears change. It craves stasis. That's why depressives like to sleep in. As we bury problems and ourselves beneath the blankets, the threatening, unpredictable outside world is kept at a safe remove. Paradoxically, we believe that no harm will occur even though we wish to harm ourselves. We're just too frightened to carry this sentiment to its logical conclusion. Death is the ultimate, self-indulgent escape, and so we brood and obsess and plot nefarious ways to achieve our very own extinction.

Acclaimed essayist Daphne Merkin wrote about her own lifelong battle with depression in the *New York Times* Sunday magazine, describing her mental burden as one that "creates a planet all its own, largely impermeable to influence from others." She called it a "thick black paste, the muck of bleakness," which isolates sufferers in their "own pitch-darkness." The worst part is that "depression, truth be told, is both boring and threatening as a subject of conversation. In the end there is no one to intervene on your behalf when you disappear again into what feels like a psychological dungeon—a place that has a familiar musky smell, a familiar lack of light and excess of enclosure—except the people you've paid large sums of money to talk to over the years."

I first began obsessing about suicide in my early twenties. A breakup with a girlfriend was one cause for a while. Periodically, I'd feel that life was meaningless, half-heartedly finding solace in Nietzsche's aphorism, "The thought of suicide is a great consolation: by means of it one gets successfully through many a bad night." Inexplicably, after I sold *Tri-Athlete* magazine at age twenty-nine, I contemplated death by my own hand. Instead of feeling positive that I had started and then sold a successful triathlon magazine, I became morose, empty, exhausted, and exhibited little interest in launching future projects. I stayed in bed a lot, reading novels and magazines, sleeping up to seventeen hours a day. I'd wake up in the morning, have a Bartles & Jaymes wine cooler and buttered toast for breakfast, then go back to bed. For lunch, I'd make myself an egg-salad sandwich, then take a nap. Sometimes, I'd go for a short run with Rockee around dusk. After dinner, I headed straight to bed.

This period of wallowing and listlessness lasted about three months. Its spell was broken when I decided to create a national literary magazine. With that impetus, my energy returned in full blazing force. The first issue came out in four months. Like a manic-depressive, I needed to completely throw myself into a new enterprise in order to experience self-validation. Why was my ego such a fragile little bird?

Other girlfriends later entered the picture, and when those relationships faltered, the suicidal tendencies would resurface, a function of low self-esteem and uncertain confrontation with serial failure. For six months, in my mid-thirties, I did see a shrink; in fact, he was one of the more famous psychiatrists in the Bay Area, having authored a bestseller about his profession. I actually had to audition to become his patient. When I passed the interview test, I wasn't sure if that was a good or bad thing. At the end of that first meeting, he said, "My job will be to provide you with a toolkit to deal with what's troubling you."

During our once-a-week sessions, I often visualized him wearing a carpenter's belt, with hammer, pliers, and a screwdriver dangling from leather hoops. I spent most of our time together trying to be charming and entertaining. I felt like a talk show guest with an audience of one. He'd never laugh at my stories, just a half-smile would crease his face, and then he'd ask, "How does that make you feel?" When he did ask me a direct question, it usually concerned my sex life, which was in working order and was *not* why I was seeing him.

The primary reason I sought his professional help was to quell a mounting fixation with suicide. Every time I'd cross the Golden Gate Bridge on my bike, I would have to ride as far away as possible from the railing because I feared that one day I would impulsively hop off my bike and throw myself into the San Francisco Bay three hundred feet below. The final leap would happen just like that, without warning or fanfare—a sudden, inexplicable act whose script had long been contemplated.

I wanted the good doc's approval and friendship, though he was distant, inscrutable, withholding. His professional mask never lowered. I paid him $170 per "hour" for those fifty minutes, so our relationship was artificially constructed and monetarily defined. How could we be on the same footing?

One positive benefit of this therapeutic hour in his book-lined Palo Alto study was that it provided a quiet bracketed window for personal reflection before and after each session. Yet I stopped seeing him because I had just launched a new multisport magazine and time was scarce. I called him up one afternoon to say that I needed to reschedule our next appointment. But I never called back. Nor did he ever call me. That was how things ended between us, almost like a lovers' breakup, when both partners walk away and nothing more is ever said again. There was no closure or final words. Oddly, we never once discussed my suicidal obsession in any of our sessions.

Throughout this period, I kept in terrific physical shape—biking and running ten hours every week. My faithful running partner Rockee was alive. My father had yet to show any signs of Alzheimer's. But when the next major bout of chronic depression crept into my life, I was in my early forties. Rockee was no longer around and my father was rapidly losing his grip on reality. I was too depressed to work out. Of course, there would be short reprieves when my mood and energy would lift for several weeks or months, but the depression would invariably return, clamping down all desire for exercise.

I persisted in thinking that I could beat depression on my own terms. Seeing another therapist seemed like a waste of money. Nor did I want to retell my personal story to a stranger, and then be judged in his or her eyes. As for mood-altering drugs, I feared the unpleasant side effects of popular antidepressants like Prozac, which can cause dry mouth, constipation, urinary retention, sedation, weight gain, insomnia, and nausea; or Zoloft, which can cause abdominal pain, agitation, anxiety, constipation, decreased sex drive, diarrhea or loose stools, difficulty with ejaculation, dizziness, dry mouth, fatigue, gas, headache, decreased appetite, increased sweating, indigestion, insomnia, nausea, nervousness, pain, rash, sleepiness, sore throat, tingling or pins and needles, tremor, and vision problems.

A somewhat similar litany of side effects is associated with most antidepressants that are actually a class of drugs called selective serotonin reuptake inhibitors (SSRIs). Serotonin is a neurotransmitter, a chemical that carries messages between nerve cells, and is believed to influence emotions. In normal circumstances, serotonin is quickly reabsorbed after its release at the junctures between nerves. Re-uptake inhibitors slow down this process, thereby boosting the levels of serotonin available in the brain. At least, that is what the medical science wants you to believe.

If I had messed-up brain chemistry, then depression wasn't my fault; the cause was organic. This left me off the hook. From my own limited layperson's perspective, a reliance on meds just seemed too voodoo. Daphne Merkin, for example, had taken antidepressants and antianxiety medications almost her entire life, including Lamictal, Risperdal, Wellbutrin, and Lexapro, but acknowledged that "none of the drugs work conclusively, and for now we are stuck with what comes down to a refined form of guesswork—30-odd pills that operate in not completely understood ways on neural pathways, on serotonin, norepinephrine, dopamine and what have you. No one, not even the psychopharmacologists who dispense them after considering the odds, totally comprehends why they work when they work or why they don't when they don't."

Meds have been shown to work treating the more extreme cases, such as schizophrenics, and for these mental-illness sufferers, pills are often their only way of to getting through the day. And a relapse of the illness, which can occur when a patient stops taking medication, doesn't mean the drugs don't work—it actually means they *do* work, though perhaps not in the most predetermined way.

Insomnia marked the worst part of my depression, and led to an addiction to sleep aids like Tylenol PM, then Advil whose toxicity—I was taking thirty or forty pills every day—royally screwed up my liver and metabolism, and was the precipitating cause, as I have mentioned earlier, of both the edema and dermatitis. When the dual skin and tissue affliction became so bad that I could barely get out of bed or walk more than a few yards, I'd lie in bed, darkly fantasizing about going off into the nearby woods one night, taking only my blue L.L. Bean down comforter, Hefty garbage bag, and roll of duct tape. I'd find a secluded place off the trail, lie down, get warm and cozy inside the comforter, and slip the plastic bag over my head, tape it shut, and wait until hypoxia, then asphyxiation claimed my last breath. Hikers or search-and-rescue wouldn't find my body for months.

I might have killed myself this way—the Hemlock Society recommends that terminally ill patients use a similar "exit bag"—had it not been for my inability to walk very far. The hike into the woods was about a half-mile, much longer than I could manage with swollen, inflamed legs. My life was thus spared by a savage irony: The mental and physical illness making me want to extinguish my life also prevented me from carrying out the very act of self-destruction.

I withdrew from friends and from a formerly active social life. I never told my closest friends what was really going on in my head. "Oh yeah, last night, I kept having these disturbing visions of my skeleton being pawed over by cadaver dogs in the woods."

Writing books was, at best, a temporary distraction from depression. Forced to work only from home, I had limited interaction with interview subjects and spent most of 2005 writing an oral history on political dissent in post-9/11 America. The phone was an invaluable lifeline as I tracked down candidates for the book. Nobel Prize–winning economist Paul Krugman of the *New York Times* or Pentagon Papers whistleblower and political activist Daniel Ellsberg, to name two interviews, had no idea that the guy on the other end of the telephone could barely sit up and was in constant discomfort.

Stress from working on a subsequent book—an edited collection of Al Gore speeches and interviews—triggered a relapse of dermatitis. This was getting old and tedious. I needed to break free of this cycle and find a new, healthier lifestyle—one that revolved around exercise. From past experience,

I knew that running would make me feel better. But I wasn't there yet with my health to start working out. So, step one was simple: I stopped taking NSAIDs, which I'd been gobbling down like they were jelly beans, and improved my diet. Within several months, my legs healed and it was now possible to go for half-hour walks several times a week. Just this simple act of regular physical activity lifted my spirits. I was finally on the road to recovery.

EXERCISE AND STRESS—WELCOME TO THE RAT RACE

Research scientists love tormenting lab rats. The furry little rodents are starved, shocked, bullied, and even water-boarded. Their torture is encouraged under the rational aegis of science—to find out how stress affects the brain. Because rats provide a fairly reliable indicator of human behavior, scientists use them to examine how stress affects overall health, including blood pressure, immune system, and depression.

In 2009, scientists at the University of Minho in Portugal discovered that chronically stressed rats acted rather un-ratlike. They'd continually press a bar for food pellets even when they had no intention of eating. The rats were stuck in a habit-forming groove of futile, non-productive behavior. It's as if their stressed brains were unable to make intelligent decisions such as, "Hey, no food, so why don't I do something else with my time?"

Speaking with the *New York Times*, Robert Sapolsky, a neurobiologist at Stanford University School of Medicine, called the Portuguese study "a great model for understanding why we end up in a rut, and then dig ourselves deeper and deeper into that rut. We're lousy at recognizing when our normal coping mechanisms aren't working. Our response is usually to do it five times more, instead of thinking, maybe it's time to try something new."

Stress had an important evolutionary role in keeping our ancestors alive. Survival in the forest or on the savanna demanded quick action when danger lurked. Stress hormones like cortisol and adrenaline would suddenly flood into the bloodstream, causing the heart to beat faster, which increased blood flow to the muscles. But after the danger passed, the "flight or fight" hormones would settle down and the body would return to its normal physiological state.

But in today's modern world, stress receptors often get stuck open in a locked position. Since the body can't function all the time like this, stress hormone production is ultimately affected. Natural defense mechanisms

(continues)

weaken. The overloaded brain shuts down critical areas such as the hip-pocampus and prefrontal cortex, which affect learning, memory, and rational thought. A stressed-out person will end up engaging in harmful, counter-productive behavior, like having three beers after work, or eating junk food when not hungry.

Given identical stressful conditions, such as losing a job or breaking up, some people are better able to cope, while others will emotionally fall apart—and remain depressed for a long time. In a 2009 *Newsweek* cover story titled, "Who Says Stress Is Bad For You?," science reporter Mary Carmichael cited several studies that pointed to genetic differences in de-termining the individual outcome to stressful situations. But which specific genes are responsible? No one knows. "The science is still young," she writes.

Yet there's good news for the stressed-out population. The Portuguese scientists found that stress-caused behavior is indeed reversible. Once re-moved from a stressful environment, the rats resumed acting like normal rats. No more pressing the food bar when there wasn't any food. Their brain circuitry had somehow rewired itself.

"The brain can grow new cells and reshape itself," says Carmichael. Fur-thermore, "meditation appears to encourage this process. Monks who have trained for years in meditation have greater brain activity in regions linked to learning and happiness." The monks grew new brain cells.

Carmichael brought up another classic rat study:

Something that should lower stress can actually cause stress if it's done in the wrong spirit. Scientists put two rats in a cage, each of them locked inside a running wheel. The first rat could exercise whenever it liked. The second rat was forced to run whenever its counterpart did. Exer-cise, like meditation, usually tamps down stress and encourages neuron growth. The second rat, however, lost brain cells. It was doing something that should have been good for its brain, but it lacked one crucial factor: control. It could not determine its own 'workout' schedule, so it didn't perceive it as exercise. Instead, it experienced it as a literal rat race.

So even too much of a good thing like exercise can turn harmful if it's controlling you rather than vice versa. It's a primary reason why many athletes get injured or sick if they train or race too hard and don't take time off. The stress switch can't indefinitely remain open.

CAN EXERCISE HELP FIGHT DEPRESSION?

Build a sweat and you increase your sense of well-being. It's why we run or ride. "It's a very clear matter," says James Watson, president of Cold Springs Harbor Laboratory, co-discoverer of DNA, and quoted in *The Noonday Demon: An Atlas of Depression,* by Andrew Solomon. "Exercise produces endorphins. Endorphins are endogenous morphines and they make you feel great if you're feeling normal. They make you feel better if you're feeling awful. You have to get those endorphins up and running—after all, they're upstream of the neurotransmitters too, and so exercise is going to work to raise your neurotransmitters."

Ah yes, endorphins. We hear and use that term quite a bit to describe that post-workout euphoric rush of happy, pleasant feelings. Many label this experience the "runner's high" (sorry, cyclists). Yet endorphins' role in affecting brain chemistry is still not wholly understood despite years of scientific research. Endorphins transmit signals to the brain and help alleviate pain or make you feel pleasure. Eating chocolate does this by releasing endorphins. So do sex and drugs. But how do you measure endorphins? Can they be quantified?

In her book *Ultimate Fitness, New York Times* health and science writer Gina Kolata spoke with several neurologists and researchers looking for clues to endorphins' relationship with exercise and well-being. Surprisingly, she was unable to locate a consensus in her attempt to pry folklore from hard science. There is a kind of Holy Grail aspect to identifying endorphins.

Research first studied opiate receptors in the brain because they thought that certain drugs were mirroring a "naturally occurring brain chemical." Solomon Snyder, a neurobiologist at John Hopkins University School of Medicine, and his colleagues were at the forefront of this field in the late 1970s. "All of a sudden, opiate receptors became a popular area," Snyder says. "The chemicals were so new that they that had not even been named." So a committee was formed, and voilà—the endorphin was born. While some researchers examined endorphin levels in the blood, noting their rise or fall during exercise, Snyder believed that this was an insignificant line of inquiry. "Endorphins in the blood are irrelevant," he told Kolata. "Your brain has so many neurotransmitters that influence so many different states."

Huda Akil, an endorphin researcher at the University of Michigan, agreed with this assessment, telling Kolata, "What people do is they conflate the change in endorphins in the blood with what might be happening in the brain."

One way to measure if these endorphins do make it to the brain is by getting a spinal tap—a painful procedure that would need to take place while the subject is exercising. Bottom line, for Akil, is that the endorphin runner's high is pure speculation, "a total fantasy in the pop culture. While exercise may elicit euphoria in some people some of the time, I think it's really simplistic to make one hormone the heart of it all. I would think it is a cocktail of goodies and that it is probably a delicate mix."

"On its own, exercise does appear to have significant effects in terms of elevating mood," Dr. Andrew Leuchter, professor of psychiatry at the UCLA Semel Institute for Neuroscience and Human Behavior, told the *Los Angeles Times*. "Physical activity," he adds, "is often used to augment treatments such as medication and cognitive behavioral therapy. If people are on medication or in treatment and haven't had a complete recovery from depression, exercise is useful in getting them all the way there."

If you like working out but are predisposed to depression, you might often find yourself on that teeter-totter of experiencing athletic highs and non-athletic lows. This does seem a bit of a paradox, and it reflects how little scientists know about the inner workings of the human brain. Most of the studies investigating the links between depression and exercise have been conducted on animals. "We don't entirely understand exactly why patients get depressed in the first place," says Leuchter. "We have theories, but it's hard to know in individual cases. And we don't have a good way of looking at [changes] in the brain. Scientists do know that exercise causes an increase in blood flow to the brain and raises the amount of energy the brain uses. And even though the link between blood flow and mood isn't known, the brain in general seems to be in a healthier state."

Depression, sadly, remains a taboo subject in locker rooms and among training buddies. We are told to keep our negative feelings to ourselves even if they contribute to a cascading effect of stress, declining performance, and low energy. Athletes feel awkward discussing their inner emotions. It's almost an unwritten rule to keep mute on this topic. A tight-lipped stoicism is required, if not admired in sports. That overused adage, "no pain, no gain," ignores its hidden counterpart: the private mental pain an athlete shields from others that has nothing whatsoever to do with anaerobic threshold and lactic-acid buildup.

In an article published in *Current Psychiatry Online*, Dr. Antonia L. Baum, of the Department of Psychiatry at George Washington University Medical Center, Washington, D.C., notes: "Some athletes' toughest opponents are depression, addictions, and eating disorders. Psychiatric illness in an amateur or professional athlete may arise from coincidence, a predisposing pathology that first attracted the athlete to the arena, or a psychopathology caused by the sport itself. Stressors unique to athletes that may cause, trigger, or worsen psychopathology include pressure to win and constant risk of injury."

Athletes resist seeking outside psychological counseling. Unlike a physical ailment such as back pain or aching knee that can be professionally treated and mended through rehab or surgery, depression remains an invisible affliction. There's a stigma attached to being labeled "depressed." Conventional wisdom says to "get over it." What's even more overlooked is that one can be experiencing symptoms of depression—irregular sleep patterns, changes in appetite, erratic energy levels—without even realizing the underlying root causes. "Illness of the mind is real illness," says Andrew Solomon. "It can have severe effects on the body."

Conversely, a healthy and active body, freed from a dependency on meds, can undo the downward spiral of lethargy and hopelessness associated with depression. A 1999 Duke University study found that exercise and the anti-depressant Zoloft relieved depression almost equally—with added self-esteem benefits for the exercisers. James Blumenthal, the psychology professor who conducted the study, explained the findings to Kolata. "We found that fifty minutes of exercise a week was associated with a 50 percent drop in the risk of being depressed. People who exercised more had a greater reduction in symptoms, but we don't know if they were feeling better and therefore they did more, or if they did more and therefore felt better."

Dr. Richard Friedman, a psychopharmacologist at Cornell Medical School, likes to prescribe his depressive patients a mix of medications and exercise. "Patients have little to lose," he told Kolata. "It's never made anyone worse. Most interventions, most medicines, have lots of side effects, but I have never seen a case—ever—where a patient complains that they are more anxious after they exercised. Nearly everyone who does it feels better, and no one says anything bad about it."

"One of the first things a clinician should do is get depressed patients on an exercise program," says Robert Thayer, PhD, a California State at Long Beach psychology professor and author of *The Origin of Everyday Mood*. He cites several positive effects: "Exercise gives you energy, whereas depression saps your energy. When energy levels are high, negative thoughts, sadness, and low self-esteem—all components of depression—decrease. Exercise increases metabolism, heart rate, breathing and decreases muscle tension. The result is a handy sense of calm, well-being, and eventually a zoned-out bliss. And, exercise provides a greater sense of efficacy—you can't change your boss, but you can control something in your life."

"YES, IT WAS ALL IN MY HEAD"

It'd be misleading to conclude this chapter with a rosy prognosis that says you won't ever experience family, financial, or job-related stress—all of which can lead to depression and then an avoidance of exercise, which only perpetuates the feeling-blue cycle of inactivity and sadness. Because chronic depression eludes a complete cure—it's not like mending a broken bone—sufferers may require counseling, support from friends and family, and of course, exercise to limit its paralyzing power.

I realized that you don't completely conquer depression, so much as refuse to let it vanquish you. Fight back. And the most optimal way, I became convinced, was by working out. No pills, no expensive talk therapy, no locked hospital ward. Exercise was my panacea.

I revisited the Mayo Clinic website to find out what it had to say about exercise and depression. While it acknowledged that "the links between anxiety, depression and exercise aren't entirely clear, research on anxiety, depression and exercise shows that the psychological and physical benefits of exercise can also help reduce anxiety and improve mood." And how is this done? The three primary ways are triggering the release of feel-good brain chemicals (neurotransmitters and endorphins); reducing immune system chemicals that can contribute to depression; and increasing body temperature, which may have calming effects.

The Mayo Clinic site also provided a number of helpful recommendations for those fighting depression through exercise. These guidelines included the following:

- *Set reasonable goals.* Focus your workout plan to your own needs and abilities rather than "trying to meet unrealistic guidelines that you're unlikely to meet."
- *Avoid thinking of exercise as a chore.* "If exercise is just another 'should' in your life that you don't think you're living up to, you'll associate it with failure. Rather, look at your exercise schedule the same way you look at your therapy sessions or medication—as one of the tools to help you get better."

- *Prepare for setbacks and obstacles.* "Give yourself credit for every step in the right direction, no matter how small. If you skip exercise one day, that doesn't mean you can't maintain an exercise routine and may as well quit. Just try again the next day."

There was no denying the fact that my new regimen of psyche-cleansing workouts had chased away the black dog of depression. Despite some bad mornings when I just wanted to sleep in and not confront the day's challenges and responsibilities, I realized that I could now compartmentalize this malaise and move right past it. I attributed this new outlook to being active. Let me restate this in another way: I never felt crummy *after* running. Even a short thirty-minute jog caused the demons to flee. My mood would brighten. This run-induced altered state was a direct consequence of endorphins doing their magical tap dance inside my brain. If I were mopey *and* didn't run that day, I knew that I would feel even worse later on. Thus it was imperative not to slip into a rut and neglect regular exercise, since that harmful route could easily become a catalyst for a long-term depressive withdrawal—and, in turn, would make it all the more psychologically difficult to continue working out. It's as if the mind has essentially two gears—forward and reverse. It was entirely up to me to remain in forward.

Yet running was only going to take me so far with a genuine fitness come-back. Something else was at play, and unless I managed to directly confront it, I would still feel like a creaky, washed-up failure. I still wasn't biking. A mental barricade blocked all desire; I kept resisting, making excuses, inventing lame reasons. What was I waiting for? Running had significantly strengthened my aerobic conditioning. Cycling would further complement and improve these fitness gains. Was I neurotically afraid that I might *not* like cycling after being away from it for so long?

The only way to overcome this self-induced anxiety was to make that two-wheel leap of faith and rejoin the sport I had abandoned. But when exactly would this transformative moment occur?

DO ANTIDEPRESSANTS REALLY WORK?

An estimated 27 million Americans take antidepressant drugs. Fifteen years ago, that figure was 13 million. Mood-tweaking drugs are big business for pharmaceutical giants with over $10 billion in annual sales. Approximately

(continues)

80 percent of all antidepressant medications are prescribed by doctors untrained in the field of psychiatry, including internists and family practitioners.

Do these numbers suggest that we are more stressed-out and anxious or that time-crunched doctors are simply more inclined to write prescriptions?

The causes of depression are complex and often unknown. Researchers point to genetic, biological, and environmental factors. Medications function by altering chemical imbalances in the brain that are thought to occur in depression. The effectiveness of antidepressants varies with individuals, and it can take up to several weeks before noticeable changes are evident.

"Only about 80 percent of depressed individuals are actually responsive to medication, with about 50 percent responsive to their first, or subsequent medication," says John Greden, director of the Mental Health Research Institute at the University of Michigan. "Plus, there's an 80 percent relapse rate within the year once someone goes off the pills." If drugs like Prozac possess a Lourdes-like aura for their therapeutic powers, we can thank the marketing and public relations folks at the pharmaceutical companies for effective consumer branding.

One recent study in the *Archives of General Psychiatry* reported, "Not only are more U.S. residents being treated with antidepressants, but also those who are being treated are receiving more antidepressant prescriptions." One reason is the high cost of psychotherapy; easy-to-prescribe pills are easier on the wallet. But in 2004, the Food and Drug Administration asked pharmaceutical companies to revise the warning labels of ten popular antidepressants to notify users of harmful side effects, including the possible risk of suicide.

In 2010, the *Journal of the American Medical Association* published a study that called into question the efficacy of antidepressant drugs. While the research team, led by Jay C. Fournier and Robert J. DeRubeis of the University of Pennsylvania, acknowledged that the drugs make a positive difference in cases of severe depression, the study found that for most patients—those with mild to moderate cases—the most commonly used antidepressants are generally no better than a placebo. "The message for patients with mild to moderate depression," Dr. DeRubeis told the *New York Times*, is that "medications are always an option, but there's little evidence that they add to other efforts to shake the depression—whether it's exercise, seeing the doctor, reading about the disorder or going for psychotherapy."

GETTING BACK ON THE BIKE

A Reacquaintance Long Overdue

Sometimes the best way to move forward in life is to take a long, sustained look into your personal rearview mirror. For me, it was riding down memory lane and revisiting the summer of 1978 when I biked solo across America. That trip irrevocably changed my life. Were there any lessons learned from that continental crossing that I could apply to the present? That would help me get rolling again after a ten-year absence from the sport?

The bike trip almost never happened. Two weeks before departure, a car sideswiped me on a training ride outside Ann Arbor, Michigan. The driver, a man in his fifties heading home after work, had failed to see me when he made a left turn. His fender nicked my leg, and I was knocked off the bike into a grassy ditch. I lay there, opossum-like, quickly taking a physical inventory of my body; surprisingly, I wasn't badly injured—only some minor pain in my left thigh from the impact. The driver walked over to me, apologetically saying that the setting sun had blinded him. I waited several moments before standing up. I wanted him to think that I was critically hurt. I told him to be more careful, then got on my bike and slowly cycled home.

Spooked by the incident, I didn't get back on my British-made Falcon until the day I actually embarked for the West Coast. If I were going to be splattered across the road, I gruesomely thought, let it happen during the trip, and not before. That way I could die a brave, foolish hero. My father wanted to buy me a handgun for personal safety. I declined his generous offer. "I'm likely to use it, so I don't ever want to be tempted," I replied.

In fact, I would have wanted to use a gun on that first day.

Around eight in the morning, I left my small studio apartment and tentatively climbed on my wobbly-with-extra-weight bike. All my gear, including an eight-pound tent was stashed into two rear panniers and a handlebar bag. I headed west—the Pacific Coast was 2,800 miles away.

An hour into the ride, a car of teenagers lobbed a firecracker at me. Then, several drivers tried to run me off the road. So much for cycling in the motor state.

I noticed a surprising number of flattened fauna on the road—squished remains of birds, skunks, dogs, squirrels. Were they grisly harbingers of my own fate? Fear of riding into the Great Unknown began to rattle my already shaky nerves. Did I really need to bike across the continent to demonstrate how tough and independent I was? Perhaps I *was* a coward. Anxiety surged. By early afternoon I had only biked forty-five miles, and was on the outskirts of Jackson, home to Michigan's fortresslike state prison. Yet I needed to escape from the road and mentally regroup. I checked into a twelve-dollar-a-day motel and watched a dialing-for-dollars matinee movie. I went to bed early without having dinner.

The next morning, I resumed riding. I had a job to do. I biked another fifty-five miles, and arrived at Holland Beach State Park, sunburned and bone-tired. I pitched my tent and went to sleep while listening to souped-up cars race their engines in the parking lot.

At dawn, I packed up my stuff and headed fifty miles north to Ludington, where I then took a several-hour ferry ride across Lake Michigan to Milwaukee.

Several broken spokes in the rear wheel had me concerned, so when I reached Madison, I went to a bike shop for repair work and spent the rest of the day walking around the bustling state capitol and University of Wisconsin campus.

I biked for another day in hilly, cow-loving Wisconsin. Twenty-five miles east of the Mississippi River, a small farm dog started yapping and chasing me. I picked up the pace, but the sudden acceleration caused the rear wheel to slip out of the frame dropouts. I crashed hard. The bike frame was wrecked. My right shoulder and hip were scraped clean and bloody.

Two kids on mini-bikes rode up to me. It was their dog. I asked them if their mother was home. She soon came out and I explained what happened. She offered to drive me to Dubuque, just on the other side of the Mississippi. We lifted the bike into the back of her pickup and drove off into the setting sun.

I thought the trip was over. I had only traveled three hundred miles. After checking into a motel, I called my father in Cleveland and told him that I had an accident and planned to take a Greyhound bus back home. The bike was totaled and inoperable. He said, "Bill, you're not a quitter. I will wire you money for a new bike."

Because of his generosity, I was able to purchase a new bicycle at the only bike store in Dubuque—a Trek that was made by a small Wisconsin bike company in its first year of business.

I rode-tested the Trek without panniers for fifty miles. My destination was a nearby Trappist monastery. Surprisingly, a member of this Catholic order—known for its vows of silence—cheerfully greeted me in the visitor's office and wanted to know all about my bike trip.

The following morning, loaded down this time with all my gear, I continued west, venturing like a seafarer across Iowa's endless ocean of corn.

Rolling ever westward, I averaged about sixty-five miles each day. By the time I made it halfway across Nebraska, I had experienced fierce thunderstorms, a locust swarm, heat, dehydration, saddle sores, hunger, nerve damage in both hands, gale-force headwinds, dogs, hills, boredom, countless flats, distracted motorists, speeding semis, and dive-bombing attacks from redwing blackbirds that were protecting their fledglings in roadside nests.

A challenging moment of truth occurred one afternoon in north-central Nebraska. It was raining hard. A plumber's van stopped, and the driver waved me over. "How about I give you a lift," he said.

"How far you traveling?" I asked.

"All the way across the state into eastern Colorado. About 270 miles I reckon."

I silently considered his offer. I was tired of riding in the rain and free mileage seemed like a great opportunity to make significant progress. Instead I blurted, "No thanks. I'm okay." He wished me well and drove off. I biked another fifteen soggy miles to the small town of Merriman, where I got a twelve-dollar room with a leaky ceiling.

A sundering of will, however, occurred one afternoon on the lifeless arid plains of eastern Wyoming, where my spirit and resolve nearly disintegrated in the hundred-degree heat. I had spent the night in Natrona, population of five, bedding down behind two gas pumps at the station/cafe/post office. In the morning, I packed up my green Eureka Timberland tent and gear, loaded them in the two rear bright yellow Kirkland panniers, and after rinsing out my mouth's morning staleness with a can of Mountain Dew—there was no running water because the pump was broken—I rolled out onto Route 20 for what I knew was going to be a long day. My destination was Riverton—ninety miles away.

By nine in the morning, the sun felt like a hot branding iron pressed against my back. Apart from the occasional motor home, there was scant traffic. A dense stillness hung over the desolate land. The next town, Powder River, just ten miles away, was a cluster of trailer homes grouped around a gas station/cafe. I rested in the shade for an hour, playing with a Dalmatian puppy. I had little interest in getting back on the bike. Reluctantly, I returned to the lonesome two-lane highway.

The day continued to heat up. It was the hottest so far on the trip. The sky was baked white. The desert seemed sucked dry of life. Even the sagebrush looked limp and lethargic in the suffocating heat. The landscape's blank emptiness was unbearable for a slow-moving traveler like myself. The earth lacked a beginning or end; it simply fused with the sky, imprisoning me within its unforgiving hell. Mentally and physically spent, I got off the bike and held out my thumb like a cocky hitchhiker who expects the first vehicle to give him a lift. Who was I kidding? The Airstreams and Winnebagos glided right by, indifferent to my exhaustion and plight. I stood there for a half-hour with my outstretched digit, until reconciling myself to the reality that I didn't want to spend the night camping in the desert. I wearily climbed back onto the bike and disconsolately pedaled west.

I began to hallucinate RVs approaching me from behind, but whenever I turned around to look, the road was empty. These phantom vehicles taunted me with their mysterious vanishing acts. I tried focusing on the white shoulder line to the right of my front tire. But the endless stripe began to jump about like a baton wildly tossed in the air. I was losing it. I felt ridiculous biking here in the desert. Why was I even cycling across America? Everything seemed absurd, a summer gone awry with escalating futility. I tried to fight off these negative thoughts by screaming at the top of my lungs. The louder I screamed, the more I hoped to suppress the despair. And the yelling worked! My pace quickened and, by dusk, I eventually made it to Shoshoni, where I found a run-down motel.

The following day, heading out of town, I was rewarded with a faraway glimpse of the grand prize that I had been looking forward to ever since I left Ann Arbor. Off in the distance poked the Rockies' faint outline—a jagged, shadowy silhouette in the blue sky. For two full days, I slowly grinded uphill, riding through open grasslands and then red sandstone canyons, before I reached the geographical high point of the trip: Togwotee Pass on the Continental Divide, elevation 9,685 feet. I camped that night by a stream near the pass. I could see the snow-capped Grand Tetons forty miles away. Though this was bear country, sleep came easy as I was lulled by the soothing sound of the moving water. Despite having another 1,000 miles of cycling looming ahead, I knew I'd make it to the Pacific. I felt that confident.

It took three more weeks to complete the transcontinental crossing. When I arrived in the small coastal town of Lincoln City, Oregon, I set down my bike on the sand and still wearing my bike clothes and tennis shoes, dashed into the cold Pacific surf. Shouting with joy and splashing in the waves, I announced to the world that I had biked across the United States! But the beach was empty on that cold overcast day. My sole witnesses were several seagulls that eyed me with avian suspicion. I walked back to my bike, disappointed that I had no one to share my triumph with. I biked to a nearby Laundromat to dry my wet clothes.

I then took a Greyhound bus to San Francisco and later hitchhiked down to Santa Cruz, where I camped on the beaches. (I had left the Trek at a bike store.) Two weeks later, I flew back to Ann Arbor, where I felt cut off from everyone on the University of Michigan campus, like I had been an explorer who had just returned from a foreign land with fantastic tales to tell that no one wanted to hear. I was in splendid shape—my legs were so strong that I felt I could walk up walls—but the real transformation had been internal, marked by a coming of age, self-reliance, newfound independence, and self-discovery. It also signified the beginning of a multi-year love affair with cycling that included bike trips in Death Valley, twice up the California coast from Los Angeles to San Francisco, Lake Tahoe, southern Utah, northern Arizona, Colorado, the Canadian Rockies, the Dominican Republic, Costa Rica, and New Zealand.

Whenever someone asked me what it was like to bike across America, I usually gave the same answer: "It was as much mental as it was physical." The daily effort required a constant negotiation between mind and body. On some days, I had to dig deep, very deep, tricking my legs into performing the most basic task of moving up and down, up and down. To this day, I wonder, if an RV had indeed rescued me in the Wyoming desert heat, what would have ensued? Would I have walked away from cycling for good?

BIKING INDOORS: HERE ARE SOME BASICS

In the early 1980s, Lon Haldeman was widely recognized as the king of ultra-cycling, notching victories in two coast-to-coast races and setting both the twelve-hour track record (264.8 miles) and twenty-four-hour track record (454 miles). Because Lon lived in the Midwest, the bulk of his winter training depended upon marathon sessions on a stationary bike in his basement. The model he used was a Monark ergometer that had a belt hitched to a furnace fan for added pedaling resistance. He'd bike between three and four hours per day, going nowhere in that cramped room.

Indoor cycling has made dramatic technological and performance advances since then. Nonetheless, two considerations remain the same for many riders: how to beat the boredom and how to maximize one's training. For those getting back on the bike for the first time in years, those who live in areas where riding during the winter months is impractical or unenjoyable, or those whose job limits available daylight hours for outdoor riding, indoor biking can make a big difference in achieving cardiovascular fitness. You won't need to grind out mega-miles like Lon did to get in shape. Just two or three times a week of riding forty-five minutes to an hour will significantly improve leg and lung endurance. Yet it helps to know some basics that will make your time in the stationary saddle much more productive while alleviating the monotony.

There are several types of indoor stationary bikes. The two most popular exercise bikes found at the gym are the upright and recumbent. The upright version is engineered to simulate a road bike, while the recumbent's seat is positioned lower and further back. Both have adjustable resistance that affects leg speed.

Spinning bikes are an enhancement of the upright version, and have a weighted flywheel that simulates the effects of inertia and momentum of a real bicycle. Spinning bikes have an adjustable seat and handlebars. The pedals are typically equipped with toe clips to allow one foot to pull up when the other is pushing down. Most health clubs offer Spinning classes. Instructors lead their sweaty troops at varying tempos and intensity, with dance or rock music blaring so that riders can synchronize their pedaling to the beat. Instructors often select specific songs for sprints and climbs for motivation.

The upright, recumbent, and Spinning bikes share one thing in common: You can't coast like you can do on a normal bike. This eliminates what Chad

Schoenauer of Asheville, North Carolina, who conducts indoor cycling classes at his local YMCA, calls "lazy legs." Writing on RoadBikeRider.com, he states that "the quality of workouts is increased because you must keep pedaling." It's like riding a fixed-gear bike (a preference among bike messengers).

Schoenauer recommends a brief warm-up to get blood to your leg muscles before going all out. He offers these additional indoor tips:

1. "Make leg speed your initial focus."
2. "Mimic your outdoor position. If you're doing a 'climbing' interval, assume the same posture that you'd have on your road bike—semi-upright, loose grip on the bar top near the stem. If doing a 'flat road' interval, get low and imagine slicing through the wind."
3. "Keep your head up. If you look at your feet or the floor, you shut down your breathing and can tense up. You can't ride this way outside or you might hit something. Focus on an imaginary road in the distance."

If you'd rather bike in the privacy of your home, you can purchase a stationary bike or stationary trainer that will involve removing the front wheel. (Rollers, however, use three metal drums and don't require removing any bike parts, though they require balance and coordination so you don't fall over.)

First becoming popular in the early eighties, wind trainers used the forward motion of the rear wheel to drive a fan that generated wind resistance. The harder or faster you pedaled, the greater the resistance and noise level.

Magnetic trainers came next, and here the resistance is produced by a magnetic field generated by the rear wheel. Unlike wind trainers, these models have adjustable resistance levels and are much quieter.

Fluid trainers use the resistance of fluid encased in a closed chamber. As the rear wheel spins, it turns a mechanism that moves through the liquid, and this is where the resistance is powered. Fluid trainers are more expensive than wind or magnetic trainers (expect to spend $300 or more), but offer a less noisy and smoother riding experience.

Of course, you can scour eBay or Craigslist for a used trainer or Schwinn Airdyne, which was one of the very first exercise bikes to hit the market in 1978 and is still being manufactured. It has an adjustable seat, pedals with a chain attached to a big fan (this creates the wind and pedaling resistance), and long, vertical handlebars that move back and forward for an upper-body

(continues)

workout. A new Airdyne costs just over $600, but you can find decent used ones for less than half the price.

Now that you have a trainer or exercise bike, where should it go in your apartment or home? You can set it up by a window or in front of the television. Keep a small towel draped over the bike's top tube since you will be creating rivers of sweat. It's also advisable to place a rubber exercise mat under your bike to protect the floor or carpet. To help cool you, park a fan right in front of the bike. This is one gentle headwind you won't mind riding into.

To stave off boredom, you can watch television, films, bike racing DVDs, or bike-travel DVDs comprised of scenic routes filmed from the rider's perspective. These travelogue DVDs come with narration and music, and are available at GlobalRide.net. For specific workout DVDs, you might consider buying either the Chris Carmichael or Spinerval training series. It's like having a virtual bike coach right there by your side, offering you encouragement to get the most out of your indoor workout.

BACK IN THE SADDLE

If the body is a machine, then mine was out of order when I stopped biking during that Lost Fitness Decade. It wasn't like I could send away for new parts. The shutdown was all inside my mind. So what would it take to get back on the bike? To make my legs slavishly and mechanically respond like well-oiled pistons?

On an early July evening in 2009, it finally happened. Without fanfare or planning, almost like going on an unexpected first date, I warily approached the abandoned Klein mountain bike that I had kept parked outside the front door all this time. It hadn't been ridden in ten years. Both tires were flat and desiccated-looking, the knobby rubber treads mottled with decay. The chain was rusted and needed replacing. The front derailleur cable was missing. I pumped up the tires, and then replaced the chain with an extra one that I found in an old gear box. I checked the brakes. They still functioned. I then wheeled the bike halfway up the dirt driveway before hopping on. The first few pedal strokes were awkward. The bike wobbled underneath my uncertain control. I felt like a six-year-old riding without training wheels for his first time.

I biked through my neighborhood for twenty minutes. This brief jaunt required making it up two small hills—the first was a half-mile long and the second was one-eighth mile. Both ascents sapped my legs and burned my lungs with rapid-breathing exertion. I was whipped when I pulled back into my driveway. I had only gone 2.5 miles. Earlier that day, Tour de France riders had covered a hundred miles in the Pyrenees in little over four hours. Yet I felt as exhausted and winded from my baby-biking effort as those pro cyclists.

The following day, I got back on the bike. Even with the padded seat, my butt was sore. I could barely sit down. My neck and shoulders felt like someone had wailed on them with their fists. I biked through southern Marin, taking frequent rest stops because my aching legs had no juice. Even on the easiest grades, I had to pause and dismount every few hundred yards—and wait for the discomfort to subside. My quads felt like Twinkies filled with lactic-acid frosting. After twelve miles, or two hours, I stopped for lunch at a small Mexican restaurant in San Rafael. A huge veggie burrito energized me, but I dreaded the ride home, since it involved going up two long hills. About a half-mile later as I biked through an industrial and warehouse section, I got a flat tire. Because I didn't have a spare tube, I called a cab and was (thankfully!) whisked home for thirty-five dollars. I tipped the driver five dollars to show my gratitude. Once upon a time, I would have walked all those miles if my bike had broken down. I wouldn't have allowed it any other way.

But wow! It was great to be riding, though my grumpy body failed to share in this unbridled enthusiasm and certainly wasn't in any mood for more cycling. It was difficult confronting the painfully obvious truth: I was essentially starting over as a beginning cyclist. All those thousands of miles from earlier years of riding meant zilch in the here and now. If I wanted to become a cyclist again, I needed to commit to biking at least two times a week, using rest days to restore vigor to my legs for the next training session. This meant that I needed to build a mileage base—judiciously, incrementally, patiently. This gradual conditioning process would take several months to achieve. There was nothing complicated or scientific about the strategy. If I were aiming to compete in a triathlon or an upcoming century, I might have rethought this plan and added high-intensity rides. But my three objectives were to recapture my former cycling mojo, rebuild leg strength, and regain a modicum of bike-handling confidence.

So, for the first two months, I rode about forty-five minutes or an hour twice a week, alternating between trails and the road. (I ran the other two or three days.) My legs were usually sore for at least a day or two afterward, depending on how much hill climbing I had done. I was still using a mountain bike; my Cannnodale road bike would see action much later, I promised myself, once my cycling comfort level had returned.

About every two weeks, I went grocery shopping on my bike. I'd strap on a lightweight backpack and ride down to the local Safeway. It was three miles to the store, and almost all downhill. I'd wheel the Klein bike inside, lean it against the large freezer with its stacks of blue bags of ice, and proceed to shop. At the checkout stand, the cashier would ask, "Paper or plastic?" I'd just nod and point to my backpack. I'd then pay the cashier and proceed to jam about thirty pounds of food and beverages into the pack. I'd cinch down the shoulder and waist straps, hoist the whole affair onto my back, and bicycle home. The first two miles were a slow, steady push. But the final mile was brutal—a steep, winding uphill torment. I would have to stop two or three times to rest. The ride gave added meaning to the word "chore." Apart from being a great heart-thumping, leg-busting workout, these grocery rides served an entirely utilitarian and multitasking purpose. It helped me get in shape and was eco-friendly. Most people drive less than five miles while doing local errands, and using your bike now and then for shopping saves gas, helps the planet a wee bit, builds a sweat, and boosts your physical conditioning.

REACQUAINTING YOUR BODY WITH THE BIKE

If you have ignored cycling for years, as I fecklessly did, or are new to the sport, you undoubtedly know that your body will experience temporary physical discomfort once you start riding. New or long-dormant muscles must be re-cruited and employed. There's a huge difference between sitting deskbound and going wheel-bound. It's not as if your Herman Miller Aeron chair mirac-ulously sprouted tires, handlebars, and pedals. The specific contact points between bike and body—hands, butt, feet—require sufficient time to adjust to these new pressure points. Your lower back, knees, neck, and shoulders will experience varying degrees of uneasiness.

How your body adapts is affected by bike fit, positioning, time spent riding, conditioning, and upper-body strength and flexibility. These factors are all interrelated. So let's see what happens to your various body parts now that you have wheels.

Bike Fit

The process of familiarization begins with bike fit. An improperly sized bike creates a cascading set of problems that can range from simply annoying to potentially troubling.

A new, expensive $6,000 carbon-fiber bike can hurt as much as a Walmart all-steel $149 clunker. Discomfort is not eliminated by price. Perched on a bike in a store is not the same as riding it. Nor will taking a few laps in the parking lot give you an accurate depiction of what to expect. Even books targeted to beginning cyclists offer in theory what can only be experienced through actual riding. Meanwhile, cycling magazine articles and websites can leave readers befuddled with complicated esoterica on body positioning and frame geometry.

Is there an easier way to understand bike fit? Paul Levine, owner of New York–based Signature Cycles, is nationally known as the "fit guru." He spends a great deal of time fitting wealthy bike owners at $200 a pop. For the average rider, however, as Levine explained in *Bike for Life: How to Ride to 100*, positioning can be neatly summarized as follows: "The proper posture to have while seated on a bicycle is like sitting on a chair that you know is about to be pulled out from under you." In other words, you should be leaning forward with your back in a neutral position. This also allows you to exert maximum pedaling power while your upper body remains in a relaxed mode.

Through further investigation into bike fit for recreational riders, I came across a website for Gregg's Cycles, a popular chain of three stores in the Seattle area. Their informative article "Your Bike Doesn't Have to Hurt You!" states that "we've been in the bike business for a long time (since 1932 in fact) and the most common complaint about cycling is that it hurts." There are three types of pain: falling off a bike and getting a terrible case of road rash; being out of shape; and "mechanical pain" caused by improper fit.

"Fit is the most important factor in purchasing a bike, new or used," says Gregg's Cycles. "Every day we get asked, 'what's the best bike for me?' and the answer should always be, 'the one that fits.' If you go to a reputable bike shop, and stay away from the big box stores that have a few bikes, you know that you will get a quality bike. So you just need to buy a quality bike that fits you. You could pay $200 and get a great bike that fits and love riding it. Or you could pay $2,000 and get a great bike that doesn't fit and never ride it. The $2,000 bike might be better, but it doesn't matter if you don't ride it because it hurts. If it fits you'll ride it, if it doesn't fit it will hang out in the garage."

According to Gregg's Cycles, the three most important criteria regarding bike fit are the following:

- *Stand Over Height:* "On a road bike you want to have at least an inch between you and the bike when you are straddling the bike and standing on the ground. You should have at least two inches with a mountain bike."

- *Saddle Height:* "When you are sitting on the seat you'll be able to touch the ground with your feet but only with your toes. As you sit on the saddle (this will be easier if someone is holding you up) you should pedal backwards until one of your feet is at the very bottom of the pedaling motion. Once it's there, stop and make sure that your foot is parallel to the ground. When your foot is in this position you should have about a 10 percent bend in your knee. No more. No less."
- *Reach:* "Reach is described by the distance between your saddle and the handlebars. When sitting on your saddle in the most comfortable position you should be able to reach forward and hold on to the handlebars with a comfortable bend in your elbows. You should also have a nice 'ready' or neutral back posture."

A good bike shop will help you find a bike that fits your body. Proper sizing might require some adjustments with the seat and height of the handlebar stem. Even the most minute change in saddle height can be critical to the discerning rider. Legendary pro cyclist Eddy Merckx used to carry a small tool to adjust his seat while he *was* racing.

MALE ANATOMY ALERT!—DOES BIKING CAUSE IMPOTENCE?

Considering that I now had a small hunk of leather and foam jammed upward into my private parts several hours a week, should I have been concerned about cycling's effect on my plumbing? Can biking, in fact, lead to sexual impotency?

A controversial article in *Bicycling* magazine in 1997 first caused male cyclists to rethink what exactly goes on between their legs. A senior editor, who consistently logged 14,000 miles per year, admitted that all this riding caused sexual impotency. *Bicycling* quoted Dr. Irwin Goldstein, director of Boston University's Medical Center urology department. Given the number of male riders who came to his office seeking relief from impotence, the urologist came out against cycling: "When a man sits on a bicycle seat, he's putting his entire body weight on the artery that supplies the penis. It's a nightmarish situation."

Goldstein believed that biking more than three hours a week was harmful to men due to potential penile and nerve damage. His tough-love message was a warning as hard and unyielding as cold-forged steel. A squashed perineum artery—he used the analogy of a bent drinking straw that stays bent—resulted from too much time in the saddle, improper riding form, wrong type of seat, or traumatic injury involving the bike's top tube. Over time, decreased blood flow can lead to erectile dysfunction (ED) or impotence, which is the repeated inability to get or keep an erection firm enough for sexual intercourse.

What got clouded in cyclists' up-in-arms reaction to Goldstein's admonition was that, as a group, male riders experience much less erectile dysfunction than the general male population whose unhealthy lifestyle factors, like poor diet, no exercise, smoking, and hypertension, all play a significant role in contributing to impotence. In fact, ED has reached epidemic proportions in this country, with 30 million American men estimated to have this embarrassing affliction.

But, as alarm bells went off in bike shops across the land, the quick-thinking bike industry refused to go entirely soft on the issue of erectile dysfunction. Several manufacturers developed a radically new bike seat with a cut-out channel running down the middle. This open-wedged design helped relieve pressure on the perineum. Specialized's Body Geometry wedge saddle soon became a top seller. Imitators flooded the market with their cut-out models. Sales soared. Men were obviously not taking chances. Today, open-wedge seats boast a sizable chunk of the saddle market. Several million have been sold.

"Much as we'd like to sell zillions of new saddles, in most cases the saddle itself is not the problem," says Mike Jacoubowsky, co-owner of Chain Reaction Bicycles in Northern California. "It's more how one sits on the saddle that is at issue here, and it really doesn't matter whether you've got a stock seat or the fanciest aftermarket urologist-approved model. If you're not set up correctly on the bike, you're going to have potential for problems down the road."

Jacoubowsky goes on to explain what a rider should know about the seat:

> First place to start is with the tilt, or angle, of the saddle. In almost no case is it a good idea to ride with a saddle that's tilted up at the

(continues)

front! This focuses the pressure on exactly the wrong areas. As you slide forward on the seat, you're essentially driving your most delicate parts into the nose of the seat if it's "up" at the front.

So do you want the seat "down" at the front? That's not a good idea either, because you're going to spend the whole ride pushing back from the handlebars, creating a lot of tension in your arms and shoulders. A level saddle is the best bet.

What if a level saddle causes discomfort? Then it's definitely time for a different saddle. The way you ride might make all the difference in the world. Most injuries don't occur instantly, but rather over a long period of exposure to whatever's causing the problem. If your riding style is such that you sit endlessly on the saddle and never stand up or stretch, you're much more likely to have problems. The best way to combat this is to regularly take a break from the grind and stand up for a bit, take a breather, stretch a bit, and then get back in the saddle.

A softer, thickly cushioned seat can also be detrimental. So says Dr. Frank Somers, an internationally known urologist and researcher from the University Medical Center of Cologne, Germany, who surveyed 1,700 German riders, as well as testing elite riders in his lab. "This is the crux of the whole issue. I have some patients who like well-padded seats very much, but they are not always healthy. Even though patients are comfortable sitting, they have diminished blood flow. And this depends on the padding. If a male rider puts down his weight on the saddle, the padding will compress because he is sinking on the saddle and the weight on the saddle is compressing very hard on the peronial area."

When I was mountain biking up to six hours a day while training for La Ruta, my crotch would often go numb. The sensation would return several hours after riding. I never considered the urological risk at the time. I blithely and ignorantly assumed that I had a good workout whenever feeling vacated the penile premises, and left it at that. Stupid me. Though I was not putting in that kind of time in the saddle during my fitness rebound, I still didn't want to become a returning member of the Numb and Number club. Because there are several prudent and preventative measures that can put the mind and crotch at ease. Allow me to share these tips:

1. Try standing up occasionally. This will help restore blood flow to the undercarriage. Even those who only use a stationary bike at the gym can be unwitting ED candidates. Get off the seat for a one-minute interval every five minutes.

2. Alter your riding or saddle position if you start feeling numb. Triathletes, take note: Don't always remain in the hunched-over aero position.

3. The type of saddle is often not the main villain. It's a combination of tilt and the drop from seat to handlebar that makes the difference.

4. Mountain bike riders are more vulnerable to penile or testicular trauma and injury, so get out of the saddle and use your legs as shock absorbers when riding over roots, train tracks, and curbs.

5. You may want to experiment with a variety of anatomically contoured saddles, but they don't come cheap. Editors at *Bicycling* tested models for their functionality and riding comfort, and shared the results with readers in the September 2009 issue. Men's saddles receiving "editors' choice" accolades went to: the Specialized Phenom SL ($150), Selle Italia SLR ($209), and Fizik Arione CX ($170).

If you still remain concerned about the possible link between impotency and bike riding, complete abstinence from cycling is certainly not encouraged or even warranted. In fact, cycling can actually enhance your sex life. You look and feel healthier. Your legs and butt are more sculpted and toned. You have more energy and endurance in the sack.

The Butt

Old-fashioned bike purists will swear by their well-broken-in leather saddles. But these seats can take several thousand miles of riding before they conform to one's buttocks. Bike seats are now made with spongy, space-age materials and flaunt other-worldly designs whose primary purpose is to make it anatomically easier on your posterior and privates. (See sidebar on cycling and impotence.)

Contrary to popular belief, a wide, thickly cushioned, gel-filled seat won't guarantee a comfortable ride. This is due to your "sit bones" (*ischial tuberosities*), sinking into the padding, thereby compressing nerves and restricting blood flow. "You want your sit bones to be on the wide part of the seat, so they're supported," Dr. Roger Minkow, MD, an ergonomics consultant and the inventor of Specialized's Body Geometry saddle, told *Bicycling*. Unused muscles in your butt cause soreness. "When you ride and get in shape, your muscle tissue gets firmer," says Minkow. "This gives you more muscle mass between your sit bones and your seat."

There really is no cure for "beginner's butt." Padded bike shorts will slightly lessen the discomfort generated by an aching tailbone. But once you get past the initial get-to-know-you riding phase, your butt should be fine.

As for the saddle, it should stay level with the ground. Tilting the nose downward will force your butt to continually edge forward, whereas tilting the nose upward will jam your private parts backward, compressing nerves and the genitals.

Another limitation with wider saddles is that they force your legs to pedal in an ineffective, splayed-out manner. You don't want to pedal bow-legged. And that's a main reason why you want to find the narrowest, firmest saddle that is suited to your type of riding. You might have to experiment and shop around, but prepare yourself for sticker shock; top saddles now cost over $200.

Long-time bike journalist Jim Langley states on his website that "the faster you ride, the more likely it is you'll want a narrow, racing-style seat. This is because a fast-riding position on a bike shifts you forward, placing more weight on the hands and feet and reducing a lot of the weight on the seat. Also, as you pedal more vigorously, you spin faster and you can't tolerate interference from the sides of the seat."

Knees and Feet

Cycling attracts a fresh, unending multitude of injured runners with blown-out knees. Unlike running, the low-impact, repetitive motion of pedaling typically won't wear down the joints and cartilage. But you still can experience knee pain on the bike. Because the knee is a complex hinge-and-pulley mechanism, it is vulnerable to stress, abuse, and overuse. For cyclists, knee pain usually results from tendonitis—the straining of hardened fibers that attach the quadriceps to the patella or kneecap and the hamstrings to the tibia or shinbone. When the tendons become stretched or irritated they can swell up, and the increased friction can cause a burning pain in the front of the knee or right below the kneecap. Too often, putting in a lot of miles on undertrained tendons causes tendonitis. Fortunately, tendonitis responds well to rest and an easy ten-minute warm-up at the start of each ride. It also helps to wear tights in colder weather.

The other most common cycling-related knee injury is chondromalacia—the irritation of the cartilage that provides joint lubrication. Chondromalacia is most often caused by lateral or unnatural movement of the knee joint, and is usually related to a seat that is too high, too low, too far forward, or pushed back too far. Unlike tendonitis, "chondro" can develop into a permanent debilitating condition once the cartilage is worn away. Sufferers can actually hear a crunching noise—bone on bone—with each pedal stroke.

Knee pain can also result from pushing too high a gear, especially on hills. You want to use a gear that allows you to pedal or spin at a rapid tempo, ranging from seventy to a hundred strokes per minute on level or rolling terrain. Don't feel like you have to be macho by trying to crank along in a big gear. Most new bikes come equipped with triple-chain rings and rear-cogs with up to eight or nine sprocket clusters. The Schwinn ten-speed of your youth is a misnomer. Many contemporary bikes are twenty-seven-speed. For those taking up biking for the first time in their forties and fifties, having a wide gear selection will save your knees from undue wear and tear.

Improper foot position on the pedal can contribute to knee pain. Because most feet have a natural angle that prefers to point either outward or inward, your foot assumes this angle in bike shoes designed for clipless pedals. Don't try to straighten out your feet in the pedal. Instead, adjust the shoe's bottom cleat to permit your foot to be at its natural angle. If your cleats are misaligned, the constant twisting or torqueing of your lower legs will create unnecessary stress on both knee joints.

Look for clipless pedals with rotational freedom, or "float," so your knees won't be locked into the same riding position. Speedplay's lollipop-looking pedals are a popular brand and provide generous float.

Ill-fitting bike shoes might lead to foot pain and numbness. Orthotics usually rectify the problem by evenly distributing the weight of the footbed. You might have to experiment with different brands and models.

Of course, you can just ride in running shoes and toe clips with straps (they provide additional power with the pedal upstroke), and though you will sacrifice some power and pedaling efficiency, your knees will be free to move about. Plus, when you are off the bike, it's easier to walk around in running shoes than in a pair of stiff-soled cycling shoes. Running shoes and toe clips make a good team for off-road riding, because you can quickly yank your foot out of the toe clips if you have to stop suddenly and are about to fall. Unlike clipless pedals, you don't have to pivot your foot for rapid egress.

Investing in a pair of clipless pedals and cycling shoes can be pricey, and some top combos will exceed $300. There's nothing wrong with using running shoes and $15 toe clips and straps. I biked 2,800 miles in running shoes and toe clips during my transcontinental ride. They worked fine. It's also what I decided to use when I started riding again, despite owning three sets of clipless pedals. If you've never used clipless pedals before, here's one very important cautionary note: Practice getting in and out of them in the parking lot or driveway. You don't want to find yourself nearing a stoplight, furiously struggling to shake a foot loose—or when the light turns green, being unable to swiftly get the foot back in.

Hands

About five hundred miles into my bike ride across America, I began to notice a loss of sensation in both hands, even though I was wearing padded fingerless gloves. It was difficult to hold a pen while writing in my journal. To open a door, I would have to clench the knob with both wrists like in a vise grip. I later came up with a do-it-yourself solution that remedied the problem. I cut off a hunk of foam from my sleeping bag pad and wrapped it around the handlebars. The numbness soon went away.

Numb hands can affect beginners as well as experienced riders. Reduced blood circulation and compressed nerves will cause a loss of sensitivity in your handlebar-clenching paws. Typically, this condition is due to hands stuck in the same riding position, hands in an overly stretched-out position on the bars, or if the body is leaning too far forward—a posture that places excess weight on the bars.

Here are several quick fixes:

1. Wrap the handlebars with an extra roll of padded tape.
2. Raise the handlebar gradually, because too-low bars (or stem) put excess weight on your hands.
3. Lower the seat, since a too-high saddle throws your upper-body weight forward and places greater pressure on your hands' contact areas.

4. Slide the seat forward or shorten the handlebar stem, so you're not too stretched-out from the rear of your saddle to the handlebars.

5. Regularly switch hand positions and make sure to limit hand time in the top-of-the-bar position.

6. Tightly squeezing the handlebars restricts blood circulation, so relax and gently rest hands on the bar (but not on poor roads or other surfaces, in traffic, or down hills—hold tight!); as long as one thumb is always under the bars, your hands can't slip and you can steer and control the bike even when riding fast with only a loose or moderate touch.

7. Avoid tight-fitting gloves that restrict blood flow.

8. Use bar ends if you mountain bike, since they provide additional places to position your hands.

9. Finally, occasionally shake out one hand at a time while holding onto the handlebar with the other hand; this action will help push blood out to the fingertips and capillaries—and restore circulation.

I never ride without padded gloves. They help cushion road vibrations and absorb sweat so your hands won't slip off the handlebars. Most importantly, gloves will protect your soft tender palms in case of a fall.

Neck and Shoulders

Neck pain is another common cycling complaint, and is usually the result of riding a bike that is too long or having handlebars that are too low. Even an awkward-fitting helmet can tire out neck muscles if the helmet sits too low in front, forcing you to tilt your head upward to see where you are going.

If the saddle slopes downward, this can cause shoulder discomfort, as your body will tend to slide forward as you ride, and then you wind up using your hands to push yourself back into position. You want the saddle level.

A good riding position is one in which the elbows are slightly bent, not straight and locked, since this allows the biceps, triceps, and forearms to act as shock absorbers.

Due to the increasing number of older riders, bike companies have come out with a plethora of "comfort bikes." These allow cyclists to ride in a more upright position. For cyclists with declining upper-body-muscle strength or flexibility, comfort bikes lessen the weight and pressure on the shoulders and upper arms.

Back

Back pain is usually caused by poor cycling posture. When riding a bicycle, the back should be arched, like a bridge, not sagging forward between the hips and the shoulders. Don't ride hunchbacked like a cycling Quasimodo. The muscles around your spine should be in a relaxed, not tense, state.

Bike fit guru Paul Levine says, "The biggest cause of back pain is a too-low handlebar. An indicator of poor bike fit for a road bike is when you can't comfortably ride in any of the handlebar positions, including the drops." Riding in a stretched-out position puts too much pressure on the back as well as the hands.

Pro riders with a high tolerance for pain can set up their bikes with low handlebars for improved aerodynamics, but it's a mistake for recreational cyclists to imitate the racers.

SOME BASICS ON TECHNIQUE AND TRAINING

Old habits refuse to die. Because I preferred riding alone and hated sucking another cyclist's wheel, I traveled at my own pace, slowed down when I wanted, accelerated when I desired. I didn't mind being passed by other riders. I understood my new, altered place in the cycling universe even as I gradually reclaimed my two-wheel fitness.

As a recreational cyclist, I seldom felt bored during these one- and two-hour rides. I was attracted by the freedom that cycling outdoors offers. It's what I sorely missed when I stopped riding for all those years. Still, it took a while to shake off the rust and work on my riding skills. I wasn't interested in speed so much as maintaining a comfortable riding style and cadence.

I was content tooling along as a lone wheelman in Lycra, but others might want to hone their technique and improve their conditioning by riding with friends, joining a bike club, or even signing up for a weekend bike-skills camp. If you know someone who is a serious rider, ask him or her to go riding with you on an "easy" day. I used to do that with a friend back in the day. Alex was a brainy, popular cycling coach who typically rode three hundred miles a week. We would occasionally ride up the northern, steeper and rockier side of Mount Tam together. I would be straining every foot of the way on my mountain bike, and he would be going along at what was for him a leisurely pace, chatting about the latest French philosopher he was currently reading. He rode a fixed-gear track bike. I learned a lot about bike handling by following right behind him. He navigated ruts, rocks, and tree roots with exquisite fluidity and supple grace. During one ride, he said something that has stuck with me to this day: "When riding over rocks, think of your tires as water flowing over them. Don't waste energy fighting the rocks or thinking of them as obstructions always to be avoided, so much as ride over them." It was terrific advice.

To help you roll your way to fitness, whether you are aiming to do your first charity ride, half or full-century, triathlon, or are simply in pursuit of fun and adventure, I have put together a brief overview of some biking basics.

The Sudden Stop

Before you start, you first need to know how to stop. John Howard, three-time Olympian and renowned bike coach, told *Bike for Life* the following:

> Sooner or later, you are going to come face to door handle with a distracted soccer mom who's talking on her cell phone and screaming at her kids. What you need is a Hot Stop. It is the nearest thing to stop-on-a-dime braking. Here's how it's done:
>
> - Shift your weight rearward. At the first sign of trouble, slide your butt very far back and low, behind the seat. This lowers your center of gravity, improving rear-wheel traction and preventing an "endo."
> - Level your pedals. This keeps you from pulling to one side or clipping a pedal on the asphalt if you do lean.
> - Grab the front brake hard, the rear easier. Apply far more pressure to the front brake than you otherwise think would be safe. The correct percentage of braking bias is two-thirds front and one-third rear; in the rain, use equal braking pressure. It will probably take several tire-sliding sessions before you can get the hang of it. If you don't lock up the wheel and catapult into a truck, you'll stop amazingly fast and under control.
> - Get ready to bail. Find an escape route or stopping point and focus on it, rather than what you want to miss. The bike will naturally follow your eyes.

BEWARE OF DISTRACTED DRIVERS!—
TEN TIPS TO HELP KEEP YOU SAFE ON THE ROAD

Unless you prefer to do all your riding indoors, on bike paths, or off-road, you'll have to deal with potentially dangerous drivers. A bike is no match for a car or truck. Here's a rather disturbing statistic I feel reluctant to include in this book, but it's something that often lurks in the periphery of my mind every time I take to the streets on my bike. According to the Insurance Institute for Highway Safety, distracted drivers kill an average of seven hundred cyclists each year. These fatalities are attributed to booze, drugs, sleeplessness, daydreaming, preoccupation with the screaming kids in the back seat, and cell phone use and text messaging.

In a 2008 study, the National Highway Traffic Safety Administration found that 5 to 8 percent of all drivers are holding "phones to ear" at any given time, regardless of the time, weather, or road conditions. The report concluded that distracted driving is involved in roughly 16 percent of all fatal crashes and 22 percent of injury crashes. It also found that handheld phone use was highest in the sixteen-to twenty-four-year-old age bracket—the demographic that is most inexperienced behind the wheel and most likely to get into an accident.

Distracted driving has only intensified given our mobile dependency on cell phones and text messaging. Several auto-safety studies have shown that a person texting behind the wheel is more careless than someone legally drunk. Even hands-free devices fail to lessen the chance of possible distraction.

About two dozen states now ban texting by all drivers. Let's hope that the rest of the states take up the ban.

So what should you do to survive distracted drivers? Here are ten useful tips:

1. Ride with traffic but ride like you are invisible. While you should expect that drivers can't always see you, that doesn't give you the right to ride in the middle of the road. Try to ride as close to the right side as possible.

2. You should wear brightly colored, even fluorescent apparel. A yellow or green DayGlo windbreaker or rain jacket is advisable even when it's not windy or raining. Many cycling tops are super-lightweight and breathable, so you won't overheat. Attach reflective strips to your bike helmet.

3. I have seen many Bay Area commuters ride with a small bright flag on a three- or four-foot pole attached to the bike's rear.

4. Buy a small LED headlight and a rear-flashing beacon. Use them even during daylight hours. They are not just for night riding.

5. When approaching an intersection, try to make sure that you can observe the driver and that he or she actually sees you.

6. Ride defensively. Drivers often assume that cyclists are a minor annoyance, so they don't always bother signaling when making a turn. Or they don't think twice about cutting off a rider.

7. Ride responsibly. You want to set a good example by obeying all the traffic laws and regulations. When drivers see a cyclist misbehaving—blowing past stoplights, riding the wrong way on one-way streets—they tend to lump all cyclists together and use that as further evidence that "we" are the enemy. Don't give drivers any excuse to treat us worse.

8. Don't chat on a cell phone or sip a Starbucks coffee in one hand while riding. You too should not ride distracted.

9. Use clearly marked bike lines whenever available, even if drivers choose to ignore them.

10. Always be extra vigilant of car doors on parked vehicles that might suddenly open on the driver's side. Getting car-doored will put a severe dent in your return to fitness.

Falling

And what about falling? The wrist and collar bones are cycling's most common fractures, because riders will typically want to extend an arm to break the fall. One word: Don't.

Falling on a road bike is usually more severe than on a mountain bike. You are going faster and asphalt is less forgiving on your body than dirt.

Once again, here's *Bike for Life*'s take on executing the ideal fall, a maneuver virtually patented by Ned Overend, the six-time mountain bike national champion and three-time world champion, who went an entire career without breaking any bones:

- Slip out fast: Set up your pedals to get out of them easily in a crash. Clean them out, keep them oiled, and you can pull your foot out quickly and avoid a knee injury.
- Soft landing: Minimize impact when you hit the ground. Resist the temptation to stick an arm out; that'll risk a broken collarbone. Instead, keep your body in and try to let the handlebar and pedal hit the ground first. Before you hit, tuck your arm in and roll, letting your whole body absorb the blow.

Climbing

Lesson number one: Stay seated as you grind up a long hill. Avoid the desire to stand up and mash each pedal downward, stroke after stroke, until the hill's crest is reached. You will probably tire and be forced to stop long before you reach the top. You want to stay aerobic, not anaerobic, and to do that, you want to maintain a high enough cadence. Keep the butt glued to the saddle and try to recruit your gluteal muscles for additional power.

If you must stand up, learn to use your upper body to assist in each pedaling stroke. To do this, you will need to employ some side-to-side rocking motion. As you start the downward stroke, tilt the bike away from the foot making the stroke. Keep your body in a straight line over the weighted foot. Lean forward on the handlebars to deliver even more power, but keep your elbows relaxed. As the weighted foot finishes its stroke, shift your weight to the opposite foot and repeat the process.

Climbing dirt hills is different from going up paved ones. What happens is that the rear tire can start to slip due to a loss of traction. Don't stand up, since this places your body weight too far forward. Instead simply scoot back your rear end on the seat. Yet with all the weight concentrating on the rear, the bike's front wheel will have a tendency to lift off the ground. All of a sudden, you're doing a wheelie. The trailside secret, then, is to keep your weight balanced—lean your torso forward as you move your rear end back. Also keep your head up, since this will lower your center of gravity and distribute your weight evenly across the bike.

On steep sections, don't wait until you can barely pedal before shifting into a lower gear. Chances are, the chain will fall off and you will have to get off and walk.

Finally, try to maintain a good line. You shouldn't be looking right at the ground by your front wheel, but keep your gaze to about ten or fifteen feet up the trail. This will give you enough time to look out for obstacles. But yanking the handlebars back and forth to bypass an obstacle might cause you to lose balance and the bike to wobble out of control. Like Alex told me, think of the wheels as a stream passing over any obstacles. Obviously, big rocks and large, exposed tree roots will stop you right in your tracks, so the best option is to dismount or ride around them.

Descending

Cyclists can be divided into two groups: those who love blasting down descents and those who are cautious by nature and approach downhills with a mixture of dread and apprehension. "Over many years of teaching cycling skills, I've found that going downhill is one of the hardest things for new cyclists to get used to," says bike coach Alex Stieda on Bicycling.com. Stieda raced in the Tour de France, with the 7-Eleven team in 1986. Why the fear? "The reason is simple: Speed scares people. There are even some pros who don't descend correctly, because they're either nervous or don't practice it enough. Personally, I live for carving turns on a descent."

Stieda offered these suggestions for the gravity-challenged on road bikes:

1. Keep your hands in the drops—the lower part of the handlebars— since this will force your center of gravity to be nearer to the ground, "like a racecar." Having your weight more evenly distributed between the front and rear wheels helps maintain traction between the tires and road.
2. Look ahead, so you can have enough time to react if there's a pothole or debris in the road.
3. Avoid sudden braking; instead lightly "squeeze both levers equally with two- to three-second pulses. Constantly riding the brakes on big descents can make rims overheat—and possibly cause a blowout."

Cornering is where most cyclists run into a brick wall of terror. "It's the biggest mistake people make descending," continues Stieda. "They wait until they're in the middle of a turn to brake. If you have to brake in the turn, you didn't slow enough to begin with. Then, push your outside pedal down (right turn, left foot down) with pressure on that foot. To initiate the turn, lean the bike—not your body—into the turn (right turn, lean bike right). The faster and sharper the turn, the more you'll lean the bike. This action is similar to downhill skiing."

Descending hills on a mountain bike offers challenges of a different sort. Just like with road cycling, choose a line. Unfortunately, tree roots and deep ruts can snag a wheel. Hence you need to have good braking skills—but go easy on the front brake, since too much pressure will catapult you right over the handlebars.

For correct body English, keep your butt back to help balance the bike. Stay low, or maintain your body close to the bike. You don't want to be sitting upright. And while front or rear suspension systems may absorb the bumps and bounces, you can use your legs and arms as shock absorbers.

Personally, I'd rather prove my courage and mettle on uphills rather than downhills. (I obviously belong to the cautious camp.) There is nothing wrong with this preference. Speed was something I cherished during my younger riding days. I remember once getting up to forty-six miles per hour on a mile-long descent in Berkeley's Tilden Park. The front end of my road bike shimmied and went all squirrelly, but I pumped my legs harder. I wanted to go even faster and hit fifty. I loved the rush, the scary dance on danger's tightrope. Fortunately, I never took a spill during these solo road-warrior contests. Now that I was biking again, I knew that I wouldn't tempt fate like that on my rides. My goals changed. I rode slower, saner, more carefully. I was just happy to be riding—and I didn't want anything to interfere with this newfound feeling.

. . .

December 27, 2009

There are too many rude, impatient, and distracted drivers in the San Francisco Bay Area. Every one seems to be in such a hurry. Time and speed are measured much differently on the bike. I am fortunate that I live in proximity to all these great riding trails in Marin County—and far away from traffic. Biking this seemingly endless labyrinth of hilly dirt paths and fire roads is a perfect way to relax. Except for all the climbing!

As I write this, I have just come back from a two-and-a-half-hour mountain bike ride on Mount Tam. I was about ten miles from home, when the chain broke. Although I had brought a small chain tool, it was cold, foggy, and getting dark. I might have been able to fix the chain, using one of my small handlebar lights for illumination, but it would have been difficult to line up the tiny metal rivet and link-opening with chilled hands. And so, without bothering to make this rather minor trailside repair, I walked the disabled bike along the remaining uphill section for about a half hour, then coasted five miles down the mountain in the dark, constantly braking and dodging roots, rocks, and ruts on the wide Railroad Grade. I didn't see a soul. When I finally made it home, I was cold, thirsty, and tired, but all I could think was, "What fun! Can't wait to go riding again after fixing the chain."

ASK THE EXPERT

TESTING LANCE ARMSTRONG IN THE EXERCISE LAB: INTERVIEW WITH ED COYLE, DIRECTOR OF THE HUMAN PERFORMANCE LABORATORY IN AUSTIN, TEXAS

Lance Armstrong redefined the word comeback. His mental toughness, physical courage, cycling prowess, and charitable accomplishments are a vivid reminder that we all have the power not to succumb to life's disappointments.

Following a three-and-a-half-year retirement from racing, he returned to the sport as lean, mean, and hungry as before. Though he didn't win an eighth Tour de France in 2009, the thirty-seven-year-old Texan placed third, showing the world and detractors that it was foolish to ever count him out. He had been there before, a long shot defeating much more improbable odds by whipping testicular and brain cancer. Several weeks after the Tour, he won the toughest mountain bike race in the U.S.—the Leadville 100, with 14,000 feet of climbing at an average elevation of two miles. (Lance's mid-pack finish in the 2010 Tour, however, was marred by crashes, bad luck, and declining performance.)

I first met Lance at a bike show in Anaheim, California, in 1997. I was the editor of a multisport magazine called Winning *and wanted to see if he'd like to be interviewed in an upcoming issue. He immediately agreed. The cancer treatment had ended a year ago, but the bike industry was not welcoming him back with wide-open arms. He had split from his team, Corfidis, in a nasty, well-publicized divorce. There was skepticism about whether he could engineer a successful return to racing. At a press conference during this period, Lance defensively said, "I don't feel like damaged goods. I just feel like I am an out of shape person, which I am."*

Lance was shorter and slighter of build than I imagined, and boyishly handsome in a GQ-model way. His eyes seemed to reflect back the hardship of a long, difficult, and painful road from the cancer ward to the present. They also gave off the glint and steely determination of a fierce athlete. Like many others, I had my doubts abut how far he could go as a pro rider. He had yet to win the Tour. He had been away from riding for too long of a time. He had almost died. Though he had won the one-day World Championships, that was BC—Before Cancer. The three-week Tour de France? Highly unlikely.

As we exchanged phone numbers, the magazine story angle I pictured in my mind would center on his recovery and racing. According to news reports, doctors had given him less than a 40 percent chance of survival following the removal of a cancerous testicle and tumorous brain lesions.

Lance surprised everyone, though he knew all along that winning the battle against cancer is like winning not one, but multiple Tours. While many skeptics and naysayers claim that illegal drugs or blood doping played a role in his victories, he's always tested clean.

Lance kept in shape during his second hiatus away from racing—he ran the New York City Marathon twice (in 2007, he went a swift 2:46:43) and Boston Marathon once. Through his nonprofit foundation, LIVESTRONG, he has raised millions of dollars for cancer research and assistance to victims. He plans to compete in the Hawaii Ironman (he started out as a top junior triathlete).

Public curiosity about his private life surrounds Lance, just like any celebrity. But what was it like to work with him at the beginning of his storied career? Before Sheryl Crow. Before he made it a yearly custom of climbing onto the winner's podium on the Champs-Élysées.

Beginning in the early 1990s, Lance began making the first of eight annual visits to the Human Performance Laboratory at the University of Texas at Austin. Lance was twenty years old and fresh off from winning the one-day World Cycling Championships and U.S. Pro National Road Championships. The lab's director, Dr. Ed Coyle, put the young cyclist through a series of exercise tests designed to measure his heart and lung capacity, fatigue threshold, and muscle efficiency.

"Lance wanted to know what he could do to improve himself," Coyle told the New York Times in 2005. While Lance obviously has a considerable genetic advantage over the rest of us—his oversized heart can beat over two hundred times per minute, thereby delivering more blood and oxygen to his legs—Coyle recognized that his overall muscle efficiency wasn't all that special. But Lance soon learned to use his muscles more efficiently by using a high-cadence riding style that meant a shift to slow-twitch muscle fibers, which are more suitable for endurance than fast-twitch fibers.

Eight months after completing chemotherapy and radiation therapy, a worried Lance returned to Coyle's lab, wondering if the damage done to his body was irrevocable. Coyle found nothing alarming. Lance tested healthy. Moreover, in time, Lance continued to improve his slow-twitch muscle efficiency, which increased by 8 percent. In other words, Lance became a stronger rider. That 8 percent amount might seem trivial, but it made all the difference at the Tour and

*contributed to the greatest return to
fitness in professional sports history.*

*As lab director, Coyle had a priv-
ileged front-row seat to what made the
superhuman tick. For over a quarter-
century, Coyle, who is also a professor
in the Department of Kinesiology
and Health Education, has studied
and tested athletes, looking at physiological factors that both limit and
enhance human exercise performance.
Coyle believes that world-class endurance athletes will continue to get
faster due to improved training and
testing methods. Unlike most cautious-
sounding academics, he cherishes
making bold, provocative statements.*

Question: Were you surprised by
Lance's comeback after cancer?

Ed Coyle: No. I think one of his
biggest accomplishments, right up there
with winning his first and multiple Tour
de Frances, was that he finished fourth
in both the road race and the time trial
in the World Championships after his
first year of serious training after cancer. We had studied Lance on his
comeback when he was partially detrained, and so we had a good idea,
knowing where Lance had been, before
he had cancer. We could then extrapo-
late what he dropped down to in performance despite being normally
inactive, but then he had been training
at low intensity and higher volume for
about two months when we made our
eventual measurement, and so we were

able to make a prediction as to what
results we'd expect regarding VO_2 max,
lactate threshold, and what heart rate
would be at different power outputs.
Our predictions were right on. Lance
had come in really to see if there was
anything permanently changed or
wrong in him as a result of not just the
cancer, but also the chemotherapy. So
that's a pretty heavy responsibility for
us in the lab. I told him that I don't have
a real way of knowing that, but "we'll
measure you."

Q: How long was he away from
cycling?

EC: It was somewhere between nine
months and fourteen months. He had
begun training soon after his chemo,
but then he stopped for a while, and
then he resumed it a little bit, so it was
on and off for a while.

Q: So what kind of training?

EC: It was low intensity. Two to
three hours a day. He started with one
hour a day and he worked up to two
or three.

Q: What did you expect to see *and*
what did you find?

EC: We published the results in a research paper, "Lance Armstrong's Physiological Maturation" in the *Journal of
Applied Physiology*. His VO_2 max had
been around six liters a minute and
that correlates to about eighty-one
new liters to kilogram per minute And
with his reduced training, he dropped
down to 5.3 liters a minute, or with his
slightly increased body weight, it was

66.26 kilograms per minute. So, sixty-six is the value for an average Category 2 or 3 bike racer. But a pretty good Category 2 or 3 rider could not have a VO_2 max of 66, if he had experienced what Lance had been through, that is, had detrained and then resumed training only a little bit. When a good cyclist detrains, he reduces his VO_2 max down to around 50, 52, Lance probably never dropped his VO_2 max below 58 or 60.

Q: You mentioned in the study that he had a large heart and low level of lactate acid, which makes him so unique, physiologically speaking. What percentage of the elite athletic population has large hearts like his? Is he an anomaly or are there others who might someday follow in his footsteps?

EC: He's not an anomaly or a freak. Regarding his heart size, Lance's values are in the same range as probably at least a hundred other bicyclists. With his big heart, he probably had a genetic head start that he nurtured with years of intense training. And in addition to that, Lance had very low blood lactate levels and very good endurance, obviously, and low fatigue-ability. So yeah, we tested a number of athletes who have the same VO_2 max as Lance, or within that range, but I've never tested anybody whose blood lactate was as low as his at the end of exhaustive exercise.

Q: Let me digress a bit. What physically or chemically goes on in your body that creates that burning exhaustion associated with fatigue?

EC: The burn is a result of the sensory fibers, almost like pain receptors, in your muscle. They're responding largely to energy availability and acid and other chemicals. They are really the sensors of fatigue and they provide feedback to your brain, and essentially the brain is deciding how much blood needs to go to muscle, how fatigued you are. That level of muscle fatigue affects heart rate in addition to your perception of the pain, so it's a very important feedback signal. And that's one of the important adaptations to training. When you're fatigued and you are highly trained, your brain doesn't respond as much to it; so even though you still are fatigued, you'll suffer a little bit less. Trained people are also able to clear that acid faster from the muscle so that the length of time the muscle is fatiguing, or the length of time it takes one to recover, is markedly reduced.

Q: You told the *New York Times*—and I quote you—"One of the reasons for Lance's success was that he appears to have increased the proportion of his slow-twitch muscles from 60 percent to 80 percent, so he was using slow-twitch muscles for his power output."

EC: Right, and that was based not on changes in lactate acid per se, but to a given level of oxygen uptake and how much energy his body's expending, and so he was able to generate 8 percent more power. His muscles were becoming more efficient, producing more power at a given level of oxygen uptake, at a given level of body stress and fatigue—and that we think was due to the change in the chemistry of the muscle fibers. That 8 percent improvement over seven years in how much power he could generate—that's a big increase.

Q: You read about endurance athletes burning fat for energy. Excuse me for my lack of knowledge about the human body, but can you help the general reader understand the difference between burning fat for energy versus getting your energy from the muscles themselves?

EC: That really is an area that's very misrepresented and the public *should be* very confused. As it turns out, during exercise, trained athletes don't use much of their subcutaneous body fat—which is the fat you can grab below the skin. They don't use very much of that for energy. So that's a misnomer. When they're exercising intensely, and certainly when they're competing, they're not really using much of this tissue fat. What they are using is the fuel that is stored directly inside the muscle fiber because when you're going very intensely, you can only get a limited amount of energy coming from the blood, that is to say, from the fats in the blood or glucose in the blood. And so you rely on what's already there inside the muscle, and what's in the muscle is

glycogen and also some fat is stored in the muscle triglycerides.

Q: Fat is stored in the muscle fiber?

EC: Yes. And when we say training increases a person's ability to use fat, well it's not body tissue fat; it's those lipid triglyceride fat droplets inside the muscle fiber that are the source of the greater fat-burning. Trained subjects will use more fat only when they're going at low intensities, you know, with heart rates of 120 to 150, 160. The reason trained subjects go faster for the most part is because they can burn more glycogen without developing as much lactic acid or fatigue. So this whole story of "trained subjects burn more fat," yeah, well, they do and it's fat from inside the muscle.

Q: Did you test Lance after he won his first Tour de France?

EC: We studied him in November of 1999 and that was not the peak of his racing season. And essentially, his VO_2 max was back to where it had been when he was in top shape. We haven't tested him officially since then. But let me begin by saying that we found that the main thing that changed in him when we tested him over that seven-year period was his efficiency. He had been training intensely for years when he was a teenager, then as a triathlete. A few years of intense training is enough to raise your VO_2 max as well as raise your lactic threshold. And then after that, we think it's improving efficiency, which takes years and is the last part. So we had seen his muscle efficiency increase aggressively in a straight line throughout that seven years. But if you're asking me, did the line keeping going up straight or did it level off? I can't answer that.

Q: Do other professional cyclists come through your lab?

EC: A few professionals. We test more amateurs who are on their way to being professionals. So that's more of interest to us as to how they get there rather than studying them when they're there. I published at least twenty studies about bicyclists before we tested Lance; that's how we develop our theories: how efficiency is related to slow-twitch muscles and lactic threshold. In those studies, we tested almost all of the best U.S. amateurs. This was before professionals were allowed to ride in the Olympics.

Q: In labs across the world, are there other athletes who tested at Lance's level, because it just seems inconceivable that someone can win the Tour seven times in a row.

EC: I don't share that feeling.

Q: Why?

EC: That is not diminishing Lance's ability and what he accomplished. But for somebody to win seven times in a row, or for somebody to win just once, they really can't have a major weakness in their physiology. They have to be pretty well-balanced in their VO$_2$ max and their muscle efficiency, and certainly have psychological toughness.

Armstrong early on in his career was not prepared to win the Tour de France because his muscle efficiency wasn't very good and he didn't understand the psychology of riding for three weeks and how you have to use your teammates to get through that. And I think what Lance demonstrated is that once he decided that the Tour de France was the race he wanted to win, he focused on that more than any other race. And then he trained specifically in the way that you need to train to win the Tour de France, and he also developed the team who could best support him. What I mean by that is to win the Tour de France, you have to be able to time trial well and you also have to be able to not make some stupid mistakes, crash, have a bad day, or misjudge, and then most importantly, you have to be able to ride up steep mountains toward the end of the [stage] races for about twenty minutes faster than anybody else. You better break away on the steep climbs at the end. He made sure that he didn't have a weakness in any of those abilities, especially in his climbing ability. And one of the important things he did is that he lowered his body weight. When you're riding uphill, you've got to carry your body weight, so you look at how much power you have relative to your body weight. Any reductions in body weight have a direct effect on allowing you to go faster on the steep hills. I mentioned that his power increased by about 8 percent because he became more efficient, and he reduced his body weight by about 8 percent by mostly losing fat. With 8 percent more power, and 8 percent lower body weight, this meant that his power per body weight increased 18 percent over the seven years we studied him.

Q: Do you think another Lance will come along in the next decade?

EC: In the next decade? Gosh, I don't know!

Q: When you studied him after the cancer, you realized that there wasn't anything debilitating from the chemo or the radiation treatment.

EC: Correct.

Q: Was that a real surprise to you?

EC: Well, I'm not a physician and I didn't really know what to expect. After we'd done our tests and found that we didn't see anything wrong, we called his physician who said, "Well, of course there's nothing wrong. He's cured." Lance and his physician selectively picked the type of chemo that wouldn't scar the lungs. "What do you mean?" we asked. He said, "It's like he never had cancer; his lungs should be fine." And I even was a little hesitant to suggest that Lance go back to full-time training as intensely as he had been. I thought he needed to protect his immune system a little longer, but that wasn't even a consideration among his doctors or Lance. That was the same week that Corfidis dropped his sponsorship contract. But I'd like to make

one further point about Lance. He's not superhuman or freakish. You know, what is very remarkable is that he did not have a weakness; that he was able to resolve and balance himself so he was proficient and strong in every area he needed to be, and once he found that formula, he was able to repeatedly apply that formula to win the Tour de France. What I'm surprised at is how the sport of cycling hadn't really changed that much. Some of Lance's competitors would ride the Tour of Italy, the Tour of Switzerland before the Tour de France. Well, you know, that's something you may need to do when you're just starting out your first couple of years of professional racing and learn how to suffer, but the last thing you should be doing is riding the Tour of Italy before the Tour de France. Lance had put in his back-to-back races over the years, but he changed his focus to just one race. I'm just surprised how some of the training methods that had been typical of bicycling are not going to be the best way to win the Tour. Lance knew exactly what he had to be producing in terms of watts. He was confident riding at those wattages and actually riding on the specific climbs.

Q: A number of pro cyclists have been caught illegally adding blood to their bodies to increase their performance. What if somebody who was once sedentary decided, "Okay, I'm going to try to be fit, so let me get more blood in my body, perhaps another liter or two"?

EC: I wouldn't recommend doing this, but it would raise the person's fitness level. Essentially when you put more blood in the body, you're able to deliver more oxygen to the muscle. The more oxygen you deliver, the faster you can go in your sport. Untrained people are just as responsive as trained people to increased blood. With untrained people, their blood volumes are suboptimal, or below the optimal amount for maintaining stroke output, or how much blood the heart pumps per heartbeat. So when untrained people expand their blood, that is, if they reinfuse whole blood or even just red blood cells, they get a lot more benefit in delivering oxygen to the muscle. There is more oxygen in the blood with their heart pumping more ounces per heartbeat.

Q: Will we see amateur athletes and weekend warriors who want to do well in a 10K or century ride begin making visits to the local blood bank and saying, "Load me up, guys, for another liter. I got a race this weekend!"

EC: [Laughs.]

Q: Athletes are always looking for an edge, you know, a more expensive pair of shoes or bike, an energy drink, the latest training gimmick. So what about blood doping? I mean, kids use steroids in high school because they want to be pumped up. I just thought that blood

would be the next frontier of craziness that athletes would want to explore.

EC: Well, put it this way. The people who train only once or twice a week and just do it without a real plan and without a coach and not very intensely, well, performance-enhancing drugs or blood doping can raise performance by 5 or 10 percent, but training intensely for three months with a good coach and teammates will raise your performance 30 to 50 percent. Your body can improve in training so much more than anything accomplished with drugs or doping, because when you train, your body naturally raises its blood volume. So why would you want to go through all the trouble of drawing your own blood and reinfusing it and all that nonsense if you can just do nine hard workouts in three weeks?

Q: Do you run or bike?

EC: I ran in high school and college with a club for about twelve years and after that, I biked recreationally for about fifteen years. And now I'm playing tennis and doing yoga and trying to get my body back in shape for, hopefully, running.

Q: How old are you?

EC: Fifty-five.

Q: Playing tennis at fifty-five?

EC: [Laughs.] The best part is to be able to bounce around. I have to learn how to get a little more spring. But this old dog is trying to learn a new trick.

⑦

MOTIVATION

Gyms, Gizmos, Goal-Setting,
and How Hollywood Stays Fit

"Of course I'm not motivated. I'm paying you to motivate me."

—Client to personal trainer, overheard at a
24 Hour Fitness gym, as reported by the San Francisco Chronicle

Motivation is a slippery eel. Some of us have little difficulty sticking to a consistent workout schedule. Others allow the slightest distraction to intrude, and exercise gets postponed. That's one reason why goal-setting is critical for long-term success. It tends to outmaneuver or override these pesky daily diversions.

A 2009 *Runner's World* reader's poll asked, "What do you most want to improve?" Over 4,500 respondents answered as follows: 43 percent wanted to better their race times; 27 percent wished to increase their endurance; another 15 percent were looking at health benefits; 12 percent were focused on diet; and just 3 percent wanted to work on their attitude.

So let's look at some potential ways to crank up your motivation since this will help facilitate your fitness and health goals. But what works for one individual might have the opposite effect for someone else. The key to motivation is finding what excites you, and then turning that emotion into a regular habit. We'll begin with the gym. Some view health clubs as a secular temple of worship and pain. Others avoid these contemporary sweat lodges altogether. Maybe it's all those mirrors and perspiring bodies.

JOIN A GYM?

The siren's call of weight loss or fitness leads many of us to the gym. But gyms are a funny place. Depending on time of day and year, health clubs either percolate with souped-up testosterone or seem quieter than a Christian Science reading room. With the "New Year, New You!" mantra annually drummed into our post-holiday egg-nogged noggin, most gyms depend on January and February as their membership dues–paying cash cow. Gym owners know from past experience that most new members will soon stop coming in for their regular workouts. So it makes financial sense to lock in memberships early in the year.

> ### DON'T MAKE ANY NEW YEAR'S RESOLUTIONS!
>
> Fortune 500 corporate motivational speaker, bestselling author, and humorist Judy Carter not only hates gyms, but the self-described "Goddess of Comedy" urges everyone *not* to make any New Year's resolutions. She explained why in an email she sent to friends and clients in late December 2009:
>
> This year I'm going to . . .
>
> 1. Lose weight! This is stupid because 90 percent of diets end in failure. You have more of a chance of seeing Paris Hilton win a Nobel Peace Prize than keeping weight off. Plus, intense dieting ruins metabolisms. After so much dieting, now I have to jog fourteen miles to work off a Tic Tac I ate in 1999.
>
> 2. Exercise more! Have you ever wondered how gyms can sell thousands of new memberships every year and they never get crowded? Because people join and don't go. Take my advice—just walk to the gym and then walk back. It's cheaper and you don't have to listen to someone breaking wind while they're doing sit-ups.

To keep that revenue pipeline flowing, health clubs typically offer three membership options:

1. Initiation fee, monthly contract, and a monthly fee that's automatically debited from your credit card or bank account
2. Initiation fee and annual contract paid in full or spread out over time
3. Pay-per-visit, often in the form of a multi-visit pass

But here's the financial kicker: Even if you've stopped going to the gym though you signed up month-to-month or annually, your membership dues will most likely continue to appear on your monthly credit card statement.

Lesson number one: Ask questions and read the fine print of any health club membership agreement so you fully understand the contractual obligations. Even that "free" monthly or weekly trial can be misleading if you are required to hand over your credit card or bank information. You might still get billed when the trial period is over. Canceling can turn into a time-consuming headache.

Many clubs rely on high-pressure sales tactics. In exchange for what appears like a great deal, that fit-looking sales consultant will often pressure you to sign up right there on the spot. By all means, don't bite. Take the contract home. Scrutinize it carefully. Try checking out the competition. Visiting a new club for the first time is not unlike stepping onto a used-car lot. Try to avoid feeling intimidated if you are a newbie. Feel free to negotiate membership terms; you might be able to receive tremendous savings.

The best health-club membership option for many is pay-per-visit. That's the conclusion drawn from a three-year study of fitness clubs conducted by University of California at Berkeley's economics professor Stefano Della Vigna. After studying the records of nearly 8,000 gym memberships in the Boston area, the academic data cruncher discovered that "gym users on monthly plans pay 70 percent more than those pay-as-you-go plans based on usage."

Vigna published his findings in the *American Economic Review* (June, 2006)—hardly the kind of sweat-stained periodical one finds stashed in the reading bin by the stationary bikes. Since consumer behavior is not always based on rational decision-making, new gym members often fail to take into account declining interest in working out. "Gym members who choose a contract with a flat monthly fee of over $70 attend on average 4.3 times per month," explained Vigna. "They pay a price per expected visit of more than $17, even though they could pay $10 per visit using a 10-visit pass. On average, these users forgo savings of $600 during their membership."

The study produced another interesting set of results that reflect consumer habits. "Members who choose a monthly contract are 17 percent more likely to stay enrolled beyond one year than users committing for a year. This is surprising because monthly members pay higher fees for the option to cancel each month."

Seeking to explain this statistical anomaly, Vigna theorized that "overconfidence about future self-control" is the reason. In other words, those signing up for an annual membership might have set unrealistic fitness goals for themselves, and when they fail to reach these benchmarks, they become less motivated and more likely to quit than month-to-month users.

Vigna found that monthly users are reluctant to quit even if they stop working out. On average, just over two entire months elapse between the last club visit and contract termination for monthly members. Which means a monthly user can expect to lose two hundred dollars or more before finally deciding to throw in the membership towel.

Meanwhile, despite the recession and cutbacks in corporate-funded gym memberships for employees, the health club industry is going strong. About 17,000 clubs are now operating in the U.S., with memberships topping 32 million, nearly double the number from twenty years ago. But that number is misleading. Mark Lipanski, a personal trainer in Menlo Park, California, told the *San Francisco Chronicle* in 2009 that "about 12 percent to 15 percent of Americans own gym memberships, and of those, 40 percent actually use them. Within that group, less than half work out regularly and vigorously."

For gym newcomers, one of the biggest obstacles to overcome is the intimidation factor. In fact, there was a *Simpsons* Season 19 episode, "Husbands and Knives," that satirically raised this point. Marge immediately feels out of place and clumsy amid all the hard, muscular bodies at her new club. Her inept bout with the treadmill is a direct reference to the smash music video hit "Here It Goes Again" by OK Go. So she quits the gym and starts her own Springfield health club called Shapes, which is solely for out-of-shape "regular women" like herself. (Writers actually based it on Curves, the Waco, Texas–based women's only gym franchise with 10,000 centers worldwide.) Shapes becomes a wildly successful international business, and in turn makes Homer insecure about his own masculinity. Afraid of losing Marge to a younger, buffed "trophy husband," he undergoes a series of radical cosmetic surgeries, including stomach stapling and pec implants. Naturally Marge prefers the old, flabby Homer, and has the doctor reverse all the procedures.

Yet gyms, generally speaking, are non-judgmental venues. It's not like stepping inside a chic nightclub. Gym regulars are fairly focused on their own bodies. If there is a pick-up scene, it usually involves picking up weights or a medicine ball. The atmosphere is democratic, and clientele come in all sizes and shapes and ages.

Even if you are a newbie, you will encounter helpful, supportive fellow members and staff who will be happy to answer your questions or offer advice. Just ask. They know firsthand that getting in shape takes time, effort, self-discipline, and commitment. The fact that you are *at* the gym is adequate proof of your desire to become fit. Remember that old Groucho Marx line—"I don't care to belong to a club that accepts people like me as members." Well, with gyms, the opposite is true.

Going to a gym will also expose you to the latest equipment gadgetry and conditioning techniques, including circuit and core training, balance balls, yoga, Pilates, boxing, and even martial arts. One ultra-fit friend refers to his gym in Los Angeles as "a candy store of fitness." When a bum knee prevented him from running, he worked out on the elliptical machines and did pool running. Another pal, also in his early fifties, lives in Boston, and when it gets too cold to run outside in the winter, he heads to his local gym and uses the treadmill. "I can only last about twenty minutes, or two miles, before I get bored out of mind," he once told me. "I'd rather run for an hour by my house." He recently took up Pilates after seeing how much his extremely toned wife benefited from it. "Pilates works my entire body—and I mean *entire*," he added. "I can barely move afterward."

The most important thing you should know about joining a gym is that getting in shape is not something you can achieve overnight. It takes a steady, consistent, and balanced approach that should incorporate all facets of one's lifestyle—diet, job, relationships, stress management, and regular exercise. Yet we live in a consumerist-oriented society in which we're constantly being bombarded by marketing pitches promising instant weight-loss results if you follow this new diet or that radical workout program. These commercials and ads delude us into thinking that a model-perfect physique is no more difficult to acquire than buying a flat-screen television.

Bottom line: A gym membership won't make you fit within thirty or sixty days of joining. It's essential that you adjust your expectations accordingly.

Otherwise, you might possibly become discouraged and uninspired. If you are the type of person who likes adhering to a regular routine in a social setting, then the gym offers the ideal motivating environment to take control of your body.

A PERSONAL TRAINER CAN HELP
YOU STAY FOCUSED AND MOTIVATED

Should you hire a personal trainer to keep you motivated? A good trainer usually charges eighty dollars an hour. And what exactly do you get by working out with a personal trainer?

A friend from my U.C. Berkeley grad school days, John Seery, regularly started working out with one when he reached fifty-one. He's married, has two super kids, and is a professor of political science at Pomona College in Southern California. He sent me an email explaining why he used a trainer:

In my twenties until mid-thirties, I played basketball, softball, racquetball. No gym exercise at all, though some cardio machine work. Mid-thirties to early-forties, it was swimming and some mountain biking. Then, fortyish to fifty-one: gym, gym, gym, including cardio, with some swimming and occasional biking. At first, I wasn't inclined to use a personal trainer. I thought that my basic athleticism and determination would suffice for a good gym workout. But one falls into comfort zones and exercise routines, and workouts can then become inefficient or unchallenging. Jack, a competitive bodybuilder, who used to work at my gym, gently challenged me at one point to take my exercise "to the next level" by doing some personal training with him. At first I thought that was a concession: Isn't exercise supposed to be an enactment of one's willful determination? Something seemed inherently contradictory about turning to a helper. But for me, I found the main benefit was exposure to knowledge about form and technique. Since I'm not trying to bulk up at my age, my results aren't visible in that sense. But I definitely have much more muscle tone and definition, much better cardio levels—and my blood work shows vast improvements, too. I also feel great for the rest of the day— and sleep deeply on a regular basis. I do work out alone now, because I've internalized or remembered many of the lessons.

Bay Area personal trainer Kelly Mills believes that "the trainer should be able to help you assess your goals (like, is it realistic to lose 20 pounds in two weeks?) and come up with a reasonable way to meet them." In an article for the *San Francisco Chronicle*, she writes, "If you are new to fitness, your trainer might help you design a program for getting in some cardio exercise that works with your schedule, and cover the basics of weight training."

When it's time to make a serious commitment and you are seeking more than instructional tips, Mills says that "a good trainer can make you do what you cannot, or most likely would not, do on your own."

Motivation comes in many hues. So having a scheduled appointment that gets your butt into the gym on a regular basis makes sense.

Selecting a personal trainer is a matter of choice, not unlike finding a dentist or hairdresser. Hire one you feel comfortable with. Look for one with good people and coaching skills. Don't be wowed if the trainer has Popeye arms or to-die-for abs. Make sure that he or she is properly certified. Three organizations—the National Strength and Conditioning Association, the American College of Sports Medicine, and the American Council on Exercise—offer correspondence courses and require a comprehensive written exam for certification.

Like any relationship, you might experience friction with your trainer. If it doesn't pan out, find another one. As Mills suggests, "You need someone who listens to you, who works well with you, who knows when to push you and when to ease up, and who can help you do the best thing for you."

Of course, a personal trainer is not unlike a shrink. In their own manner, both persuade you to consider options that reside beyond your natural comfort zone. But two significant differences separate these professions: A shrink will tell you to get *on* the couch, whereas the trainer will demand that you get *off* the couch. The shrink often asks, "What are you *feeling*?" The trainer says, "*Feel* the burn!"

WORKING IT OUT IN HOLLYWOOD:
GETTING IN SHAPE FOR THE BIG SCREEN

Gyms and personal trainers are big business in Hollywood. Trainers often show up on film sets. They don't come cheap either. The top ones charge $500 per hour to motivate their clients. Former super-agent Mike Ovitz's martial-arts personal trainer actually ended up a movie star. Yes, him!—hulking, ponytailed, Buddha-buddy Steven Seagal.

(continues)

So let's roll tape for a quick look at some notable Hollywood fitness success stories.

Kirk Douglas wowed moviegoers in 1960 as the bare-chested, muscular slave in *Spartacus*. That well-oiled, chiseled body was sculpted with the assistance of personal trainer Harold Zinkin, who invented the Universal Gym Machine. Douglas continued using a personal trainer for daily workouts into his nineties.

A trainer helped Linda Hamilton acquire her shapely upper arms in *Terminator 2* by having her do countless pull-ups.

A weight-training coach assisted buzz-cut Demi Moore so she could strut her buff stuff as a Navy SEAL in *G.I. Jane*. (I have a friend who is a Navy SEAL, and he actually played Charlie Sheen's double in a movie about the SEALs. I asked him about the grueling physical on-screen punishment that Moore is forced to endure, such as carrying logs on the beach or experiencing near drowning. "Yes, it's tough," he said, "though there was a lot of Hollywood phoniness in *G.I. Jane*. But no, they don't have to do one-arm push ups.")

Jane Fonda's workout videos sold millions and inspired the aerobics craze in the early 1980s. Later came the film *Perfect*, which focused on soap opera hijinks inside a health club and a magazine loosely based on *Rolling Stone*. While Jamie Lee Curtis made a credible aerobics instructor, her buns of steel were not firm enough to save this cinematic dud.

Arnold Schwarzenegger leveraged his Mr. Universe bodybuilding physique into a number of '80s and '90s box-office hits, including *Conan the Barbarian* and the *Terminator* franchise.

Boxing and Hollywood have long gone hand in glove, dating back to the 1930s, but the genre was transformed when Sylvester Stallone launched *Rocky* and its moneymaking sequels. In a curious career move, Stallone went against casting to play an overweight cop in *Copland*, which required packing heat and a paunch. The film fizzled. The Italian Stallion quickly got back in shape to reprise his long-in-the-tooth Rocky and Rambo roles.

Robert De Niro, one of the most self-disciplined method actors, played boxer Jake LaMotta in Martin Scorsese's *Raging Bull*. He worked out constantly, gaining twenty pounds of muscle, and boxing 1,000 rounds at a New York City gym. When it was time to portray the retired, overweight LaMotta in this Oscar-winning performance, he gained sixty pounds in four months.

Hillary Swank, a top junior gymnast, also won an Academy Award as best actress for her realistic portrayal of the boxer Maggie Fitzgerald in *Million Dollar Baby*. To prepare for this demanding role, she gained nineteen pounds of muscle and trained for months in the ring.

Ditto with perennial big-screen hit-maker Will Smith in the biopic *Ali*. The popular actor put on forty pounds of hardened muscle with the help of a personal trainer. End result? A flawless impersonation of the Greatest's foot-shuffling, rope-a-dope style.

Russell Crowe went from being a pudgy cigarette-industry whistleblower in *The Insider* to kick-ass killer slave in *Gladiator*. In *Cinderella Man*, his boxing prowess shined with pugilistic perfection.

Mickey Rourke temporarily gave up acting to become an amateur boxer, then muscled his way back to a starring role as an aging professional grappler in *The Wrestler*.

Christian Bale wins honors as the reigning champ of fasting and bulking-up. He starved himself for *The Machinist*, losing over sixty pounds; then the human skeleton retooled his physique for *Batman Begins*. With the help of a trainer, the Welsh-born actor gained a hundred pounds of mostly muscle in six months. He then starved himself again to play a light welterweight in a boxing flick called *The Fighter*, which co-starred Mark Wahlberg, another actor and former Calvin Klein underwear model who takes his workouts seriously.

Yet too many bulging muscles can be a bad thing in Hollywood. Times change. Audience tastes change. Today's public wants its male stars cut and well-built, but not too pumped-up. Brad Pitt sported a smokin' hot bod in *Fight Club* and *Troy*, where soldiers wore short leather skirts in battle.

Former party animal Robert Downey shed twenty-five pounds and turned into a weightlifting ironman for *Iron Man*. His trainer, Brad Bose, devised a special workout regimen that involved wheeling a 600- to 800-pound wheelbarrow through an obstacle course, kettlebell swings, and pounding on tires with a sledgehammer. When it was time to depict a leaner look for his starring role in *Sherlock Holmes*, Downey switched to more traditional circuit-style training and higher reps.

Ben Stiller got pumped up in *Dodgeball*. But he didn't want too much bulk for his role as Tugg Speedman in *Tropic Thunder*, his trainer Sebastien Lagree told the *UK Telegraph*. "He is really fit, but he has really weird proportions—

(continues)

these long legs and short torso. Ben is really conscious of that, and he never wants to work his upper body too much because if you work his back and make his back too wide, it's going to make his torso look even shorter than it is."

According to two other celebrity trainers interviewed by the *Telegraph,* the chiseled physique male actors now want to copy is Daniel Craig who wore blue swimming trunks in one scene in *Casino Royale.* His 007 performance left female moviegoers feeling both shaken and stirred.

Motor-mouth Jeremy Piven, best known for his role as super agent Ari on *Entourage,* mixes it up with yoga and four-times-a-week gym sessions with a trainer who employs a variety of core and strengthening exercises.

A-list actresses Jessica Alba and Nicole Kidman used personal trainers to help them lose weight following pregnancy.

Talk show diva Ricki Lake melted away 127 pounds with a 1,200-calorie-a-day diet and by going on ninety-minute hikes, along with weight training, three times a week.

Renee Zellweger is Hollywood's workout queen. She swims, practices yoga, jogs up to five miles several times a week, and regularly hits the gym with circuit training.

But like with all things in Hollywood, there is a definite gender divide when it comes to fitness. "Men want a six-pack and abs," says Lagree. "The gut is the male obsession, while women are looking at their inner thighs, arms, everything—they want to be taut, but they really don't want to be manly."

"LIVING BY THE NUMBERS"— ## KEEPING TRACK OF YOUR PROGRESS

Long before there were GPS devices, mobile phone fitness apps, and do-it-yourself personal training websites, most athletes kept track of their training and racing in cheap spiral notebooks. I did for years. Each diary was dog-eared, and sported bike chain grease and spilled Gatorade.

With the digital age, the world of number crunching is at your nimble fingertips. Slip a Nike sensor chip into your shoes, and go for a run. Mileage data gets transmitted to your iPod Nano or iPod Touch. When you get back home, walk over to your computer and sync the data with iTunes and it automatically uploads the information to Nike servers. Click over to NikePlus.com and presto: you can view your entire running history—mileage, distance, calories burned. Over 1.2 million users currently track themselves on Nike's website, making it the world's most popular online destination for runners.

Wired magazine called Nike's mass data collection "living by the numbers—the ability to gather and analyze data about yourself, setting up a feedback loop that we can use to upgrade our lives, from better health to better habits to better performance."

Here's a list of additional motivating gizmos and websites that will assist you in monitoring workouts:

- The Garmin's GPS watch, the Forerunner, lets you store data that can be sent straight to your desktop.
- RunKeeper Pro is the iPhone's mobile fitness center. Using the GPS chip, the application tracks speed and distance.
- WeEndure is a social network site for runners that allows users to log data and compare their numbers with others.
- Fitbit records how many steps you take each day and the calories burned. The data gets wirelessly uploaded to its website. Similar portable fitness tracking devices are the DirectLife and BodyBugg.
- The Buddy Runner on T-Mobile's GI phone effortlessly charts your route, distance, time, and pace. Another one of its apps, the Cardio-Trainer, works like a virtual training partner as it records past runs and compares them to the present.
- Blackberry's AllSport GPS allows your mobile phone to track speed, distance, and elevation gain of bike rides, runs, and hikes.
- The *Men's Health* fitness app for the iPhone and iPod Touch includes eighteen workouts and instructions for 150 exercises. It's like having your own personal trainer at the gym, providing cues on proper weightlifting form.
- The McMillan running calculator, on the McMillan running website, estimates the pace of your training runs and uses your current fitness level to predict your race pace. The astonishingly precise calculator also lets you know your optimal running pace during training, including long runs, tempo runs, and recovery jogs.
- The ithlete is an ingenious iPhone app and iPod Touch device that measures heart-rate variability in a sixty-second test, and is a far more accurate gauge of health and fitness than checking your resting heart rate or pulse.

But while the technology has changed, the fundamentals of keeping a training log haven't. The journal should act as your conscience and personal coach. Just make sure that the journal doesn't take over your life, that it doesn't become more important to reach your weekly quota of miles or hours than to remain healthy. For example, say that you don't want to have this week's mileage fall off from the previous week, but you are nursing a slight fever and the weather is wet and cold; nonetheless, you feel compelled to go for a short run in the rain to make the week's goal. But this run makes you even sicker, and you then spend the next several days in bed. Let common sense, not guilt, be your guide. Your fitness log, whether displayed online or documented on paper or an Excel spreadsheet, can be forgiving and tolerant like a caring parent.

"A journal helps you grow by increasing motivation," notes Joe Friel, author of *The Cyclist's Training Bible* and *The Triathlon's Training Bible.* "Motivation comes from recording successes such as training goals accomplished through higher levels of training, subjective feelings of achievement, and personal race performance records." But, Friel continues, "Be forewarned. Training diaries can be abused. I have known athletes who realized on Sunday afternoon they were a few miles or minutes short of their weekly goals and so they went out for a short ride to reach their magic number. This is how you go about building 'junk miles.'" He recommends that you use the log or journal as a diary, not as a scorecard. Another area where training-journal obsessives often falter, in Friel's opinion, is improperly recording mental comments, which "should include unusual stresses in your life. Visiting relatives, working overtime, illness, sleep deprivation and relationship problems all affect performance."

PERSONALLY ASSESSING YOUR LEVEL OF FITNESS

Nothing better ramps up motivation than having specific fitness goals. Personally, one of my primary objectives was running up Mount Tam. But there are many other ways to test your fitness level that don't require running up a mountain. You can enter a 5K or 10K, or sign up for a charity bike ride. Think of these challenges as personal fitness report cards. You will most likely graduate to longer and more physically taxing events. This natural evolution is a pleasing byproduct of getting back in shape. For a quick self-assessment, try the President's Challenge "Adult Fitness Test." In 2008, the U.S. government launched an online test—www.adultfitnesstest.org—that focuses on aerobic

LOSE WEIGHT OR PAY UP!

Diet betting is in vogue. Here's how it works: You make a signed wager with one of your pals that if you don't lose a certain amount of weight by a set date, the other person collects on the bet. A study in a recent issue of the *Journal of the American Medical Association* discovered that those who had financial motivation to lose weight were much more successful at shedding pounds than those who did not. The likelihood of losing or gaining money was a powerful incentive for dieters. "The very simple fact [is] that people do not like to lose money," says the study's co-author, Dr. Kevin Volpp, an associate professor in behavioral economics at the University of Pennsylvania School of Medicine and the Wharton School.

The website StickK.com motivates people to make changes in their lives by signing contracts: If you fail in your goals, it costs you money. With over 20,000 users, the most common commitment contracts involve losing weight. StickK takes your credit card information and charges your card if you fail to meet your goal. Obviously, the site depends on the honor system, or you can select a third party to act as your referee. Users can choose a charity or friend who can collect on the bet should they fall short. But here's the interesting part: You can also choose a "foe or anti-charity" as the intended recipient. The website cheekily asks, "Wouldn't it just kill you to hand over your hard-earned money to someone you can't stand?"

---

fitness, muscular strength, and flexibility. The tests involve a one-mile walk (or running 1.5 miles), sit-ups, push-ups, "sit-and-reach" flexibility test, and body-fat composition. Once you've inputted your data, the site provides you with a national fitness ranking.

Many health clubs also administer private fitness tests. Some even sponsor club-wide competitions. Or you just might feel more comfortable testing yourself, though it's helpful to have someone else with you checking on your form or counting out reps. Fitness tests have long been part of America's phys-ed landscape. These exercise exams range from exceptionally difficult to moderately challenging. Some are mandatory for those seeking jobs in law enforcement, military, or firefighting. Minimum standards must be achieved to prevent washing out. Here are the most popular ones.

- *Marine Corps:* You'd expect that the Corps would demand tough conditioning standards for its fresh-off-the-bus recruits. Think again. Guys between the ages of seventeen and twenty-six must only be able to do three pull-ups, forty sit-ups in two minutes, and run three miles in twenty-eight minutes, while ensuring their body fat doesn't exceed 18 percent. *Semper* Sigh.

- *Army Physical Fitness Test:* The APFT is a three-event physical performance test used to assess endurance and strength, while providing a baseline for Active Army soldiers and Active Guard/Reserve who are required to take the APFT at least twice each year. The test uses a 100-point measuring system per event. Planning to score a perfect 100 in each of them? Then, if you are say, between the ages of twenty-seven and thirty-one, you must be able to do seventy-seven push-ups, eighty-two sit-ups, and run two miles in 13:18. (Fancy that—the Marines make you run an additional mile!) For age and point scoring info, go to http://www.benning.army.mil/usapfs/Training/APFT/.

- *Harvard Step Test:* Decades before StairMasters and VersaClimbers began showing up in gyms, this five-minute step test was developed at the Harvard University Fatigue Laboratory during the Second World War. The test is simple: you step up onto a bench (forty-five centimeters high) and back down continuously for five minutes. One minute after finishing the test, take your pulse for thirty seconds to count beats per minute (BPM). This is Pulse 1. Two minutes after finishing the test take your pulse for thirty seconds. This is Pulse 2. Three minutes after finishing the test take your pulse for thirty seconds—Pulse 3. The changes in heart rate over these three periods show your heart-rate recovery time; a fit person experiences fewer BPMs and quicker recovery. To calculate your score, go to the test section of http://www.brianmac.demon.co.uk and enter your results.

- *Cooper Institute's "Fit for Duty":* Dr. Kenneth H. Cooper coined the term "aerobics" in 1968 to measure healthy and harmful levels of exercise. The Dallas-based Cooper Institute later devised a "Fit for Duty" testing standard that is used by law enforcement agencies. To place in the top 99 percentile (according to a recent single-norm database survey of 2,400 law enforcement officers from twenty agencies), you must be able to have a 28.1-inch vertical jump, run three hundred meters in thirty-six seconds, sit and reach 22.7 inches, crank out sixty-two push-ups and forty-five sit-ups, single bench press 1.07 times your weight, and run 1.5 miles in 9:07 (www.cooperinst.org).

- *Navy SEALs*: Many of the nation's best-conditioned soldiers are Navy SEALs. Combined with sleep deprivation, the physical testing is so rigorous that only twenty-five out of a hundred recruits pass—an astonishing 75 percent failure rate. When a candidate can't take it anymore, he rings the infamous bell near the beach and his SEAL dreams are toast. Here are the absolute minimums for BUD/s (Basic Underwater Demolition) SEAL training physical testing, with average competitive scoring numbers following in parentheses: five-hundred-yard swim using breast- or sidestroke in 12:30 minutes (8:00), 10 minute rest; minimum of forty-two push-ups in two minutes, two minute rest (100); minimum of fifty sit-ups in two minutes, two minute rest (90 to 100); minimum of eight pull-ups with no time limit, 10 minute rest (15 to 20); run 1.5 miles wearing boots and fatigues in 11:30 (9:00 to 10:00). After successfully passing these physical hurdles, SEAL hopefuls are then required to pass more difficult training segments such as the land-warfare phase in which they must run fourteen miles and swim 5.5 miles.

- *Smokejumpers:* They are the airborne elite of wildlands firefighters, parachuting into the hottest hot spots with their gear. To be eligible for this prestigious yet hazardous position, all smokejumper candidates must have substantial firefighting experience and be able to pass the standard smokejumper physical training (PT) test on the first day of smokejumper training. Candidates must do a minimum of seven pull-ups or chin-ups, forty-five sit-ups, twenty-five push-ups, and run 1.5 miles in less than eleven minutes. The test is taken in one time frame with five-minute breaks between specific exercises. Smokejumper candidates must also be able to carry a 110-pound pack a distance of three miles in ninety minutes or less, over a level course.

TAKE THE STAIRS

Ever since Rocky Balboa immortalized the steps at Philadelphia's Museum of Art, athletes have flocked to other steps in cities. These vertical-challenging workouts are outdoors, free, and guaranteed to turn your legs into pudding. One of the oldest running races in America, the 7.4-mile Dipsea in Mill Valley,

California, begins with a quad-tiring 671 steps. Each year, an invitation-only field of just over three hundred runners races up the stairs of the Empire State Building. Competitors must climb eighty-six floors, with the winner finishing in around ten minutes. The rest of the year, due to post-9/11 security concerns, the building's stairwell is off-limits to the public.

If you want indoor steps, the gym is one venue. The StairMaster used to claim a popular place in the health club until it was replaced by the elliptical trainer, which is easier on the lower body. Only fit masochists attempt the VersaClimber for more than ten minutes. But if it's a free indoor workout you want, nothing beats climbing the stairs of your favorite high-rise—condo, hotel, or office building. Some places require permission from the property manager. One cautionary reminder: Going up the stairwell like a billy goat is much better for your knees than going down. You should take the elevator down.

"Stair climbing will give you a little more bang for your buck because of the vertical component," said Cedric Bryant, chief science officer for the American Council on Exercise, in an interview with the *New York Times.* "Compared to jogging or cycling at a moderate pace without much of an incline, stair climbing will be a bit more challenging and therefore allow you to burn more calories for that same amount of time."

According to the *Times,* a growing number of running events, many of which benefit charities, are held in skyscrapers in Taipei, Milan, Chicago, Las Vegas, Denver, and, yes, Philadelphia.

Doing stairs is ideal cross-training for the heart and lungs, and will help strengthen the gluteus, quadriceps, and calf muscles. Bryant told the *Times* that "walking up stairs at a moderate intensity should burn 5 calories a minute for a 120-pound person, 7 for a 150-pound person, and 9 for a 180-pound person. The impact on knees and feet is relatively low, with the pressure equivalent to two times one's body weight walking up stairs. The pounding on the body going downstairs, however, equals six or seven times one's body weight." Hence, the elevator will save your joints and give you time to rest before you tackle the stairs again.

GO WITH THE GROUP

You might want to join a bike, running, or triathlon club; masters swim team; or fund-raising organization. Wall Street trader Bruce Cleland founded the Leukemia Society's Team In Training (TNT) in 1988 after his youngest daughter, Georgia, then two, was diagnosed with leukemia. Looking for a way to raise money for the local Leukemia and Lymphoma Society chapter, Cleland came up with the idea of combining fund-raising with his personal dream of running the New York City Marathon. Out of shape and overweight, the former rugby player recruited other former jocks to join his cause, which he named Team In Training. Coached by New Zealand running great Rod Dixon, Cleland's group of thirty-eight aspiring runners completed the 1988 marathon while raising $325,000.

Under the direction of the Leukemia and Lymphoma Society, similar TNT fund-raising efforts rolled out in other cities. Participants receive coaching in running, triathlon, and cycling. The goals are to raise money and get in shape for a big-city marathon, half-marathon, century ride, or triathlon. Team In Training has trained over 400,000 participants and raised over $850 million. Cleland himself has raised over $1 million, the most of any individual. Currently, Cleland, fifty-eight, speaks at pre-marathon TNT pasta parties throughout the country, and lives in Towson, Maryland, with his family, including Georgia, who is twenty-one and cancer-free. "A lot of people who join TNT don't have an athletic background," he says, "but they have big hearts and amazing spirits."

Launched in 1983 in Dallas, Texas, with 800 participants, Susan G. Komen for the Cure 5K fitness runs and walks promote breast cancer awareness. It's now the largest series of 5K runs and fitness walks in the world, in over a hundred cities and with over 1 million runners and walkers since 2005. For the super-motivated, there are three-day walks that cover sixty miles. Participants often train together in their local areas. Coaches are available for training assistance.

TIME MANAGEMENT

What often erodes motivation is a self-defeating loop of procrastination. Who hasn't used this excuse: "I don't have time to run or go to the gym because I have too much to do at work." But sacrificing your workout so you can answer all those emails is a mistake. Instead of carving time out of your busy week for training, you create even more reasons not to get on the bike or go for a run. This will only jeopardize your return to fitness. Your goal is to pry yourself away from the desktop, BlackBerry, iPhone, or iPad.

"The reality is that most people don't need more time, they just need to re-prioritize the time they've got," says Jeffrey Gitomer, author of *The Sales Bible* and *Customer Satisfaction is Worthless, Customer Loyalty is Priceless.* The basic underlying principle of time management is "do what's important first." Make that in-box so yesterday. Ever notice that CEOs in Hollywood movies have desks the size of aircraft carriers but with nary a scrap of paper in sight. Maybe a Mont Blanc pen holder, but that's it for the clean-desk club. Learning to prioritize your workload streamlines productivity and saves time.

You need to unshackle yourself from superfluous information and data overload, or to empty what is known as your "collection buckets," says David Allen, productivity guru and author of *Getting Things Done.* The best way to make that happen is "do it, delegate it, and defer it" so long as it appears later on an action-item list.

A time log is also an effective way to see where time escapes your grasp. Looking to find not just extra minutes in the day, but extra hours? All that downtime spent on Facebook, Twitter, or Hulu can add up to large chunks of wasted productivity. To help manage digital distractions, there's a software program called RescueTime that records everything you do on the computer. For those lacking self-control when it comes to the keyboard, you might want to try LeechBlock. You tell this stern net nanny which sites you should be prohibited from seeing, and it won't let you visit these selected websites during certain periods of the day.

"CREATIVE" WALKING, RUNNING, AND CYCLING

Try treating your hikes, runs, and bike riding as if you were on an adventure. Sample new trails and back roads. It's awfully boring to remain trapped inside the same workout cage that confines you to an inflexible workout. If you only run on a treadmill or ride on a stationary bike, your training will inevitably grow stale. Instead, strive to make connections with the natural world in a myriad of ways—through exploration, curiosity, and beauty. The average recreational cyclist can benefit by viewing the bike as a means, not as an end in itself. Of course, reaching your destination is important, but you don't want to be so hard-pressed by this goal that you miss out on all the interesting things you might notice along the way.

If you like riding, use your bike to commute or do local errands. You don't need to be a five-days-a-week bike commuter. By simply integrating one or two commute rides per week, you can find yourself getting stronger on the bike; work and working out make an ideal tandem. A bike commute of five or ten miles in the morning will energize you better than a jumbo latte, anyway. You'll be luxuriating in an endorphin high while your colleagues are swilling the black stuff to stay alert. The ride home will do wonders to help alleviate job stress. You don't have to worry about traffic. You'll sleep better.

NEED VERSUS WANT

During my own return to fitness, I'd often turn to my pal Tim, an endurance sports journalist who used to be a serious marathoner (3:24 PR) for either a motivational pat on the back or swift kick in the butt. He knew me when I was fit and we competed in triathlons together, and we frequently talked on the phone during that long, barren, ten-year stretch when I stopped working out. But as I climbed out of the hole of inactivity, he was there in spirit and as a sounding board. Sometimes, I would call him after I went on a long run, feeling giddy with a sense of accomplishment. Then there were the darker days when I'd tell him that I didn't feel like exercising, and he would berate me, saying that I was still in a precarious, fragile state and that I *needed* to run or bike, or else the entire house of cards would collapse. It was a matter of necessity to keep to a routine. He wanted me to succeed—as a friend, or maybe even vicariously since he had fallen off the fitness wagon. Who knew exactly?

One morning, several months into my comeback, as I was loping along in the middle of an easy forty-five-minute run, I thought about that word *need*. This made me wonder, "How is *need* different from *want*?" Because when I woke up that morning, I *wanted* to go for a run. There was no inner conflict or fierce tug-of-war between guilt and desire. I just felt like running.

Seeking clarity about these dueling concepts—need and want—I called Tim when I got back from the run, and asked him to help parse the difference.

Here's a summary of what he said:

"You may need to work out. Desperately need to. But you won't work out until you want to. You may know intellectually that you enjoy working out and you want to. Getting from need to want may be the hardest challenge in sports. Because it's a mental challenge to set up the mind-set. You have to build a habit."

Tim then used a metaphor. "A habit is like a NASA space suit. You can't survive in space without it. Likewise you cannot survive an exercise or running program without being equipped with a habit." (I liked where he was going.) He continued, "A habit is like self-hypnosis. You know you will enjoy working out. But you need to create that knowledge, a hunger, in your subconscious. Someone beginning a fitness regimen after a prolonged period of neurotic inactivity is like a crack addict tiptoeing past a drug-buying alley. One or two days off, your body craves the old drug of inertia. When the habit is self-sustaining, you have hurdled that chasm from need to want. It's a good place to have arrived at." Tim's brief riff was strong motivational medicine.

A DOG'S LIFE: ROCKEE WAS THE PERFECT TRAINING PARTNER

I've had only one utterly dependable training partner: a golden retriever named Rockee. We were joined at the hip for fourteen years and 7,000 miles of running together. Rockee was a seventy-pound bundle of crazy canine love, with a white clown face that turned even whiter as he got older.

His death on May 10, 1996, as I mentioned earlier, set into motion my long fitness decline. In the absence of his woof, my motivation went poof. Several friends often asked, "Bill, why don't you get another dog?" One part of me really wanted to, but the prospect of losing another long-time companion like Rockee was simply too painful to relive. I preferred moping about with a tail between my legs.

But the truth was, I missed having a terrific workout pal like Rockee, especially on Mount Tam's trails. He never once complained if we ran too far, or if I was going too slow. I never heard him go on and on about an injury, like so many runners do. He never bellyached if the weather was too hot or too cold. He just loved to run. His limitless energy and unflagging enthusiasm were inspiring to behold.

While a Jewish mother can slay a son with guilt, she doesn't even come close to the emotional manipulation generated by looking into the large brown eyes of a golden retriever. Those soft, imploring orbs forced me into my running shoes and out of the house on countless occasions when all I wanted to do was relax indoors with a book or magazine. It was impossible to let him down. Rockee was like having my own full-time, live-in personal trainer, though one who constantly shed blond hair and liked sleeping in my bed. That was one reason why getting back in shape had initially been such a challenge. Without Rockee's importunate stare prodding me to get off my butt, I had to locate and act upon the motivation from within.

Perhaps you will want to get a dog if you honestly believe that it will help you become fit. By all means, please do so. Certain breeds and mixes are better suited for hiking and running. Don't expect a pug, bulldog, or dachshund to run a 10K with you.

Suzi Thibeault, elite ultrarunner and dog trainer, told *Runner's World* that not all dogs are naturally born runners. "A great running dog depends on three things: genetic temperament, socialization and training. Some dogs are born with easygoing personalities. That's how some people get away without training or socializing their dogs. But if your dog doesn't have the temperament, you've got an uphill battle ahead of you. In the worst-case scenario, you'll see someone running with a loose large dog who likes to clip people on the knee and bowl them over. Much more often, you'll see a dog dragging someone down the trail or the road."

I always ran with Rockee leashed if we were running on city streets or bike paths. He trotted at my right side, and I would try to ensure that there was some slack in the leash—but he invariably would want to run ahead, so it often turned into a battle of wills—me pulling back on the leash, him straining against his collar. On hiking trails, it was an entirely different story: He ran unleashed, also by my right side, just behind my right hand. If I raised it high and said "Go Rockee," that command meant instant freedom and he could go wherever he wanted, and that usually meant fifty or a hundred yards ahead to check out new smells—and away from me! Who could blame him? A dog's sense of smell is two or three hundred times more powerful than a human's. Would you like to run next to someone for two hours whose body odor overwhelmed your olfaction? The only thing I didn't like about Rockee's freedom romps was his eagerness to roll in cattle or horse dung. I was never able to curb him of that disgusting habit.

If you are keen on having Fido as your fitness partner, Thibeault suggests first asking yourself these important questions: "Does the dog want to run, and, two, can you train the dog to run safely with you and around other dogs in public? The best running dog wants to be with you—not chasing squirrels or deer."

So which breeds does Thibeault favor? "Any dog that's been bred to work athletically and to respond to people is likely to make a good running partner." These include labs, retrievers, Doberman pinschers, German shepherds, collies, and shelties. And the one she runs with? Boston terriers. "They've got it all," she says. "An 80-pound dog in a 15-pound package."

· · ·

(continues)

If you've never had a dog, and are seriously thinking about purchasing one, then allow me to be of some assistance. Owning a dog will change your life. It did with me. Rockee was my first dog. Or rather, he was my birthday present to my girlfriend. Costing just sixty-five dollars, Rockee was the last claimed pup from a litter of eight. But when she left me two years later, she said, "He's *your* dog; you take care of him. I won't have time in law school." All those nights of Rockee crammed between us in bed, either as a barrier or bridge to affection, were replaced by new, less crowded sleeping accommodations: a man and his dog.

A dog's life can be either good or bad. It all depends on who's in charge. I was Rockee's boss, the pack leader, though his response to my alpha status wavered between rapt obedience and sly rebellion, like in the kitchen where he remained a criminal at heart. Sticks of butter marked his favorite scores. He liked misbehaving because he knew he'd get away with it. I was a slack disciplinarian who tolerated his wayward antics. I never wanted his unruly independence corralled or choke-chained—indoors or outdoors.

He knew more about me than I knew about him. He was willful, indulgent, spoiled, and always happy. Dark moods were foreign to him. He never held a grudge or faulted me for anything. I never once heard him scold me for not doing the dishes or forgetting to take out the garbage.

I liked to dress him up in T-shirts, swim caps, and sunglasses. He attended numerous triathlons. He once appeared in a local charity dog fashion show that aired on MTV.

I nearly lost my life protecting him from a vicious, unprovoked assault by a rottweiler in Oakland. It was past midnight and we were walking by the train tracks near the warehouse loft where we lived amid artists. Out of the darkness skulked this Cujo demon dog. I found out later that it belonged to a night watchman at a nearby office building. As the menacing beast moved toward us, I grabbed Rockee's collar and waited for the worse. The rottweiler went straight for Rockee's throat, clamping down hard with its powerful, wide jaws. I knew that Rockee would be dead in seconds. Still holding onto Rockee, I tried shoving my hand into the attacker's mouth, but it wouldn't let go. It was a death grip. I thought that I was going to die as the three of us rolled around on the ground. I started screaming for help. I really don't know what happened next because everything flashed by in a blur, but a neighbor, who heard my cries, came over and struck the rottweiler with a stick. The beast finally let go of Rockee and walked off into the darkness.

I don't have any children, but on that terrifying night I was ready to sacrifice my own life for Rockee. An ambulance took me to the hospital for an overnight stay (I got a broken nose and bloodied scalp and fingers) but Rockee was safe and alive.

• • •

Let's return to that sixty-five dollars for a moment. In fourteen years, that figure telescoped into excess of $20,000. Money went to vets, kennel boarding, extra-large airline travel cases, forfeited security deposits from landlords, leashes, collars, ruined clothes, dry cleaning bills, ripped window screens, trashed doors, flea and tick shampoo, flea and tick defogger canisters, dog sitters, anti-barking electronic device, water and food dishes, approximately four tons of dog food, doggie treats, one pound of fresh hamburger meat from Safeway, Domino's pizzas, Slim Jim beef jerky, arthritis medicine, dog tags, two-foot-long jumbo rawhide chew toys, a carpeted dog house, two new sofas, water bowls, combs, and blankets. Rockee was worth every one of these monetary indulgences.

I took Rockee running the second day he entered my life. We managed only one mile since it required a great deal of coaxing and gently tugging on his leash. But then I noticed that his tender puppy paws had become abraded from the rough texture of the sidewalk, so I ended up carrying him home. Yet within several months, he became my regular running partner, which was especially useful since I was training for the 1982 Ironman. Each time I took out my Asics shoes, running shorts, or bandana, he'd go into wild paroxysms of insane delight, bouncing up and down, twisting and corkscrewing in midair like a demented acrobat.

Rockee was an Irondog. While living in Boulder, we liked going on weekly two-hour runs in the foothills. One of our more memorable runs was an eleven-miler during a blizzard. Wind chill had lowered the temperature to around zero. Orange plastic booties protected his paws, but the footwear became frozen and useless. Every mile or so, I'd stop to remove the caked snow between his paws. As we battled our way back home through the icy teeth of the blizzard, it felt like we were living inside a Jack London story.

(continues)

Rockee ran until he was about thirteen-and-a-half years old. Then arthritis made it too difficult. His rear legs would sometimes buckle during short walks, or he'd procrastinate more than usual near his favorite bushes. He could no longer jump up into the passenger seat of my jeep. I would have to lift him each time. It was sad to witness his physical decline. Old age had snared him.

Even though he could no longer walk very far, it didn't mean he still couldn't enjoy and experience Mount Tam. I called several local bike stores, and found one in Mill Valley that had a two-wheel children's bike trailer in stock. The person on the phone said it could accommodate a child up to eighty pounds. I didn't mention that it was for my dog. I would tow Rockee up Tam on my mountain bike.

As soon as I got home with the Burley trailer, I hitched it behind my bike and lifted Rockee onto the seat of his new set of wheels. "I'm your beast of burden now," I said. The uphill pedaling was hard due to the excess weight. But I was in good biking shape. We gradually inched up the mountain. Rockee sat upright in his off-road chariot, beaming like a proud Roman general. A number of hikers stopped and said things such as, "That must be a special dog," or "You must really love your dog." I basked in the praise.

Rockee and I never made it to the top. We still had three miles to go. It was getting dark and the cycling was more tiring than I had imagined. I apologized to him that we would have to turn around and go home. Rockee didn't seem to mind. He was thrilled by the speed and rushing air during our half-hour descent.

The following morning, Rockee had trouble standing. His nose was dry and he was panting. He then went into a minor convulsion. His breathing became more rapid. I put down the buttered bagel I was eating and quickly carried him to my jeep. We drove to the Mill Valley Pet Hospital. It wasn't yet opened so we waited on the front steps for an hour. I cradled Rockee in my arms. He was growing weaker.

As soon as the vet arrived, we hurried into the operating room. The vet lifted Rockee onto a stainless steel examining table. His once bright red tongue hung listlessly off to the side, a gray ugly thing. His raspy panting lessened to slow, quiet breathing. I pleaded for him to hold on as he disappeared to a faraway place. He had run away many times in the past, but this time I knew that he wasn't returning home.

The vet jabbed a needle into his hindquarters and dark blood quickly filled the syringe. "It looks like his spleen has burst," he said. "He's lost a lot of blood. The likely cause is probably from an undetected tumor. Unfortunately, it's too late to operate."

I had trouble comprehending his words. I strained to hear something else, a different prognosis that would offer hope.

"Let's just make his last minutes peaceful."

I tearfully nodded okay.

The vet slipped a small green oxygen mask over Rockee's nose. His labored breaths came slower, then finally stopped. He died with his eyes wide open. His body was still. Rockee was dead. Without saying anything, I dashed out of the pet hospital and sat in the parking lot by my jeep. I wept for over an hour. An emptiness spread inside me and just kept increasing. An unfathomable sadness, I realized, would be my new companion.

I wanted to dig a hole in the ground and hide inside it. I wanted to howl in pain, cruise the neighborhood and lift my leg at Rockee's regular marking spots. I wanted to be stroked and petted and comforted. I didn't know what to do. Instead I checked into a San Francisco motel for several days because I didn't want to return to an empty house and see his red leash hanging by the door or his orange water dish on the kitchen floor.

Later in the week, I went back to the bike shop with the Burley trailer and explained to the manager why I no longer needed the $300 trailer. He accepted the trailer and issued a credit card refund. "Sorry for your loss," he said.

A decade later on Tam's trails, now that I was running again, I often imagined seeing Rockee trotting at my side. We sure made a great team, I'd reminisce. Every now and then, if I happened to run past one of his favorite streams, I'd pause and see him charge into the shallow water. He would plop down into the creek bed and look back at me with his wonderful smile. "You won't mind if I linger here a bit?" he seemed to ask.

Memories are man's best friend.

⑧

BUILDING AN AEROBIC AND STRENGTH BASE

Doing It the Right Way

"Do my exercises every day, I do. Push ups and bends, all that sort of thing. And when I'm in the shower, I do a good bit of shouting, singing, and poetry reciting."

—*Richard Burton*

I was perplexed. Despite several months of biking and running, averaging four or five hours of training per week, I required frequent rest days. My legs needed recharging between workouts. For example, if I biked ninety minutes, it meant a minimum of two or three off-days before I felt rested and ready for another workout. The same thing happened after running for forty-five minutes. I wondered why my muscles weren't recovering more quickly. Was the fatigue and lingering soreness due to age? Or was there something I was doing incorrectly with my training?

To solve this predicament, I once again turned to wellness guru and multisport wise man Dr. Phil Maffetone. "What can I do to ramp up my fitness?" I asked him. He responded with just three words: "heart-rate monitor." Not that I was listening. I never wore a watch while running or biking. Nor could

I see myself becoming entangled in technology's seductive web. But I wondered if I were just being stubborn for all the wrong reasons by rejecting a monitor without ever trying one. Perhaps using a heart-rate monitor would improve my training. So one day, I went online to Amazon.com, and after reading a number of monitor reviews, I bought a Timex T5J031 Unisex Digital Fitness Heart Rate Monitor. It cost sixty dollars. I emailed Phil news of my purchase. He immediately replied, "That's cheap for all the fat-burning, muscle-strengthening, endurance-generating, aerobic-developing, stamina-producing, health-promoting, and fitness-forming benefits."

To learn about the basic principles of a heart-rate monitor, I read the chapters on heart-rate monitors in the most recent edition of Phil's book, *In Fitness and In Health*. Here's a summary of the three major points:

1. As important as it is to keep most workouts aerobic, most people do just the opposite. Instead of programming their bodies to burn fat and spare sugar, they are developing their anaerobic systems to burn more sugar, and less fat. Normally, the body produces oxygen-free radicals in response to many stresses, including anaerobic exercise. Too many of these free radicals contribute to degenerative problems such as inflammatory conditions.
2. The level of exercise intensity will dictate how your body reacts to that exercise session during the next twenty-four hours.
3. Performing aerobic exercise is a key to developing the aerobic system. [But] how can you be sure your exercise is aerobic? Trying to monitor your heart rate by stopping to take your pulse is often not very accurate. If you are just one or two beats off in a six-second count, that's a difference of ten to twenty beats per minute!

Phil first began training endurance runners with bulky heart-rate monitors in the early 1980s. Based on performance data, he devised the "180 Formula" to accurately find the optimal heart rate, which, when not exceeded, will give one optimal aerobic and fat-burning benefits. He explains:

Many athletes are familiar with the 220 Formula to calculate heart-rate intensity; you subtract your age from 220 and multiply the difference by a figure ranging from 65 to 85 percent. The resulting number supposedly provides you with the training heart rate. But this formula contains two serious errors. It assumes that 220 minus your age is your maximum heart rate. In reality, most people who obtain their maximum heart rate by pushing themselves to exhaustion (I don't recommend you do this) will find it's probably not 220 minus their age. The second inaccuracy is the percentage multiplier. This arbitrary figure doesn't consider a person's overall health or fitness. Most people opt for the no-pain, no-gain approach and guess at a number that offers a higher heart rate. Rather than guess, it's best to use a formula that is not only more sensible, but has a proven success record and is more scientific: the 180 Formula.

This method also considers physiological rather than just chronological age. To find your maximum aerobic exercise heart rate, first subtract your age from 180. Next, find the best category for your present state, as follows.

Calculating Your Maximum Aerobic Heart Rate:

1. Subtract your age from 180.
2. Modify this number by selecting one of the following categories:
    a. If you have, or are recovering from, a major illness (heart disease, any surgery or hospital stay, etc.) or if you are on any regular medication, subtract 10.
    b. If you have been exercising but have been injured or are regressing in your efforts, or if you often get colds or flu, or have allergies, or if you have not exercised before, subtract 5.
    c. If you have been exercising for up to two years at least four times a week without any injury, and if you have not had colds or flu more than once or twice a year, subtract 0.
    d. If you have been exercising for more than two years without any injury, have been making progress, and are a competitive athlete, add 5.

I calculated my maximum aerobic heart rate: 180 – 52 = 128. This now meant that while running or biking, I needed to keep my heart rate at 128 beats per minute or lower in order to remain aerobic. (My resting heart rate was 71). Any higher and I would be entering into the counterproductive, non-fat-burning anaerobic zone.

RUNNING WITH THE MONITOR

My maiden road test with the monitor was a 2.5-mile hilly loop in my neighborhood. The first half-mile was a steep downhill, and I had difficulty keeping my heart rate at 99 beats per minute, nearly thirty beats lower than my target of 128. The next half-mile segment was a steep uphill grade, and here the monitor held steady at 132, just a few beats higher than what the 180 Formula dictated. I noticed that my breathing was labored, but I maintained an okay rhythm. The next section—and longest—was mostly flat, and once again, I was running below my target rate, averaging 117 beats. I needed to go faster. The final quarter-mile was straight uphill, and as expected, my heart rate averaged 132, then shot up to 140 toward the end of the climb. I later checked with Phil for his analysis.

He promptly emailed back:

> Congratulations for incorporating this very simple but effective biofeedback component into your training. You seemed to grasp the concepts and application right away. Remember the warm-up and cool-down, when the heart rate should slowly increase and decrease, respectively. Running fast downhill is different from running hard. The difference is stride length. Keep your stride length "normal" on the downhills (like you were on the flats). This will increase your cadence and speed (a great addition to the workout) without increased pounding. And, 128 is your maximum aerobic training heart rate, so don't exceed it. In some people, going above even by two or three beats triggers a mildly anaerobic response in the body, which is something you want to avoid right now if your goal is to quickly build significant aerobic function, endurance, and good health.

On my next run with the monitor, I chose the same 2.5-mile loop. I was still going too slow on the downhills, but my heart thumped a few beats lower on the uphill grades. And I needed to pick up the pace on the flats. The monitor's audible two-note beeps reminded me to either slow down or go faster whenever I went outside the target zone. These beeps had a musical, incantation-like quality, almost soothing and meditative in their auditory effect, and made this run one of my most enjoyable in months. (I have never run with a Walkman or iPod.) And so it went with my new workout partner—the monitor. Running with it brought back sweet remembrances of Rockee trotting by my side. Then, his red leash connected us; now I was tethered to a digital fitness device manufactured in China.

After just one month with the Timex heart-rate monitor, this former Luddite became a true believer in his new biofeedback gadget. Though I was running slower, I was running farther—and without taking rest breaks. An hour hilly run became a twice-a-week workout. I got fitter faster by remaining in an aerobic state. I wasn't concerned with seeing how fast I could run; I was simply excited that I could easily run for an hour nonstop. My resting heart rate even dropped five beats. I took fewer rest days. I could now work out four days a week. An added bonus was that several unwanted pounds melted away because my body had reprogrammed itself to burn fat for sustained energy. I was glad I heeded Phil's recommendation.

Occasionally, I used the monitor while biking and noticed that my heart rate spiked on uphills at my usual pace, and thus I was forced to pedal slower to remain in an aerobic state. Conversely, on flat and downhill stretches, I had to bike faster to get the heart rate up.

After three straight months of using the monitor, I was amazed by how cooperative my body had become—no adrenal fatigue or burnout from overtraining. My weekly long run averaged between ninety minutes and two hours, almost always done on Mount Tam's trails and fire roads. I made sure that my heart rate never edged past 128, and whenever it did on steep sections, I'd stop to allow my heart rate to settle back down and then I'd resume running. Speed, as always, was never a concern. Movement was bliss, with legs and lungs taking me to secluded sylvan places that had become half-forgotten during my lethargic, dysfunctional past.

I was building a strong, viable aerobic base with the monitor. An easy day was a half-hour run. I was now able to work out on consecutive days—I'd go on a two-hour mountain bike ride, and then the next day, I felt sufficiently refreshed for an hour run. Compare this progress with my shaky, sputtering fitness foray in the beginning when a two-mile run sapped my energy for several days. I had come a long, long way.

"That's the beauty of biofeedback," Phil told me one day. "It provides an accurate assessment of where your body is at."

BUILDING STRENGTH: IN PRAISE OF THE PUSH-UP

As I became increasingly satisfied with the positive results of my improved conditioning, I realized that it was time to embark upon a new chapter in my return-to-fitness crusade: rebuilding upper-body strength. Because you begin to lose 1 percent of muscle mass each year after the age of thirty, there's only one way to slow down the decline, and that's with weight training. By defying gravity's obstinacy when you raise a slab of iron, you don't necessarily turn back the clock on aging, but your body won't turn into squishy flab either. You are also strengthening your bones.

During my lost fitness decade, I squandered any and all interest in doing chin-ups, pull-ups, or push-ups. These existed off the grid. I never went to the gym. So when it came time to work on the muscles, I could only manage one chin-up, a half pull-up, and twenty-five push-ups. Those pitiful numbers marked the upper limit of my upper-body strength. And to think that when I was in my twenties and thirties, I would regularly rattle off fifty push-ups or fifteen chin-ups first thing in the morning.

I decided to first focus on doing push-ups. Many fitness experts believe that the push-up is the perfect strength-training exercise because it builds strength in your back, shoulders, and arms. It also revs up your heart rate. When done properly, the push-up engages the body's core, including abdomen and hips.

"You are just using your own body and your body's weight," Steven G. Estes, a physical education professor at Missouri Western State University, told the *New York Times*. "If you're going to demonstrate any kind of physical strength and power, that's the easiest, simplest, fastest way to do it."

"One of the reasons the push-up has endured so long is it's cheap, it's easy, it doesn't require any equipment, it can work multiple parts of the body at the same time—and pretty much everyone, from beginners to athletes, can derive benefits," says personal trainer Jonathan Ross, a spokesman for the American Council on Exercise, on WebMD's website.

The American College of Sports Medicine recommends using the push-up to measure endurance and upper-body strength. The push-up is a fitness staple of the military. Ask any Navy SEAL recruit about push-ups, and you'll get a thousand-yard stare in return. These warriors-in-training learn to worship the almighty push-up. Tough love doesn't get any tougher.

You can do push-ups in the living room, office kitchen, parking lot, hotel lobby, or dance floor at your nephew's wedding. The under-appreciated push-up is the ideal exercise in a down economy; it doesn't require a gym membership or personal trainer. It's just you, your upper body, and a few square feet of floor space. Fitness legend Jack LaLanne entertained television viewers in the 1950s and '60s with fingertip push-ups.

So why did the push-up fall out of favor? Did it remind us too much of gym class? Judging from the recent popularity of websites like http://hundred pushups.com and www.1000pushups.com, the push-up is once again gaining traction. As well it should be. The human species is indebted to the push-up. Three hundred and fifty million years ago, the *tiktaalik,* a type of extinct fish, used its modified fins to push off from the muddy bottoms of shallow creek beds to search for food on dry land. Paleontologists and evolutionary scientists believe that human DNA is directly descended from the *tiktaalik.* Those fins eventually evolved into limbs.

Based on national averages, a forty-year-old woman should be able to do sixteen push-ups and a man the same age should do twenty-seven. By the age of sixty, those numbers drop to seventeen for men and six for women. These are minimum numbers.

There are several types of push-ups—fingertips, hands spread far out, kneeling and against table counters (for beginners), raised legs, clapping, knuckles, one-handed—but the one I prefer is the basic push-up except with one variation: I use metal U-shaped push-up bars for greater arm extension.

It's easy to do a perfect push-up when you are only doing several. But the more you do, the harder they become, as lactic acid builds up in the muscle fibers. Thus, it's important to maintain proper form, otherwise you aren't maximizing the push-up's strength-enhancing benefits, or worse, you can risk injury.

To get you pumped, here are several push-up pointers, courtesy of "7 Weeks to 100 Push-Ups," by Steve Spiers:

- Your chest shouldn't touch the floor; there should be an inch or two of space.
- Each push-up should be done in a consistent, deliberate manner rather than in a herky-jerky fashion; no bouncing! Try to maintain full control of your body at all times.
- Inhale during descent and exhale on the ascent.
- Keep your head in a neutral position—neither looking up, forward, or down at your navel.
- At the top of the movement, your arms should practically be straight but don't lock your elbows in the "up" position, even if you need to rest.
- Finally, because your muscles are being stressed, you need to take days off for their recovery and rebuilding; start with a three-day-a-week push-up plan.

I actually enjoyed doing push-ups because each time I dropped to the floor, I was reminded of all those years when I neglected doing them. In eighth grade, I held the school record with seventy-three push-ups. Nearly forty years later, it took several months to reach that number. On more ambitious days, I would do two or three sets of fifty, sixty, or seventy. If I were waiting for a bagel to brown in the toaster oven or a bowl of soup to heat up, I'd do a quick fifty. (This reinforces my long-standing belief that one shouldn't store workout equipment in a separate room like the den or garage; instead keep it in the kitchen!)

One morning, I cranked out five hundred push-ups—ten sets of fifty each. But this deed came with a small price: It made typing on the computer keyboard difficult for several days. The neuromuscular electrical signals traveling from my brain to the fingertips were sluggish and unresponsive.

KETTTLEBELL

To augment the almighty push-up, I bought a kettlebell, which looks like an undersize bowling ball with handles. Originally made from cast-iron cannonballs, kettlebells were used in the 1800s by Russian soldiers, and then later by fitness clubs in America. Because there's a mass of iron located below the handle, the weight is unbalanced and unwieldy, requiring the deft use of underutilized muscle groups.

The three basic lifting movements—swing, clean and jerk, and snatch—should be performed with speed and a fluid, graceful motion. Even though it's also popularly known as a "handheld gym," the kettlebell focuses on whole-body conditioning because lifting and controlling a kettlebell's motion works the body's core. That's also a primary reason why kettlebells are showing up in more gyms. Reintroduced into the United States in 1998 by ex-Soviet Special Forces physical trainer Pavel Tsatsouline, kettlebells have gone mainstream; marathoners, triathletes, and Hollywood celebrities have even taken up this old-school workout. A high-intensity five- to ten-minute workout will leave you utterly breathless. "You gain strength without gaining weight," says kettlebell coach Chris Hartwell at CrossfitCentral.com.

Some kettlebells can weigh over a hundred pounds, and there are now kettlebell competitions all over the world in which muscular men and women swing and lift these heavy metal spheres as if they were made of styrofoam. Fact: Valery Fedorenko, Russian émigré and head coach for the American Kettlebell Club, holds the unofficial world record in the sixty-kilogram (132-pound) kettlebell jerk with fifty-three total repetitions. Impressive.

There is, however, a big downside to the kettlebell. If it's used incorrectly or the weight is too heavy, it can cause joint or muscle injuries. Because movement patterns are much different from those of traditional weight lifting, the kettlebell takes some coordination and time to master. My initial kettlebell mistake was that I bought one that was too heavy. With my twenty-five-pound kettlebell, I could only do about five reps of the military press and with steadily decreasing form. Having locked elbows at the end of each repetition wasn't happening. On downward single-arm swings—with the kettlebell passing through my opened legs in swooping arcs—I feared that the big iron ball would collide with my two smaller ones. Realizing that I was flirting with testicular disaster, I purchased a lighter kettlebell from GoFit.net—a fifteen-pound version.

Even this smaller weight offered a terrific five- and ten-minute workout. Just one set of ten reps got my heart pumping. The primary thing to remember with a kettlebell is to use your butt and legs—not your back—as leverage when swinging the metal orbs, so you are employing both the upper and lower body. While a DVD and small instruction booklet came with my kettlebells, you might want to read *Enter the Kettlebell: Strength Secret of the Soviet Superman*, by Pavel Tsatsouline, to learn more about how you can develop all-purpose strength.

MUCH ADO ABOUT ABS

Anatomically speaking, the abdomen refers to the part of the upper torso that lies between the thorax and the pelvis and encloses the stomach, intestines, liver, spleen, and pancreas. A thesaurus suggests similar names like belly, gut, middle, tummy, maw, breadbasket, pot, and paunch. No other body part receives as much attention in men's and women's fitness magazines. Practically every issue flaunts cover blurbs like "Lose That Gut!" "Flatter Tummy!" "Banish That Bulge!" or "Rock Hard Abs in Six Weeks!"

You'd think there's a national *absession.* Because who doesn't want washboard abs? But to achieve this aesthetic goal, all the sit-ups and crunches in the world won't make much difference unless you first focus on losing body fat. In other words, you can't spot-reduce belly fat. The body is unable to lose fat in a particular area by solely engaging the muscles in that region. Nor will those ab gizmos advertised on late-night television do the hard work for you. If you crave six-pack abs, then you must lay off the six packs of soda or beer and go easy on the carbs.

I nonetheless bought a padded incline sit-up and crunch board because lurking underneath my gut were dormant muscles waiting to be drafted and called into action. Once the slant board was assembled, I set the incline at forty-five degrees, and proceeded to crunch. I could only do twenty. There was fire in my belly—but the one that says quit.

Seeing that I needed an ally in this endeavor, I poked around the Internet and came across a site called Flat-Stomach-Exercises.com. It recommended "that your ab crunches are done in small quantities of controlled movements with short rests in between." The site also offered these two critical tips:

1. "Place your hands crossed on your chest. You should always bend your knees because it provides necessary support for your lower back."
2. "Some people like to place their hands behind their head but this is not the ideal position because you can strain your neck. What happens is when you get tired you have a tendency to pull on your neck (rather than your abs) to complete the exercise."

The point is not to zip through several hundred crunches since your form will tend to become increasingly sloppy. Instead, do sets of twenty-five or fifty reps with ninety-second rests between each set.

Crunches, I discovered, can only accomplish so much in strengthening the body's core or mid-section. Many fitness trainers suggest adding "the plank" to one's exercise regimen. Unlike a conventional crunch or sit-up, the plank is a static isometric exercise that works the entire mid-torso and both the external and internal abdominal muscles to assist in better posture, improved balance, a stronger back, and, of course, a flatter stomach (provided the days of being a chowhound are over).

There are several plank variations. The basic front plank requires getting into a push-up position on the floor but with your weight balanced on your forearms and toes. Lift your body in a straight or plank position, keeping the back flat and diagonally to the ground; your butt should be neither drooping nor pointing to the ceiling. Now hold the plank. A good starting point is thirty seconds or one minute. On my first attempt, I got up to two minutes. My immobile body was practically quivering from the strain and exertion. It felt like torture—yet I couldn't wait to plank again in a few days.

During subsequent plank sessions, I listened to music to pass the time, choosing three- and four-minute folk-rock songs with an up-tempo beat because it was better than staring at a Timex Ironman watch while waiting for the seconds to digitally flit by.

Side planks are designed to work the side abdominal muscles or obliques. Here, only one elbow and your toes support your body weight, while your free arm can be held straight up in the air for balance or folded across your torso. Other variations include the basic plank with one leg lifted and side plank with a raised leg. For advanced plank exercises, you can rest your toes on a chair or medicine ball.

The popular RunnerDude's Blog heartily endorses the plank, especially for runners:

> When you do crunches, you actually work out your hip flexors more than your abs. If you're a runner, you're already giving your hip flexors plenty of attention and sometimes doing a ton of crunches on top of that can be overkill and even lead to injury. The problem with a crunch is that it's only one movement—crunching forward. Think about it. How many times during the day do you crunch like that? Now think about how many times you twist up, down, sideways? Your core exercises need to include more of a full-range of motion. Incorporating the elements of stability and balance into your core exercises is also great. This "extra recruitment" helps develop a stronger core as well as better balance and stability. One of the best core exercises a runner can do is so simple, yet extremely effective—the plank.

Additional web sleuthing led me to the American Council of Exercise (ACE), a San Diego-based outfit that certifies personal trainers. In 2001, ACE commissioned a study with the Biomechanics Lab at San Diego State University to examine thirteen of the most common abdominal exercises, ranking them best to worst. Using electromyography (EMG) equipment, researchers monitored each participant's muscle activity as he or she exercised. The study found that exercises that require constant abdominal stabilization, as well as body rotation, generated the most muscle activity.

Topping the list of the most effective exercises was the bicycle maneuver. "Lie flat on the floor," says ACE, "with your lower back pressed to the ground. Put your hands beside your head. Bring knees up to about a forty-five-degree angle and slowly go through a bicycle pedal motion. Touch your left elbow to your right knee, then your right elbow to your left knee. Keep even, relaxed breathing throughout."

Coming in second was the captain's chair, which looks like an infant's high chair with side rails for your arms and hands. "Stabilize your upper body," says ACE, "by gripping the hand holds and lightly pressing your lower back against the back pad. The starting position begins with you holding your body up with legs dangling below. Now slowly lift your knees in toward your chest. The motion should be controlled and deliberate as you bring the knees up and return them back to the starting position."

As for crunches, these came in third place but only while using an exercise ball to sit upon. Reverse crunches all scored significantly higher than traditional crunches. Ranking dead last in the study was the Ab Rocker. Why fork over $100 for an ineffective piece of exercise equipment that does little to retool your abs.

MAKING PROGRESS

Several times a week I was doing a hundred push-ups and twenty chin-ups—all nonstop. I had never reached these numbers before in the gym. My routine of crunches and planks (I got up to three minutes) were definitely plating the midsection with muscular definition. I now had a two-pack.

I now liked flexing in front of the bathroom mirror. Biceps humped parabolically. Gravity had reversed direction with my chest; the man boobs were gone. Pecs had returned.

Even though I still had a long way to go in reaching my fitness goals, I had achieved what at one time seemed nearly impossible. My upper-body strength had come back. And with my overall aerobic conditioning base nearly in place, I began to feel that my inner jock had finally come alive.

All of this was made possible with a bare-bones home gym arsenal that included a chin-up bar, thirty-pound dumbbell, kettlebells, sit-up bench, and resistant stretch cords. Since I was making real progress with my stay-at-home regimen, I didn't feel the pressing need to join a gym. My last gym membership was in 1998. The 24 Hour Fitness Center was six miles from my home—just far enough away to make driving there a minor inconvenience—but because it was open twenty-four hours a day, I liked scheduling workouts just after midnight when there were few people around. I never had to worry about someone else's sweat left behind on a Cybex station. My exercise routine was fairly straightforward: ten minutes on the treadmill or stationary bike to warm up, followed by a single circuit of upper-body exercises, topped off with sit-ups and some free weights.

Perhaps some day in the future, I will reconsider going back to the gym. There are a number of muscle groups that could definitely use specific attention. And who knows what other exercise and weight-lifting tips I could come across in the gym.

• • •

Journal Entry
December 15, 2009

It was rainy and cold all last week, and I was getting antsy. I took a day off, then another. Yes, it can be a downward slippery slope. Days of inactivity can expand into a week, then two, and so on, until apathy hardens—and you no longer feel like working out. For the past four months, I made sure not to take more than two consecutive days off from training. Yet here I was on day three, doing nothing but climbing the walls. My last workout had been a half-hour nighttime run in the cold drizzle. Since I was unable to tolerate the guilt of having done zilch over the weekend, I decided to run for an hour early Sunday evening. The rain had somewhat abated; it was more like thick mist. (I simply refuse to run on a treadmill or use a stationary bike. Exercise is hamstery enough.) I bundled up like I was heading to the Arctic—tights, rain pants, polyester long-sleeve shirt, down vest, rain jacket, and winter gloves. I think the temperature was only in the high forties, so I had obviously overdressed. That fact soon became apparent as I was slowly chugging downhill when a woman runner was coming up the hill—lean, blonde, ponytail pulled tight and clad in only a singlet and shorts. Boy, did I feel foolish. But it gets worse. Overheating, I removed the vest and T-shirt and gloves and stuffed them in my rain pants and jacket pockets. I now felt like the Michelin Man—all puffed up.

As I circled back home along a two-mile uphill stretch, I noticed a guy with an umbrella hiking about a hundred yards behind me but gaining! I tried to pick up my speed but he kept pace. I tried to run faster, but my legs felt fatigued and listless from the previous two days of inactivity. I wasn't wearing a heart-rate monitor, but I could sense that my heart was thumping much too fast. I did my very best not to let Umbrella Man catch me, but it was getting more difficult. So I ducked into a long driveway, feigning that I reached my destination, and glumly watched him power-walk past. I felt humiliated. I wanted to quit running.

Who cares about fitness anyway? And why should I? Nonetheless I trudged home at a slow jog, demoralized and defeated. Nine days earlier, I had run for three hours on Mount Tam, and yet, this 4.5-mile, Sunday run symbolized that I was more sissy than Sisyphus. Had all those months of maintaining a consistent workout routine been a waste of time? An experiment in self-delusion and fantasy-mongering?

As soon as I got home, I emailed several friends about my crummy run. I needed emotional support and some psychological propping up. I felt that the return-to-fitness edifice I had so painstakingly built was in great danger of collapsing. My friends all promptly emailed me back. Each offered his own advice to my woe-as-me email:

1. *"You need to remember that your motivation is really high, even if it lags (and geez, give yourself a break—rainy weather is a bummer). It doesn't mean that you've spiraled downward completely, or will. My only point of comparison about motivation is with my own exercise routine: I don't try to do as much as you're doing, and so I'm not pushing toward major goals and peaks, but I'm also not experiencing the lows. Steady eddy. That would be my fifty-two-year old wisdom."*

2. *"I know exactly how you feel. It gets to be such a struggle. I feel good for a few days and then I can barely run a couple of miles. I ran thirteen miles three or four weeks ago, but yesterday I ran three miles on the treadmill and I could barely walk afterward. Getting old ain't fun!"*

3. *"Shrug it off, all athletes experience days when they feel good and days when they feel like shit, especially older athletes."*

4. *"U inspire me! Goin' for a five-hour bike ride. It's scary how fast we lose fitness."*

This last response came from a hard-core endurance junkie who obsessively trains fifteen to twenty hours a week. But I was somewhat cheered by their collective pat-on-the-back encouragement. They were all quite familiar with my struggle to get back in shape. And they certainly didn't want to see me quit.

The next day, when there was a brief break in the rain before another series of storms rolled into the Bay Area, I biked for an hour. It felt like I got my groove back. And the following week I ran for ninety minutes on the mountain. I didn't see any hikers with umbrellas. I felt much more energetic. Legs were strong.

Then why had I been so fearful of losing fitness because I didn't work out for several days in a row? Was I overreacting or responding to a deeper insecurity and frailty? In retrospect, I guess that being anxious was a good thing. This meant that the motivational well hadn't gone dry.

Bad days might come and go, but I was able to get through this short dismal stretch because I ultimately believed in what I was doing. Failure wasn't an option. Plus I still had to run up Mount Tam. Its summit was waiting for my arrival.

ASK THE EXPERT

PERSPECTIVE ON HEALTH AND FITNESS: INTERVIEW WITH NEW YORK TIMES "PERSONAL BEST" COLUMNIST AND MEDICAL REPORTER GINA KOLATA

Gina Kolata is one of the most influential health, fitness, and medical reporters in the nation. Her biweekly "Personal Best" column in the New York Times *brings to a mainstream readership new findings on exercise, aging, weight-loss, and injury prevention. Her most recent book,* Rethinking Thin: The New Science of Weight Loss and the Myths and Realities of Dieting, *explained why diets don't usually work, and that a person's weight is pretty much a function of genetics, and not necessarily a result of diet and exercise. In response to one reader's question about weight loss on her* Times *blog, Kolata wrote, "Decades of research, including genetic studies, twin studies, animal studies and clinical studies, indicate that there is a limit to how much weight an individual can lose."*

Question: Over a thousand people work at the *New York Times*. If you could place its entire staff on a bell curve in terms of health and fitness, how would your colleagues compare with the rest of America?

Gina Kolata: People are always judging themselves by what somebody looks like, but the truth is that you really can't tell. I was at a brunch yesterday and there was a woman whom I would have said looked fine, the picture of health. I found out afterward she's recently had a bone marrow transplant for leukemia and was having chemotherapy and wearing a wig. What I've noticed is that people tend to zero in on people that they think don't look fit. So, for example, there was a picture in the *New York Times* of some kids running and immediately my eye went to a fat boy in the front. I thought, "Why am I doing this? There are twenty kids in this picture and who do I see? The fat one." So I said to my husband, "Look at this picture, what do you notice?" He said, "There's a fat kid." So when you say how do people compare in terms of health and fitness, we focus on the people who are fat. We tend to confirm our prejudices when we do.

Q: It's like having fat radar or *fadar.*

GK: I think everybody has it. My husband and I were in Italy on a bicycling trip. It was fantastic, but two things happened. First of all, I looked at the group and said, "They don't look fit. These people are never going to make it." Before we signed up, we looked at the website. Andy Hampsten, who ran the tour, was trying to scare everybody off by telling them, "You should be riding ninety miles a week and riding up and down hills."

But actually, even though most of the riders in our group did not do all that training, a lot of them did fine. I was really surprised. I even wrote an article about how people who are a little bit heavier—they weren't fat, but they weren't skinny either—could actually do okay on a bike because it's more forgiving than an activity like running. Heavier people even have an advantage going downhill.

Q: Your book *Thinking Thin* seems quite revolutionary because it reminds me of what Woody Allen wrote years ago about fat. He said something like, "Why are fat cells inherently evil? What is it about fat that makes it so despicable?" With your book, you basically say that we have a natural body weight that we tend to gravitate to, and that no matter what kind of diet we choose, and there's plenty to choose from these days, and plenty of diet books to read, it's a losing battle.

GK: It's also hard because everything you read, see, or hear tells you that you should be judgmental [about being overweight], and it's something you have to fight all the time. If people could be thin, there wouldn't be a fat person on this planet. It's so hard to go through life being fat.

Q: *Thinking Thin* is an evisceration of the diet industry. What was the response?

GK: I found out that I've become a hero with the Fat Acceptance Movement. That was nice! I've mostly heard from people who said "I'm so glad you wrote this book. Nobody ever understood why I am so fat or what I've been going through." Scientists loved the book and thought that it was really important and that people have to hear this message. And then I would get people who would write these emails, "I haven't read your book, but I know about it, and don't you tell me that people have to be fat." Or somebody would say, "I'm the living example of why you're wrong. I've lost all these pounds and kept it off for blah, blah, blah." But I'd always write back and say, "Well, that's really great for you. A lot of people have a lot more trouble and they wish they had whatever it was that made it work for you."

Q: You see these late-night weight loss infomercials like Hydroxycut. Who are those people who lost all that weight? What happens to them? Where do they go?

GK: My daughter used to be a personal trainer and she knew a guy who looked really great and he was approached by one of these companies and they wanted to pay him a bunch of money; they would take pictures of him looking really terrific, very cut and then he would stop going to the gym, and gain a bunch of weight and then they would take the "before" picture!

Q: Say someone wishes to return to fitness. He or she is between forty and fifty, has stopped exercising due to injury, illness, or inactivity, and wants to get back in shape. Do you find that people who get in shape want to be healthy, or just want to be fit, or want to lose weight, or all of the above? I mean, what is the driving motivation for people to start going to the gym?

GK: I don't know whether anybody has studied that enough. My own impression is that for a lot of people, it's always, "I want to lose weight, I want to lose weight, I want to lose weight." And then, my feeling is that people who stay with [working out] discover that after the initial pain, they're starting to like it. If you don't like it, you'll never stay with it.

Q: What sports do you recommend?

GK: I think people should find out what they like. In a recent column, I wrote about how much fitness you really lose when you get older and how to manage to *not* lose as much. And I talk about this woman, Imme Dyson, who's actually [*the physicist*] Freeman Dyson's wife, and she started running when she was forty-eight. She's now seventy-one. But anyway, she told me, "You're sore for the first two weeks," but she loved it from the very first day. Her daughter Esther [*the well-known technologist*] told her how to train. She

said, "Mom, if it doesn't hurt when you finish your workout, you haven't worked out hard enough." She loved it so much that she stayed with it. But for people who don't find something they really love, they'll never stay with it. You've got to find something you at least enjoy or like for some reason. And then you've got to ask, what is your goal? Why are you doing this? Your goal will determine what you do. If your goal is to be muscular, then, of course, you have to lift. If your goal is to be healthy, then you can walk.

Q: Dies exercise have its own built-in addiction?

GK: I don't feel good unless I move that day. When my daughter was a personal trainer, she used to think it was just a matter of getting to a certain level of fitness where it could be fun for you. And there is something to that. But then she discovered that some people just never enjoy exercise. One woman whom my daughter trained got fit but never liked working out. Eventually, she just gave up. But if you do love working out, you will put up with a lot just to get that good feeling back. For example, I couldn't run for about a month because I had an injury and so when I got back to running, I had to tell myself, "You've just got to get through that initial period where you're getting a little bit reconditioned again." Sure enough, the feeling I crave, the exhilaration, came back.

Q: How did you get injured?

GK: I was running with my friends. We were doing this eight-mile loop and it has this one really long hill. That night my forefoot hurt. Two days later, I went running again and I thought, "Oh, jeez, I really did something." I could hardly even walk. So then I went to a podiatrist who said, "Oh, you're on the verge of having a stress fracture. You've got to stay off it for a few weeks." I wasn't convinced; actually, I'm never convinced. But anyway, I went to the gym and I did either the elliptical or intervals on the Spinning bike. And by coincidence, I had just written my Personal Best column that said that if you have to have a layoff, you can't maintain all the specific muscles that you need for that sport unless you're doing that exact exercise. But to maintain almost everything else in terms of fitness, you have to work out really hard, you have to push yourself. So I did a lot of hard workouts for a month and then I came back to running. I didn't start out at thirteen miles for my long run. The first week back my long run was eight miles. The next week it was 12.3 miles, and I was running more than thirty miles a week, increasing my distance every week. So it wasn't that bad. I'll never really know why I got the injury. Injuries are such mysteries. And if you can't figure out why you got one, it's hard to figure out how to prevent yourself from getting it again.

Q: If runners just focused on half-marathons instead of marathons, the injury drop-off rate would decrease and more people would probably stay with running.

GK: I'm not sure. It may not be distance. Maybe it's intensity that leads to injuries. I just saw this movie, *Spirit of the Marathon*. It's mostly about the Chicago Marathon and they have ordinary people training for it, and they also show the elites. The elites are like a different species. There's no comparison. After seeing that movie, I totally believe that anyone can run a marathon. And if you give yourself plenty of time to train for it, you are likely to do fine and not get injured. Many ordinary people just want to run a marathon and their goal is not to set a time record. Success is finishing; and if that's your goal, it's not that hard because you can go very slowly, you can walk if you have to. And, at least in this movie, these ordinary people were exuberant when they finished. When people talk about a marathon, it's an endurance event, but it's not that intense for most people. It really isn't. It's hard to be on your feet for five or six hours running, but the slower runners are not running like the elites run. I think it's a good thing because the ordinary people are the ones who pay for the marathons and who generate the crowds, both on and off the course.

Q: There are two kinds of people who cross the finish line: those who immediately look at their *Timex* watch and frown because they wanted to go faster, and those who look up to the sky and rejoice that they have done something fantastic and soul-affirming.

GK: For those who do have a time goal, the temptation is always to say, "if only." If only I had started out a little faster, or if only I hadn't made that pit stop. My ultrarunner friend says it's the rationale of submaximal performance; you know that however well you did, you could have done better, if only. That, of course, motivates you to try that race again.

Q: Were you ever a personal trainer?

GK: No, as I mentioned earlier, just my daughter. I'd come to the gym and she'd lift with me. But even though I never had a personal trainer, I wouldn't mind working out with one. I just never did. Not that there's something wrong with it.

Q: Some people feel like they can't work out without a trainer?

GK: Once again, it depends on what your goals are. I know how to lift. This is going to sound ridiculous, but I have cuts and all that stuff. I have what I want. And I can maintain it, but my goal is not to be a bodybuilder. So for me, a personal trainer might be fun, but it's a lot of money and a real time commitment. And I'm not sure lifting helps with distance running. It may even make your times worse. My goal is to be a fast distance runner. So at this point, for the first time, I actually am

working with somebody. I have a distance training coach who reins me in. He tells me how far to run and at what pace.

Q: In your book *Ultimate Fitness,* you did a thorough job investigating the origins and causes of endorphins. Nobody knows exactly how they trigger that feel-good reaction within the body. Can we train our body to be addicted to endorphins?

GK: I just can't imagine people missing out on them through exercise. But everybody reacts to everything differently. We see colors differently; we taste things differently, smell things differently. And I guess we react differently to exercise.

Q: You've gone through different athletic episodes in your life. Spinning, bicycling, long distance running. Have you found a difference between those three activities?

GK: I loved Spinning for a while. You can get a great workout in just forty-five minutes to an hour. In a Spinning class you're pushing your heart rate the whole time. But when I got a custom road bike, it changed my life. It was like I suddenly realized what cycling was all about. The problem with serious cycling, though, is that it takes a lot of time. You have to be devoted and I am to a certain extent. I try to train for a century ride every year. But I don't devote the time to it that I devote to running. I just discovered that I have this talent for distance running. What got me started racing was my son asking me, "Are you running for a reason or do you have some goal in mind?" And I said, "Oh, I guess I should have a goal, huh?" Then I tried to train for a 5K two weeks in advance and my time really plummeted and I won my age group (fifty-five to fifty-nine).

Q: Do you train with a heart rate monitor?

GK: Not with running, I only use them on a Spinning bike or elliptical cross trainer, because your heart rate is the only indication you have of how hard you are working. You can't look at your time and distance like you can with running, or riding outside. And you sweat no matter whether you are working moderately hard or really hard. Elliptical machines vary from manufacturer to manufacturer, and even from machine to machine made by the same company. You can't go by the level or resistance or even the machine's calorie counts. All can be misleading.

Q: You once wrote something in your column that posed the question, "Is running safe for you?" Every year it seems that someone dies in the New York City Marathon, and at the 2006 San Francisco Marathon, a former magazine colleague died. He was in his late forties, athletic, lean, in peak shape. But you mentioned that you have a greater chance of dying *driving* to a marathon than in a race. Is fitness a guarantee for longevity?

GK: Fitness helps your cardiovascular system, but people often think that if you're fit, you'll live forever; if you eat some special diet or something, you'll live forever. I think there's just only so much that you can do. When somebody who's fit dies suddenly, everybody who's not fit says, "See what fitness gets you." It's a silly argument, but that's what people do.

Q: Are you an advocate for moderation rather than excess when exercising?

GK: I'm an advocate for excess when it comes to me! That's just my personality. It's not everybody's. One time I was writing this article about this scientist. I was looking at what life is like for a high-powered scientist who was on a lecture circuit. He went from meeting to meeting with his PowerPoint, gave talks, and that's all he did, while the graduate students were back in his lab getting all the data. He had this one graduate student whom he thought was really coming along. He told the student, "Some day you could be like me." The graduate student looked at him and said, "I would *never* want to be like you." And that's what I always think of.

Q: In a review of your book *Ultimate Fitness*, there was a great quote at the end. It said, "Exercise is more often a marker of health than its cause."

GK: I think that's true. If you're not healthy, there's no way you're going to be able to exercise anyway.

Q: Anything you want to say about aging and the athlete?

GK: One exercise physiologist did this twenty-year study of runners. He said that it showed that they needed a sports psychologist more than a sports physiologist for the study because people would say, "I just can't stand to see my times go down." And times go down because you lose muscle and cardiovascular fitness even if you continue to train. So yeah, it does drive people crazy. On the other hand, as you get older, every five years, you get into a new age group. I wrote about this one guy in my column, who was doing really fast marathons but then got slower and slower and finally, the last one took him almost four hours. He's sixty-seven years old. He said he couldn't have worked any harder; it wasn't that he didn't try. He said he's giving up running; he's taken up mountain biking. He said that so far he hasn't slowed down yet. There are people who do really well, and actually if you look at some of the older people now, they're doing better than people used to do in the old days before people knew how to train.

ALL ABOUT AGING

How Our Bodies Change Over Time

"The world was made to be wooed and won by youth."

—*Winston Churchill*

Whether one ages gracefully with the bronzed aplomb of George Hamilton or ventures into the opposite Keith Richards or Marlon Brando direction, it's smart to follow Dirty Harry's advice in *Magnum Force:* "A man's got to know his limitations." Granted my body wasn't the same one that got me through my twenties and thirties. And one of the main purposes behind my desire to get fit again was to re-experience that former athletic vitality and potency.

Yes, my body had slowed down, like a forty-five record going at thirty-three. Even though I was in the process of successfully rebuilding aerobic endurance and muscle strength with the help of a heart-rate monitor and commitment to regular exercise, I was running and biking at a syrupy pace that I would have once found laughable.

I began to wonder how much of this general slowdown had anything to do with natural aging. To address this lingering curiosity, I decided to delve deep into the literature of aging and exercise in the hopes of acquiring additional guidance that would facilitate my own fitness return. Is it even possible to turn back the age clock through diet and exercise?

What follows here is a brief summary of Father Time's uncompromising grip on our body—and its relevance for both the active and inactive individual.

. . .

Here's what happens as we age: Muscle mass shrinks, maximum heart rate and lung capacity decrease, joints grow stiff, flexibility wanes, and bones become more brittle.

Going slack and being inactive only makes things worse by speeding up age-related deterioration.

The natural fall-off rate with the heart and lungs is the same whether one is active or sedentary. So why bother exercising when the same fate awaits both the 10K runner and the couch potato? The answer is simple: Aerobic exercise combined with strength training will help prevent age-related problems. Just working out three times a week for about an hour each session—and this can include only walking—will help reduce the risk of heart disease, stroke, diabetes, obesity, osteoporosis, depression, and several types of cancer. Your heart and bones will grow stronger. You will have more red blood cells to transport nutrients and oxygen, helping muscles work longer and harder. You will have improved mental alertness. You will want to eat healthier foods. Your body will burn fat more efficiently. Your immune system will be given a natural boost, providing better protection from common ailments like colds or allergies.

Exercise clearly benefits the body, even for those with serious ailments like heart disease and certain types of cancer. "The data show that regular moderate exercise increases your ability to battle the effects of disease," Dr. Marilyn Moffat told *New York Times* health reporter Jane Brody. Moffat is a professor of physical therapy at New York University and co-author with Carole B. Lewis of *Age-Defying Fitness*. "In years past, doctors were afraid to let heart patients exercise. When my father had a heart attack in 1968, he was kept sedentary for six weeks. Now, heart attack patients are in bed barely half a day before they are up and moving."

The *Times* article also quotes from the *Journal on Active Aging*, which says that "with every increasing decade of age, people become less and less active. But the evidence shows that with every increasing decade, exercise becomes more important in terms of quality of life, independence, and having a full life. So as of now, Americans are not on the right path."

"Contrary to what many active adults seem to believe," writes Brody, who quotes several other aging experts, "physical fitness does not end with aerobics. Strength training has long been advocated by the National Institute on Aging, and the heart association has finally recognized the added value of muscle strength to reduce stress on joints, bones and soft tissues; enhance stability and reduce the risk of falls; and increase the ability to meet the demands of daily life, like rising from a chair, climbing stairs and opening jars. Improving balance and reducing the risk of falls is critical as you age—if you fall, break your hip and die of pneumonia, aerobic capacity will not save you. Ten minutes a day stretching legs, arms, shoulders, hips and trunk can help assure continued mobility, and daily exercises like standing on one foot and then the other, walking heel to toe or practicing tai chi can improve balance."

TIME TO GET ACTIVE—NO MATTER YOUR AGE

In 2007, the Department of Health and Human Services commissioned an expert panel to review the data and literature of exercise science, wanting to separate fact from fiction as well as gauge the effect of exercise on health and disease prevention. The results of its two-year study is a six-hundred-page report whose findings can be summarized as follows:

- Even a little exercise has significant health benefits. A half-hour walk five days a week at a moderate pace will contribute to a lowered risk of heart disease, diabetes, and other ailments lumped in a category called "all-cause mortality." You don't need to spend hours at the gym, hire a personal trainer, or devote your entire Saturday bike riding. Your sole investment in time and money can be walking. Walk at lunch. Park far away from work. Walk to the store. The study adds that the health benefits accrue even if you are overweight.
- Moderate amounts of exercise can contribute to overall health benefits, but if you need to improve your fitness level, you will need to increase duration and intensity in order to enhance cardiovascular endurance and muscle strength. That moderately paced walk should double in length, to an hour. Plan B is a minimum of thirty minutes a day of sweaty, heart-pounding exercise. It doesn't matter what the activity is: biking, running, jumping rope, are all fine.

- To lose weight, you need to work out about an hour or more a day. And proper nutrition is critical.
- Regardless of your age, resistance or weight training will strengthen your bones and joints. Your aim is to slow muscle loss, which is especially important after you reach middle age. You don't necessarily have to go to the gym. Buy some resistance bands or weights and work out at home. Your objective is to induce muscle fatigue in each of the major muscle groups.

Too often, though, exercise isn't prioritized as we grow older. (It's regrettably becoming even less relevant for children in schools faced with budgetary cutbacks.) Habits take root, family and work obligations increase, and resistance to physical activities hardens over time. If the aging athlete notices a gradual decline in strength and conditioning, just imagine the health and fitness deterioration of a forty-five-year-old who eats poorly, is overweight, and hasn't worked out in twenty years. A simple task like climbing stairs must feel like making that final summit push on Everest.

"The common fitness declines that occur with aging include changes in body composition with increased body fat and decreased muscle mass, loss of height (sometimes due to osteoporosis), diminished cardio-respiratory capacity and muscle atrophy," says Dr. William G. Raasch, director of the Division of Sports Medicine at the Medical College of Wisconsin and company physician for the Milwaukee Ballet. "Additionally, it's estimated that much of the physical declines associated with aging aren't inevitable but are due to a detraining or deconditioning effect that comes from a decrease in exercise levels, frequency or intensity. [But] older athletes are often able to compete in endurance exercise because they often have higher proportions of slow-twitch fibers." That's good news for all middle-aged weekend warriors. You have many fruitful years of fitness remaining in your future. You just need to remain active.

CHRONOLOGICAL AGE VS. PHYSIOLOGICAL AGE

Given the nation's growing graying population, American scientists are spending more time and money investigating the aging process. Essentially, there are two types of aging: your chronological age (when you were born) and your physiological age (how healthy you are). Looking beyond cosmetic factors like hair, skin, and teeth, a fifty-year-old male who exercises regularly, practices healthy nutrition, doesn't smoke, and limits his drinking can have a body of someone ten or fifteen years younger. This is what is known as "successful aging." It also works in reverse. A fifty-year-old male who is sedentary, eats junk food, smokes, and loves hitting the bottle might have the body of someone two decades older. This is called "poor aging." In the second example, the poorly aging person might experience any one of several life-debilitating diseases: obesity-related diabetes, hypertension, arteriosclerosis, emphysema, or arthritis.

In 2004, a fit and youthful-looking New York City attorney by the name of Chris Crowley, seventy, teamed up with his internist, Dr. Henry Lodge, forty-five, to co-write a "turn-back-your-biological-clock" book called *Younger Next Year: A Guide to Living Like 50 Until You're 80 and Beyond.* Folksy and engaging, Crowley described an active personal lifestyle involving skiing, sailing, windsurfing, cooking, and enjoying his wife's company. Lodge, the more austere member of the writing duo, was alarmed by "the downright bad health that seems to be the American lot these days. Some 70 percent of premature death and aging is lifestyle-related. Ailment and deterioration are *not* a normal part of growing old." All this can be dramatically altered, the physician insisted, with sufficient willpower, rejection of sedentary behavior, good nutrition, and exercising six days a week. "The fact that exercise reduces death from vascular disease is not a surprise, but how about the fact that cancer mortality falls with exercise and lifestyle as well? It is now clear that cancer is an immune, inflammatory lifestyle disease." *Younger Next Year* went on to become a *New York Times* bestseller. And Crowley today, at age seventy-five, still powers down the ski slopes and rides the waves on his windsurfing board.

The consistent message emphasized throughout *Younger Next Year* is to treat the human body with respect so you can avoid harmful aging. Evolution gave humans all this cunning, inventive cellular machinery that was like "inheriting a biological fortune." You must go back 3.5 billion years to witness the first stirrings of life. Out of this primordial goop emerged our "direct ancestors—algae, yeast, and then bacteria. That pedigree is not humiliating. It's awe-inspiring, and we should be grateful for it. About half of your basic metabolic machinery comes directly from bacteria, unchanged, ticking along perfectly for millennia." All these cells communicated and conspired with one another, adapting, evolving, growing ever more complex. About five hundred million years ago, our invertebrate ancestors arrived on the scene—snails, jellyfish, worms—whose primitive nervous system contains the same genetic blueprint as our own. (Fish came later on the Darwinian docket, followed by reptiles, then mammals.)

AS THE WORM TURNS

Scientists involved in age-related research like studying the lowly nematode worm. In 2008, researchers at the Buck Institute for Age Research in Marin County identified biomarkers of nematode aging that can help predict with 70 percent accuracy both chronological and physiological age. Active, non-stressed worms have an average lifespan of three weeks, but when their similarly aged slimy brethren are placed in inactive, stressful situations, they show signs of premature aging. According to the online edition of *Aging Cell*, the senior-citizen worms exhibited "a lack of symmetrical appearance, uncoordinated motion, and the need to be prodded into movement."

So what do geezer nematodes have to do with humans? The website http://esciencenews.com explains: "The analogy for people would be to take people and keep them all in the same house, feed them the same food and give them the same amount of activity over their entire lives. Some of them will age well and others will not and we could determine who had the best genes for that environment. But we live in a world with lots of change and variation. So the key is to understand the genetic factors and adjust/optimize your lifestyle to minimize risk." In other words, you can't change your genes, but you can improve the probability for disease-free longevity by making smart lifestyle decisions that include proper diet and exercise. Neglecting your body's well-being, to use an apt metaphor, is like opening a can of worms.

Just as 80,000 nematode species have successfully adapted to almost every ecological niche, ranging from the Arctic to the tropics, humans have shown a similar ability to acclimate to diverse environments, including the Internet, now home to countless anti-aging sites. The most popular one is RealAge, which asks users: "Are you older or younger than your calendar age?" You have probably seen ads for RealAge splashed across the web. Twenty-seven million people have taken its online test featuring 150 questions about diet, lifestyle, and family history to calculate a "biological age." These questions address the following: whether you smoke, drink, own a pet, live alone, commute to work in a car, eat breakfast, income, blood pressure, resting heart rate, cholesterol level, if your biological father and mother are still alive, and so on. According to the site FAQ, RealAge experts developed its survey metrics by reviewing 25,000 medical studies that revealed 125 different factors that can influence rate of aging. Yet one survey question left me puzzled regarding its particular relevance: "Do you attend church, synagogue, temple, mosque, or other places of worship at least one time per week?"

I took the RealAge test twice. The first time was before I started working out and scored 51.8, which was nearly two older than my real age; the second time, I had been exercising and eating better for three months, and my real age dropped to 48 years. It could have gone lower if I'd lied while answering some of the questions. (Hey, guys do that all the time on online matchmaking sites. "Of course that's a recent photo of me. I still have all my hair. . . .")

RealAge's real moneymaking purpose is to provide pharmaceutical companies access to its membership database. The firm was co-founded in 1999 by Charles Silver, a former Michigan resident who had created the largest independent quick-oil-change franchise business in that state. He sold RealAge to the Hearst corporation in 2007 for close to $70 million. While the site is a decent informational starting point for anyone taking the initiative with his or her own self–health care, try to ignore all the ads and special diet and vitamin offers. Then afterward, shut off the computer and go for a 30-minute walk.

EXERCISE PHYSIOLOGY 101

It might have been a while since you cracked open a biology textbook in high school or college, so let's briefly review some basics about the human body and exercise.

The human body contains 25 trillion red blood cells carried by 60,000 miles of vascular highways and 280 million hemoglobin molecules that mix our food with oxygen to fuel the body's 650 muscles. The average heart weighs just 1.2 pounds and beats 100,000 times a day and almost 40 million times a year to move 38.3 million gallons of blood during the average seventy-five-year lifetime.

Whether you're climbing stairs or running for thirty minutes, your heart circulates and pumps additional blood to your muscles, lungs, and stomach to fuel working fibers, produce more oxygen, and transport glycogen, lipids, and amino acids to the mitochondria, the body's little factories of energy located in our cells. Mitochondria are the tiny power plants that generate adenosine triphosphate, or ATP, the main source of energy for cellular functions and the catalysts that transport chemical energy for metabolism. The mitochondria also perform other functions, such as controlling cell growth.

(continues)

For most people, regular aerobic exercise increases the size of the heart's left ventricle, improving stroke or pumping volume while increasing the power of the contracting muscles. Exercise also thickens the walls of the heart's chambers so the muscles can sustain a higher-intensity output. After months of training, a previously sedentary person's resting heart rate might decline from seventy beats per minute to forty or fewer as the blood stroke volume increases.

While serious athletes are familiar with the concept of VO_2 max, most of us have a hard time defining the term. Briefly put, VO_2 max refers to maximal oxygen uptake—how much of the stuff we can take into our lungs during each breath. The number is usually expressed as a relative rate in milliliters of oxygen per kilogram of bodyweight per minute (ml/kg/min). A large VO_2 max means you can hold your own on a hilly run while your pals are sucking wind. A sedentary person's VO_2 max normally ranges between 20 and 50. Exercise can increase VO_2 max up to a certain threshold, and results in increased performance. An especially high capacity is due to genetics and bolstered through high-intensity training. For example, Lance Armstrong's VO_2 max registers in the low 80s. (A non-human's VO_2 max, like a sled dog's, can go as high as the mid 200s; no wonder they love endurance running.)

The body's circulatory system carries waste products, including carbon dioxide and lactic acid, away from working muscles and redistributes exercise-generated heat, where it is pumped to the skin surface and dissipated via heat loss and sweat evaporation. When faced with the positive stress of consistent training, the body's energy systems respond with amazing adaptations. Hard training can increase the number of capillaries that serve specific muscles by as much as 40 percent. Activities like running also stimulate red blood cell production and increase hemoglobin, the iron-protein compound that boosts the blood's oxygen-carrying capacity. Exercise allows blood to flow more easily to the muscles; this means more power and endurance.

Consistent training causes adaptation to occur in the heavily used muscles of the legs and arms and, to a lesser degree, in the body's core area. The two most common muscle fiber types are fast twitch and slow twitch. Fast-twitch fibers contract rapidly and have a high capacity to produce more anaerobic or quick-burst energy for activities like weightlifting or sprinting. Slow-twitch fibers, which are used at well below their maximal contraction strength, can sustain low levels of exertion for long periods of time, such as walking, jogging, or cycling. Aerobic exercise consumes a mixture of fat, protein, and carbohydrates for energy, uses large amounts of oxygen, and produces little lactic acid. Generally speaking, humans have a fifty-fifty ratio of fast- to slow-twitch fibers, though genetics affects this ratio; with aging, however, there's an increase of slow-twitch muscles (where fat is burned for energy) as well as a corresponding decrease in muscle mass and strength.

Delayed onset muscle soreness from working out generally subsides within two to three days. The soreness is due to micro-tears in the muscle fibers. Muscle stimulation or stress occur during exercise; muscle growth takes place afterward when the muscles are at rest. Muscles need time to recover and rebuild. Sustained overuse can lead to tissue inflammation, cellular damage, and injury. A good night's sleep will do wonders for muscle recovery. Go for a moderately brisk walk if you still experience fatigue.

A DECADE-BY-DECADE LOOK AT HOW WE AGE

Our bodies morph over time, with changes reflecting diet, exercise, stress, health, and lifestyle choices. Where we start our journey in life is a result of genetics and prenatal circumstances, and from that point forward, we are at the mercy of our family environment, upbringing, society, career, chance, and our own free will.

The Twenties

In terms of strength, agility, and muscle mass, your twenties is a good decade. You feel strong and invincible. Your heart and pipes are working great. You will be pleased to know that your VO_2 max, which is the maximum amount of oxygen that your body can process, reaches its high point during this decade. Your main concern, however, should be keeping limber and flexible, because the cartilage in your joints begins to show signs of breaking down, even from lack of use. Tendons, which connect muscles to bone, and ligaments, which keep your joints together, become less elastic and are also easier to tear due to overtraining or muscular imbalance.

Back when you were a teenager, an aching shoulder or knee would feel better within several days. Badly twist your knee snowboarding in your mid-twenties, and you'll probably be making costly visits to a sports orthopedist for treatment of a torn ACL. Sports like football and basketball that stress the joints through bone-jarring impact and constant stop-and-go motion are known for eating their athletes through injury. But low-impact aerobic activities like running, cycling, or swimming will make these your wonder years, since you will achieve speed and endurance.

Your muscle mass is at its peak, and the same goes with fast-twitch muscle fibers (great for sprinting or dashing across the tennis court for a drop shot). But you still need to be kind to your joints, especially the knees. The tendons, ligaments, and cartilage can only take so much abuse. So if you are a runner averaging more than twenty or thirty miles per week, it would be sensible to start cross-training. Invest in a bike and substitute running with two-wheel workouts at least once a week.

What about healthy grub? It must not just be Red Bull and Carl's Jr. "Runners in their 20s tend to either eat poorly or eat just to get by; they don't make the connection between food and performance," sport nutritionist Lisa Dorfman told *Runner's World.* "When you're running, you want your body to tap into easily accessible carbs for fuel, not drain your protein stores. Not only does protein aid in muscle repair, it also contributes to your immune system, the upkeep of your hair and skin, managing your hormones and water balance." The same goes for cyclists or gym regulars. For those simply returning to fitness and not trying to win a bodybuilding contest, there's absolutely no need to gulp down performance-enhancing supplements advertised in the men's magazines. Instead, eat healthy and snack regularly—but without the junk food. Your body will take care of the rest.

The Thirties

Unless you're careful and consistent in your exercise, this decade marks the beginning of rapid fitness decline. Specific action is required because muscles without regular maintenance begin their countdown to meltdown—biceps go blubbery, pecs turn into pudding. With a steady decrease in muscle mass, you will only be able to lift 1.5 percent less weight each year. Meanwhile, your aerobic capacity continues to ratchet down another 1 percent every year. A slower metabolism means gradual weight gain. Calories from that morning latte or muffin will sneak up on you. Gaining two pounds every year might not like seem like much, but when your twentieth high school reunion arrives, you'll have a gut.

Those who liked nothing better than cranking out high-intensity miles running or cycling in their twenties are in for a rude awakening. Rest or easy days are as critical as hard ones. By going all out in your training nearly every day of the week, you increase the risk of injury, falling performance, or general burn-out. Athletes who continue high-stress training while ignoring fatigue eventually produce high amounts of cortisol and adrenaline, two stress hormones that, in excess, have many negative effects on the body such as depression, inflammation, insomnia, and joint injury.

Many endurance coaches thus recommend periodization, in which you physically peak at different times throughout the year. These periods can last up to twelve weeks; then you need to back off and decrease the hours and intensity. So take up a new hobby like fly-fishing or bird-watching. The short-term effects of detraining or deconditioning are minimal as long as you don't go to complete rest. Your heart will shrink somewhat in size, and less blood will be flowing through your capillaries, but this fall-off is only temporary. Nor will you lose much muscle mass. Still, it's prudent not to entirely eliminate strength training.

By being kindler and gentler to your body during this decade, you will reap significant rewards, especially in aerobic activities like cycling and running. The average age of a marathoner is thirty-eight. Same with triathletes. The Spaniard Carlos Lopez won the marathon at the 1984 Los Angeles Olympics at age thirty-seven, having broken the world 10K record the previous year. The 2008 Beijing Olympic Games women's marathon winner was thirty-eight-year-old Constantina Dita-Tomescu, of Romania, who lives and trains at altitude in Boulder, Colorado. Mark Allen won his sixth Hawaii Ironman triathlon at age thirty-seven.

Low-impact, low-intensity aerobic exercise will also keep the pounds off, as you learn how to make more efficient use of slow-twitch muscles, which burn fat for energy, rather than fast-twitch muscles, which are used for sprinting. This is why many coaches recommend using a heart-rate monitor—not to see how fast you can rev up your ticker but to ensure that you are exercising within the slower, fat-burning range.

Your thirties can be productive years. Just be extra vigilant about your body's changing needs. If you have been idle for years, then getting a preliminary medical exam is strongly recommended.

The Forties

Good news first: The body can accomplish amazing things during this decade. Jack Nicklaus won the Masters at forty-six. Priscilla Welch, a British marathon runner, took first place at the New York City Marathon in 1987, just shy of her forty-third birthday. She had only begun to run competitively at thirty-five after giving up her pack-a-day cigarette habit.

Of more recent athletic vintage, American swimming wonder woman Dara Torres nabbed two silver medals in the Beijing Olympic Games at forty-one. The mother of two defied convention by practicing less in the pool, down from ten to twelve water workouts per week in her teens and twenties, to just five times. "My body definitely takes longer to recover," she told the *New York Times*. "I have my good days when I feel like I'm twenty, and then I have my days when I can't lift my arms out of the water." It's on dry land where Torres put in long, muscle-aching hours, with ninety-minute weight room workouts and sixty minutes of vigorous resistance stretching that flushed out toxins and lactic acid, lengthened muscles, and sped up recovery time. Of course, Torres didn't attempt all this on her own. She spent $100,000 on a sprint coach, strength and conditioning coach, dietician, two full-time personal stretchers, physical therapist masseuse, and nanny.

Endurance athletes—ultrarunners, triathletes, swimmers, cyclists, and adventure racers—prosper in this decade only by changing training methods, specifically by learning to use the body's fat-burning stores for sustained energy and stamina.

For the rest of us, these years can be either friend or foe. "Muscular strength is well-preserved to about forty-five years of age, but thereafter deteriorate by about 5 to 10 percent per decade," says David Nieman, an exercise physiologist at Appalachian State University and author of *The Exercise-Health Connection*. "Because your metabolism is slowing down, you will need 120 fewer calories per day at age 40 than at 30."

Due to less joint mobility, you should use core exercises and weight training to strengthen the small muscles that keep the upper and lower back, shoulders, hips, and knees flexible. Yoga or Pilates will help you stay limber and flexible.

Runners—at their own peril—often overlook setting aside time for rest and recovery. "If you are in your 40s," says marathon training guru Jeff Galloway, "you had better take three days off from running per week." Your muscles need to take a break. Otherwise you risk fatigue or injury. "The older the runner, the longer he or she has to pay for the excessive training."

Cross-training and active physical recovery are critical if you get injured. Complete rest will delay, not hasten, a fitness return. Runners should bike to lessen the risk of knee injury due to repetitive-motion impact; cyclists need the heavy impact of running to help prevent a decrease in bone density that might lead to early-onset osteoporosis.

The Fifties

Just before you reach fifty, you might get in the mail a solicitation to join AARP. It's absolutely the worst birthday present a fifty-year-old will ever receive. With this make-it-or-break-it decade, success or failure is all in your hands. Even those returning to fitness after years of little or no exercise can discover how forgiving and malleable the body is. You can take up running, cycling, and even triathlon for the first time. You might not set age-group records, but you can get really fit. A 2007 study by Carl Foster, a professor in the Department of Exercise and Sport Science at the University of Wisconsin, La Crosse, discovered that people over fifty could achieve significant fitness by combining intense cardio, strength training, and additional rest.

But the decline in muscle mass has already begun to accelerate. Steadily decreasing levels of testosterone for men mean less strength and power. With women, the danger is a decrease in bone density, which is triggered by a rapid decrease in estrogen following menopause. This increases the risk of osteoporosis. Since men and women need to prevent muscles from weakening further and bones from becoming more brittle, there are three words to remember: lift, lift, lift. Strength or weight-bearing resistant training should not be ignored because of an addiction to the elliptical trainer or stationary bike.

Outside magazine recommends the following weight exercises for strength-building:

Work the whole body—chest, back, shoulders, stomach, and legs. Studies show that in only two months, you'll gain two and a half pounds of muscle and could lose more than four and a half pounds of fat. "Make sure to vary the weights and reps with each workout to prevent your muscles from adapting to the loads," advises William Kramer, professor of exercise physiology at the University of Connecticut. One day, lift heavier weights for six reps. The next day, lift lighter loads for fifteen reps. The next workout should be a normal day of pushing out ten reps.

If you are gym-phobic, do push-ups at home.

Runners and cyclists should scale back their training intensity by inserting additional rest and recovery days. Galloway counsels, "If you're over 50, it's best to run only every other day." Recovery is his mantra here. "By preventing extra fatigue and taking rest at even the first hint of slower recovery, you can maintain a steady performance increase without being forced to take a week or more off because of injury or over-training."

With less muscle mass, speed should be less of a concern than endurance. Your diet might also have to adapt to your changing body as the joints continue to become less flexible. Consider taking vitamin C for collagen formation; Omega-3 oils (from nuts, seeds, fish oil) for anti-inflammatory effects, and antioxidants (vitamin E) for protection against the damaging free radicals that proliferate in the body with age.

It is a mistake to go to complete bed rest or inactivity if you are experiencing aches and pains in your joints, knees, lower back, or hip. You want to keep moving, even if you are worried about something more serious and chronic such as arthritis. Substitute fast walking for running if you are experiencing common injuries such as knee tendonitis or illiotibial band syndrome, which is caused by poor biomechanics, muscular imbalance, or poor flexibility. Stay active and your ligaments and tendons will be grateful. Plus the increased blood flow enhances metabolic activity. If you're experiencing lingering problems, make an appointment with a physical therapist to see what's wrong. It could be the wrong running shoes that are causing knee or foot pain, or awkward biking form or fit that's making your back ache. Don't wait until it's too late and surgery is required. If your car breaks down and won't start, do you leave it parked in the garage and hope that one day it will miraculously restart? You take it to a mechanic to see what's wrong. The same goes for your body.

Still, with all these modern breakthroughs in medical science, many aging athletes often turn to surgery to extend their careers. Knee joint replacement is generally successful with minimal risks. The latest trend for those with faulty hips is not complete replacement but a medical procedure called hip resurfacing, which repaves the worn-out ball-and-socket part of the hip with a steel alloy or titanium cup-like device. But where back pain is concerned, don't immediately start thinking about going under the knife to repair a dislodged disc. Try ab and core exercises that will support and strengthen your back.

SHOULD MEN TAKE "FOUNTAIN-OF-YOUTH" DRUGS—HUMAN GROWTH HORMONE (HGH) OR TESTOSTERONE?

It's freakishly rare to see a sixty-year-old man climb into the boxing ring. But cinema distorts expectations of what's possible. Here's what *New York Times* film critic Stephen Holden said about an aging Sylvester Stallone in his sixth installment of *Rocky*: "[His] body is a sight. A weightlifter's slab of aged meat, knotted with tiny hard veins popping out of the shoulders, it is just this side of muscle-bound and somewhat grotesque. It is something you might see hung in the window of a steak house and wonder what kind of carnivore would order such a leathery, sinewy carcass."

Thirty years after he made the first *Rocky*, Stallone is still widely known for his punishing workouts and strict adherence to a healthy diet. But he's also publicly admitted that he takes human growth hormone (HGH) and testosterone, two substances that supposedly promote a lean, muscular body. In 2007, he was busted at the Sydney Airport for concealing forty-eight vials of Jintropin—a HGH drug manufactured in China—in his personal luggage. Though he avoided Down Under jail time, Stallone was ordered to pay $10,651 in fines and court costs. To make further amends, he submitted the following written apology to the court: "I made a terrible mistake. I have never supported the use of illegal drugs or engaged in any illegal activities in my entire life. I wish to express my deepest remorse and again apologize for my actions."

Yet here's what the Italian Stallion later said in a *Time* interview: "Human growth hormone helped me to get up to 209 pounds for the new Rambo movie, which is 40 pounds heavier than I was for the last one 20 years ago. Human growth hormone is nothing. Anyone who calls it a steroid is grossly misinformed. Testosterone to me is important for a sense of well-being when you get older. Everyone over 40 years old would be wise to investigate it because it increases your quality of life. Mark my words, in 10 years it will be available over the counter."

It's doubtful whether HGH or testosterone will be found anytime soon in drugstores, but testosterone has long been used by bodybuilders, weight lifters, and football players to pump up. The Mayo Clinic estimates that over 3 million people in the U.S. take anabolic steroids, which are artificial or synthetic versions of testosterone.

(continues)

The recent surge of popularity in HGH (which is not a steroid) is owed in large part to marketing by anti-aging clinics, where it's promoted as promising the restoration of energy, increased muscle mass, and enhanced sex drive. Eight thousand physician members of the American Academy of Anti-Aging Medicine treat back-to-the-future-minded patients with HGH. Over 100,000 American males now spend up to $1,000 a month for their injections.

According to *Sports Illustrated*, "a serious academic and research war rages between those who say that HGH and testosterone are natural substances that need to be replenished when the body's supply runs low and those who proclaim such a philosophy as quackery. 'There are very basic questions we're trying to get answers to,' says Gary Gaffney, associate professor of psychiatry at the University of Iowa's College of Medicine. He is against doctors prescribing HGH and testosterone for anti-aging reasons, and even dislikes the term. 'Is aging a disease? Should it be treated?'"

And it's not just the gents who are juicing. Even female high school cheerleaders, looking for buff Madonna arms, are getting HGH injections. The wife of retired baseball star and seven-time Cy Young Award winner, Roger Clemens, was alleged to have received an HGH injection right before being photographed in a two-piece swimsuit for *Sports Illustrated*.

Testosterone builds bone density and muscle mass. While classified as an androgen, or male sex hormone, testosterone is produced by both men and women, though the average male produces ten times more than the average female. That is why men, generally speaking, are bigger and stronger than women. Starting around age forty, the body produces less testosterone; this decline picks up speed in your fifties and sixties.

Testosterone therapy, which can be rubbed on the body, injected, or swallowed, can seem like an ideal anti-aging formula, just as Stallone maintains. Here are the potential benefits: It will increase your muscle mass and strength, sharpen memory and mental focus, boost your sex drive, and improve your energy level. But what are its health risks? It can cause a litany of woes: adverse skin reaction, fluid retention, baldness, sleep apnea, non-cancerous growth of the prostate, worsen urinary symptoms, enlarge male breasts, shrink testicles, and reduce sperm production.

"While studies show that testosterone therapy can restore your testosterone level to that of your youth," says the Mayo Clinic on its website, "it isn't clear that there's any benefit to this. And it isn't clear if a higher testosterone level can help you live longer."

Is HGH a better path to anti-aging? Human growth hormone, critical for normal bone development as well as stimulating muscle growth and facilitating cell reproduction, is naturally produced in the pituitary gland—the pea-sized "master gland" that sits at the base of the brain. Unfortunately, HGH levels start falling once you reach age thirty. Then, the decline accelerates by over 20 percent per decade, which corresponds to an increasing loss of muscle mass.

Medical researchers first harvested HGH from cadavers, then began manufacturing a synthetic variety for clinical use twenty-five years ago. The Food and Drug Administration approved injections of artificial HGH in 1996. Under FDA regulations, human growth hormone is a controlled substance that can be administered only by a physician.

In a short time, competitors in a variety of sports began using HGH instead of anabolic steroids, which are easily detectable in drug tests. At the 2004 Tour de France, cyclists were not yet tested for HGH because it had not yet been given World Anti-Doping Agency approval, but athletes were tested for it for the first time during the 2004 Athens Olympics.

Marc Blackman, associate chief of staff for research at the Washington, D.C., VA Medical Center, has conducted many of the definitive studies on growth hormone and aging. He told *USA Today* that "these are not yet ready for prime time. This is still research; it is not to be recommended for clinical practice. And neither the long-term effectiveness nor the long-term safety have been shown."

HGH's unwanted side effects can include aching joints, fluid retention, and swelling. Long-term, the picture is bleaker: It can cause diabetes, arthritis, carpal tunnel syndrome, heart disease, cancer, and even abnormal growth of breast tissue in men. "HGH should not be handed out like candy at these anti-aging clinics," Dr. S. Mitchell Harman, formerly of the National Institute on Aging and now the director of the Kronos Longevity Research Institute in Phoenix, told the *San Francisco Chronicle.*

There is, however, a natural and cheaper way to increase HGH levels that doesn't require expensive visits to the anti-aging clinic. It is sleep. "Growth hormone and testosterone production peak during sleep," Richard Auchus,

(continues)

a professor of endocrinology at the University of Texas Southwestern Medical Center in Dallas, told *USA Today*. "You can actually get people to test pathologically low for growth hormone by waking them repeatedly during the night. I always tell people that if you want to maximize your growth hormone, get a good night's sleep."

The Sixties

This has the potential to be the "uh-oh" decade. You have an increased loss of bone density and reduced muscle mass. Plus you are carting around a higher percentage of body fat. Happily, there's positive news. It's never too late to start exercising—and experience positive gains. Surprisingly, this is when you have the most to gain by working out. New studies suggest that people in their sixties, despite being out of shape for years, can become aerobically fit. In fact, it's been medically documented that a fit sixty-year-old is as healthy as a relatively inactive twenty-year-old.

"Although VO_2 max normally declines 8 to 10 percent per decade after 25 years of age," says exercise physiologist David Nieman, "much of this can be 'recaptured' when older people begin regular exercise programs." It's a much different story with muscularity, since you will continue to lose muscle mass. This is all the more reason to keep going to the gym. Yoga, Pilates, or cross-training will help keep your joints from getting stiff and brittle. If you only bike, you run the risk of an increased loss in bone density, since your legs need to experience the weight-bearing impact associated with walking hills or running. You should also do squats or lunges.

Additional recovery days for cyclists and runners are critical. Your muscles demand the extra rest and pampering. As he approached his sixtieth birthday, Dr. George Sheehan, the late philosopher king of running, dealt with his declining marathon times by cutting back on the frequency of runs per week. Instead of going five miles a day, six times a week, he reduced that amount to running three times a week while boosting his distance to ten miles per run. He was still running thirty miles per week, but it was offset by additional rest days. He stuck to this training regimen for three years, and at the age of sixty-two, Sheehan set a personal best in the marathon by going 3:01.

Sheehan is probably an exception to the norm of slower times as we age; declining performance is inevitable. But active sixty-year-olds can find inspiration by visiting the website of the World Masters Athletics Association or World Association of Veteran Athletes (WAVA). It produces detailed age-grading tables for each distance and age. Consider this amazing factoid: The men's record in the Boston Marathon for seniors (ages sixty-plus) is Clive Davies, of Oregon, who went 2:43:20 in 1981; and the women's senior record holder is Barbara Miller, of California, who clocked 3:11:57 in 2000.

As Sheehan successfully proved, recovery days are as important as maintaining a fixed workout schedule. Unfortunately, old lingering athletic injuries that never fully healed might continue to plague you in your sixties. Minor aches in your joints shouldn't be ignored; instead they should put you on constant alert about not pushing too hard. No pain *is* gain. But don't go to complete rest. "Resting is the wrong piece of advice," longevity expert Dr. Walter Bortz, told *Runner's World*. Keep active, even if this means brisk walking or gardening.

Continue your dietary modifications from the previous decade, including vitamin supplements. You might need to see a trained nutritionist. Get through your sixties fit, active, and healthy, and retirement will take on new meaning, such as biking in Spain or hiking in the Alps.

The Seventies and Beyond

Let's first acknowledge the very fit life of Jack LaLanne, also known as "the godfather of fitness." In 1985, he celebrated his seventieth birthday in customary media-savvy fashion. Handcuffed and shackled, he swam 1.5 miles in the Long Beach Harbor while towing seventy boats with seventy people. Even into his early nineties, he continued working out every morning for two hours, spending an hour and a half in the weight room and a half hour swimming. There's no excuse, in his mind, for people not to exercise vigorously.

"What helps you get out of a chair or go up and down the stairs?" LaLanne asked out loud in an interview when he was ninety. "It's muscles, right? These old people—they quit doing things. They sit on their big fat butts, thinking about what they used to do, and pretty soon their muscles atrophy. You've got 640 muscles. They all need their share of work." His other anti-aging weapon is proper nutrition. Every day, he eats five or six raw vegetables as well as the same number of fresh fruit servings. "When you get your dog up, do you give him a cup of coffee, a doughnut, and a cigarette? People think nothing of giving themselves that for breakfast, and they wonder why they don't feel good."

Today Jack might not have the same bulging biceps that he had at age forty-two when he set a world record of 1,033 push-ups, but he remains a splendid role model of how to age gracefully. He is not alone. There are plenty of active cyclists, runners, and triathletes still going strong in their seventies and eighties. Of the nearly 1,700 triathletes who compete in the Ironman World Championship in Hawaii each year, there are usually between twenty and thirty men and women battling it out in the 70–74 and 75–79 age groups.

Another example of someone who won't slow down is John Keston, eighty-three, of Sunriver, Oregon, who started running at age fifty-five. He holds world records for the 80–84 age group in the half-marathon (1:39:28) and indoor mile (6:48:02), and he ran a 2:58 marathon at age sixty-nine. "I started running because my doctor told me I had high blood pressure," he told *Runner's World*. "I had two treatment options: exercise or medication. I work out with weights three times a week and also cycle and hike. I've had to modify my training. I used to run 70 miles a week. Now I stay in the 40- to 50-mile range, which I don't find strenuous. The day after a long run, I'll walk 10 miles, and it works very well for my recovery."

Certain concessions and adjustments are required during these late-in-life years, especially for the average person. The rapid decrease in muscle mass affects one's running and walking stride. Both have shortened. Speed will dramatically decrease. You might concentrate on pool running, which gives you an aerobic workout without the road-jarring impact on your joints. Light lifting of weights is recommended to maintain balance and agility. Going idle is a mistake. In fact, regular physical activity will reduce the risk of cardiovascular disease and can increase life expectancy by up to two years. As for additional nutritional requirements, make sure you eat more protein, to help promote muscle and tissue regeneration.

Like Jack LaLanne states on his website, "Long live living long!" Staying physically active is quite common in retirement communities all across America. And we're not talking shuffleboard. There's biking, walking, swimming. As a *New Yorker* cartoon recently quipped: "70 is the new 50."

Athletic bragging rights have no age ceiling. In fact, the Senior Olympics attracts plenty of athletes in their eighties and early nineties.

THE BABY "BOOMERITIS" GENERATION

Ever wonder why the "Just Do It" generation has become the Can't Do It generation?

"Baby boomers are pushing their frames to the breakpoint," Dr. Nicholas DiNubile, a nationally known orthopedic surgeon from Philadelphia, told the American Academy of Orthopedic Surgeons and the National Athletic Trainers' Association in 2006. "Baby boomers are falling apart—developing tendonitis, bursitis, arthritis and 'fix-me-itis,' the idea that modern medicine can fix anything. It's much better to prevent things than to have to try to fix them."

Seeing firsthand the effects of aging and athleticism, DiNubile coined the term "boomeritis." The neologism neatly explains why there's a price tag associated with middle-aged fitness. Sports medicine is big business in body-conscious meccas like San Francisco, Los Angeles, San Diego, Boston, Atlanta, Chicago, Seattle, and New York City.

Human evolution didn't expect that science and medicine would lengthen our lives. Nor did it prepare for the explosive growth of 10Ks, marathons, century bike rides, and health clubs. Our bodies were meant to naturally break down as we age. Muscles, bones, joints, and cartilage deteriorate over time. So staying fit as you glide or limp through each decade becomes ever more challenging if you fail to pay attention to critical warning signs from your body.

So what's the best way to slow down age-related problems that affect your bones, muscles, and agility? That is the primary question addressed in the book *Age-Defying Fitness,* by two physical therapists, Marilyn Moffat of New York University and Carole B. Lewis of Washington, D.C. The co-authors provide a checklist to assess the current state of five key indicators of your body's overall health and fitness: posture, strength, balance, flexibility, and endurance.

Posture is the first to go if you sit at the computer all day. Muscle strength begins to decline once we reach our thirties. Balance and flexibility weaken as muscles shrink or tighten, while joints are not as pliable. And endurance can depart unless you engage in regular aerobic exercise. "The antidote to aging is activity," counsel both therapists. "Inactivity magnifies age-related changes, but action maintains and increases your abilities in all five domains."

To assist measuring your own fitness, the co-authors provide a simple quiz. See how you fare.

- Are you not standing as straight and tall as you once did?
- Is walking up a flight of stairs a strain at times?
- Are you getting up from a chair more slowly than you used to?
- Is it getting harder to look to the left and right while backing up?
- Do you get stiff sitting through a long movie?

- Is standing on one leg to put on your shoe difficult or impossible?
- Do you trip or lose your balance more easily?
- Does walking or jogging a distance take longer than it used to?

If you suspect that you are a likely candidate for "boomertitis" or exhibit any of its age-related symptoms, there is an engaging website that will brighten your day. With its cheeky name, SportsGeezer is anything but. Billed as the site for "health, fitness, and lifestyle tips for men and women over 40 who still like to play hard," SportsGeezer deftly offers an up-to-the-minute compilation of useful information for weekend athletes as well as serious competitors. You will find breezy summaries of sports science studies, the latest health and medical news, equipment reviews, and exercise techniques to keep you moving deep into old age. SportsGeezer's creator and sole editor is veteran Boston journalist Art Jahnke, fifty-eight, who loves the outdoors, still plays soccer, and swims nearly every day.

HOW OUR BONES AND JOINTS AGE

Finally, any discussion of aging must include what happens to our bones. They aren't the body's strongest parts. That distinction belongs to the teeth's enamel. We take care of our chompers by going to the dentist, so shouldn't we be equally concerned about our bones? The human skeleton matures around twenty years, but all the bones continue to be active vital tissue (while producing blood cells) throughout life. Contrary to popular belief, bones aren't cement-like solid structures, but porous like a honeycomb. These holes enlarge as bone density decreases, and are the cause of osteoporosis or thinning bones. It is why older people are more susceptible to fractures when they fall.

Women are likely candidates for osteoporosis because they have naturally thinner bones than men. After menopause, women's bone density decreases even further due to a loss of estrogen that helps transport calcium and other minerals to bone cells. But osteoporosis can also strike men once they reach their seventies, due to a decrease in testosterone.

The way to stave off brittle, thinning bones is not chugging down quarts of milk and hoping for the best. It's through weight-bearing resistance exercise. You don't have to lift mammoth barbells to achieve bone-building growth. "Just thirty minutes of weight-bearing exercise a week is all you need to maintain and build your bone density," writes Dr. Michael Roizen and Dr. Mehmet

Oz in their *New York Times* bestseller *You: The Owner's Manual.* They recommend lunges, squats, and push-ups that can easily be done at home. Stretch cords work exceptionally well for added resistance. "Bone will form in response to stress, so when muscles pull on the bones, they stimulate the bone to increase in density." Walking can even suit this purpose. Depending on your diet, strong bones also need a helping hand from plenty of sunshine and additional supplements: calcium, vitamin D, and magnesium.

Joints help allow the bones to move like well-engineered mechanical levers. These complicated structures are an orthopedic sport surgeon's best friend. Hips, knees, and shoulders are prone to overuse, traumatic injury, and age-related deterioration. Tendons and ligaments are especially vulnerable; even a misstep off the curb can land you in the ER. Your cartilage acts as a "slippery shock absorber" for the joints, in the words of Roizen and Oz. But with age comes a thinning of the absorbers' surface area, which causes the bones to lose their cushioning. With less protection, the bones can grind against one another—not the most pleasant feeling or sound. As the joints become further inflamed from bone-on-bone irritation, you have bona-fide damage. Yet you can prevent joint deterioration through good nutrition, weight-training within watchful moderation, and backing off from overuse.

HOW TO SUCCESSFULLY PLAY THE AGING GAME

The body inevitably slows down due to natural aging, but the athletic desire can burn as bright as it once did in one's youth. Enjoy and cherish where you are now in life rather than obsess over diminished times in the 10K. Perhaps this is the time to take up a new sport. If you're a runner, cycling will successfully carry you far into your golden years.

It's expected that you will want to keep up with the young whippersnappers. But suppress that natural inclination and keep reminding yourself that you are doing these activities for yourself.

The ornery and finicky part about aging is that we prefer to craft deceptive funhouse illusions about ourselves. The result of this chronological sleight of hand can be confusion, mid-life crisis, or self-loathing, as we seek to create a willful avoidance of aging—some through plastic surgery, hair transplants, drugs, or through willful denial. A better and less costly alternative is by getting and staying fit. This will make one feel young again. It did for me. It can do for you.

10

DIET AND NUTRITION

What You Need to Know
for a Healthy Body

Any discussion about health and fitness must lead directly to food. What we put in our bodies affects how those calories are utilized—how we burn energy, how it's stored as fat, which foods are best, which foods to avoid.

In theory, I knew which foods were nutritious and good, but what I often speared with a fork or scooped up with a spoon lived on the naughty side of the dietary ledger.

My diet used to be a lot worse.

You've heard of muscle memory? The following incident involved stomach memory. In 1997, I entered a solo twenty-four-hour mountain bike race. I joked to a colleague that I wasn't "a glutton for punishment; it's that my gluttony needs punishing." I only lasted twelve hours—seven laps—on that nine-mile hilly course in Monterey, California. It was a tiring, exhausting, absolutely brutal experience. Part of my downfall was due to lousy food management. Before the race, I downed two cupcakes and a half-pound bag of M&Ms. From noon to midnight, I ate a half-pound bag of Raisinets, two GU packets, one

Snickers bar, half a bagel, a small plate of chips, cheese and jalapenos at a rest stop, and drank four bottles of Gatorade, half a bottle of Coke, and one Heineken beer. Yeah, it must have been the beer that did me in, because I stopped riding just after midnight.

If I have been more Goofus than Gallant regarding diet, I could always levy partial blame on a mother who disliked cooking or a father who was a candy salesman. Our house was filled with sample boxes of Chunky, Baby Ruth, Butterfingers, Milk Duds, licorice whips, Jolly Ranchers, peanut brittle, Fleer bubble gum. It was only to be expected that I had a warped, maligned attitude toward good nutrition. Yet since my early twenties, I have been primarily a vegetarian with a lamentable preference for junk food.

My aversion to eating meat began shortly after spending several months on an Israeli kibbutz where one of my jobs was shoveling chicken shit five hours a day in several hot, stinking cavernous aluminum buildings that were home to 20,000 white-feathered fiends. Because these smelly creatures liked nothing better than to peck one another to death, one of my primary tasks was rounding up ten to fifteen birds at a time, so that their beaks could be severed with a red-hot iron blade.

Sugar has been my vice. While I seldom eat candy anymore, I crave the soothing ambrosia of fruit juice and delicious pleasantries of warm chocolate chip cookies and brownies. (I just experienced a phantom sugar rush writing that sentence.) I probably exceed the average American's consumption of 150 pounds of sugar a year. Of course, all this sugar messes up my blood-glucose levels, leading to roller-coaster energy levels.

Even though my gustatory history has been embarrassing, I knew how critical it was to practice proper nutrition during my health and fitness rebound. Muscle growth and tissue recovery are two important aspects of dietary improvement. Before I decided to get back in shape, my diet revolved around Coke, root beer, and pizza several times a week. That menu plan would be disastrous if I wanted to achieve successful results. Thus I made every effort to begin eating lots of veggies, eggs, and salmon. I also eliminated all soda since there are seventeen teaspoons of sugar per twenty-ounce serving.

JUST STARTING OUT—HOW HEALTHY ARE SPECIAL DETOX DIETS?

Anyone eager to jump-start his or her way back to health and fitness might think, "Aha! Time for that two-week detoxification!" Would a juice or fasting diet be the best way to rid one's body of harmful toxins—the yucky sludge that resides deep inside the gut? Hollywood celebrities, for example, looking to lose weight before a movie often go on detox diets such as the Master Cleanse, which is a concoction of lemon juice, cayenne pepper, maple syrup, and water. Beyoncé dropped twenty pounds prior to the filming of *Dreamgirls* on the Master Cleanse.

Some of these do-it-at-home detox regimens don't come cheap. The Fat Flush kit costs $112 and is made with herbs and nutrients like dandelion root, milk thistle, and Oregon grape root.

So what does the medical community think of these detox brews? Not much, actually. "It is the opinion of mainstream and state-of-the-art medicine and physiology that these [detox] claims are not only ludicrous but tantamount to fraud," Dr. Peter Pressman, an internist with the Naval Hospital in Jacksonville, Florida, told the *New York Times* in 2009. "The contents of what ends up being consumed during a 'detox' are essentially stimulants, laxatives, and diuretics. There is absolutely no scientific basis for the assertion that the regimens popularly defined as 'detox' will augment the body's own capacity for identifying and eliminating your own metabolic wastes or doing the same for environmental toxins."

The fluids in your body constantly pass through the liver and kidneys; these organs serve as the primary heavy lifters when it comes to removing toxins and wastes. In addition to being in the waste-disposal business, the liver is key to hormonal balance, fat regulation, digestion, and blood circulation. It performs over five hundred different chemical functions and metabolizes the proteins, fats, and carbohydrates, and even controls triglycerides, cholesterol, and other blood fats. This critical organ can regenerate itself but only if you avoid drugs (including over-the-counter NSAIDs like Advil) and eat healthy foods such as spinach and broccoli, which contain *sulforaphan*, an important compound for natural liver detox because it helps produce *glutathione*—the most powerful antioxidant in the body.

Understandably, the public is always hungry for a quick detox fix or the next superfood like the acai berry, whose health-curing properties have not been fully investigated. Fifty-four new food and beverage products debuted in 2008 with the word "detox" in their descriptions. Many of these fasting kits and juice regimens promote short-term weight loss because there are fewer calories being consumed, but the pounds usually return afterward. Some detoxers even believe that bowels should be irrigated several times a day, and suggest colonics, enemas, and herbal laxatives to hurry things along. This practice, however, can cause long-term harm to one's gastrointestinal system. Laxatives can contribute to fainting, muscle cramps, and dehydration.

The body is pretty good at flushing out the toxins on its own, provided you avoid nicotine, caffeine, sugar, and alcohol. And for those with lactose intolerance or who have an allergy to gluten-based foods, keeping away from dairy and wheat makes affordable, nutritional sense. Your gut and wallet will thank you.

Dr. Ronald Strum, medical director and founder of the Center for Integrative Health and Healing in Delmar, told the *New York Times* that "eating whole foods always trumps fasting or juice diets—and that education overrules everything. People are getting their info from the massage therapist or the clerk at the health food store who may not know the potential risks." These whole foods include plenty of leafy green vegetables, especially spinach and kale, apples, onions, and carrots, and don't forget to drink a lot of water throughout the day, because the body needs fluid to transport toxins to the kidneys and liver for elimination.

THE HUMAN DIET

As you make that return to healthy fitness, it is a good time to re-evaluate your personal eating habits. But where should you start? There is a plethora of good and bad information. New diet books are constantly being published, each one promising the latest breakthrough in weight loss. So a good place to begin is to step back in time to see what kind of foods humans used to eat and why we prefer the kind of foods we now do.

The human diet witnessed a radical change when our ancestors migrated from the African savanna—and a meal plan that depended on hunting and gathering for sustenance. The move to more northern regions in the Middle East eventually contributed to the development of farm-based grain economies and livestock. And this is where the trouble begins, asking the body to revamp a digestive tract that took millions of years to evolve.

The modern 40–30–30 diet, for example, attempts to mimic the pre-grain eating habits of early man. "Following a prehistoric, or Neolithic, diet is simple. If a food is perfectly edible as it grows in the wild, it's okay," says Ray Audette, author of *NeanderThin*. "But the diet forbids foods that require man's intervention to grow or make edible. So, you can hunt, gather or buy fruits, vegetables, meats, fish, roots, berries, eggs, legumes and nuts. But, throw away your alcoholic drinks, refined sugar and such mainstays of the modern diet as potatoes, wheat, corn, rice, beans, soy, peanuts, milk and cheese."

Corn is one of the chief contributing factors for obesity in America. We live in a world where corn is king, and the corn that now fuels our ethanol-based vehicles is also the main ingredient for high-fructose, which is found in many of our prepackaged foods, fruit juice, and soft drinks. Before a high-carb hybrid type of corn spread across the Midwest, corn used to be a healthy source of protein in Mexico and Native American culture. There used to be many varieties of corn, but agri-business giants like Monsanto have narrowed the farmers' playing field with high-yield, nutrition-deficient corn that is fattening.

It's just as bad with wheat and other grains. "Our over-reliance on grain-based nutrition is especially problematic," says exercise physiologist Loren Cordain, PhD, author of *The Paleo Diet*. "The best path for avoiding diabetes, heart disease and other diseases of civilization is to follow the hunter-gatherer diet that mankind spent two million years adapting to. Other beneficial pre-historic habits include eating leafy vegetables, low-sugar fruits, constant grazing instead of bingeing."

All this seems simple and elementary. Then why do we need a zillion diet books to tell us what to eat—and what *not* to eat? For athletes, however, the primary concern is not worrying about staving off obesity, but finding the right healthy diet for improved performance. Before modern scientific measurements were available to athletes and coaches, diets were pursued through instinct, myth, and faith. In ancient Greece, Olympic athletes ate the meat of oxen for strength.

The science of nutrition was born about a century ago when chemists were able to break down food into its major components of carbohydrates, protein, and fat. They also discovered accurate ways to measure calories. During the last several decades, a subcategory known as sports nutrition has come out of the kitchen cupboard, spawning a mini-industry of claims and counterclaims. New studies debunk old studies with increasing regularity. When sports nutritionist experts debate conflicting dietary regimens and theories, they bring to the training table all the fierce partisan flavor and fervor usually reserved for politics and religion. The two overriding questions involve quantity and quality: One, what should be the ideal dietary breakdown of carbs, protein, and fats? And two, just what kind of carbs, protein, and fats should they be?

How we think about nutrition mirrors social trends. "Ours is a culture where a meal is measured by how fast it's served or how many grams of fat it may contain. We ignore, to our detriment, the wonderful social aspects of a long leisurely lunch that one experiences in other parts of the world. We have become, in the midst of our astounding abundance, the world's most anxious eaters," wrote Michael Pollan in a *New York Times* essay aptly titled, "The National Eating Disorder," which later became the basis for his first bestselling book, *The Omnivore's Dilemma*. "*How* we eat, and even how we feel about eating, may in the end be just as important as *what* we eat. So we've learned to choose our foods by the numbers (calories, carbs, fats, R.D.A.s, price, whatever), relying more heavily on our reading and computational skills than upon our senses. Indeed, we've lost all confidence in our senses of taste and smell."

Carbs

Let's start with carbohydrates. Carbs are processed in the digestive track and converted through various biochemical processes into blood sugar (glucose). Simple carbohydrates have a basic molecular structure and are easy for the body to metabolize; they have a high caloric yield and generally have what is known as a higher glycemic index (GI)—which refers to a ranking of foods on how they affect our blood glucose levels. The higher the ranking, the greater the fluctuations in blood-glucose and insulin levels. Complex carbohydrates, however, are slower to metabolize, have a lower glycemic index, and are digested to blood glucose at a slower release rate. This stabilizes one's blood-sugar levels.

Not all carbs are equal. Bad carbs are those simple carbs that cause a sudden spike in your blood sugar for instant energy. So stay away from candy bars, fruit juices, and soft drinks in the company lunchroom. You might get a quick energy boost, but you'll soon crash afterward, requiring another trip to the vending machine. Good carbs, on the other hand, are the low GI-complex ones, like grapefruit, peanuts, lentils, peaches, and barley. These carbs provide a more sustained energy effect with a less dramatic rise in insulin levels. You won't experience that blood-sugar roller-coaster ride.

In *Get the Sugar Out,* nutritionist Ann Louise Gittleman writes that "the refined sugars that we consume in such vast quantities might seriously be screwing with our insulin response. In addition to the caloric density of high-sugar foods and processed carbohydrates, their rapid breakdown releases high levels of sugar into the bloodstream, which in turn triggers the secretion of insulin, a hormone that regulates blood sugar. The more refined carbohydrates we eat, the higher our insulin requirement, and the more out-of-whack our blood-sugar levels."

The backlash against carbs, both good and bad, was prompted by the popularity of the Atkins diet, a yummy regimen rich in protein and tasty fats. But two recent studies published in the *Annals of Internal Medicine* found that the Atkins low-carbohydrate diet outperformed traditional low-fat diets in the short term but offered no weight-loss advantage after one year. Furthermore, an over-reliance on a low-carb diet can overtax the kidneys and contribute to minor health problems like constipation, muscle cramps, diarrhea, general weakness, and headaches due to a lack of fruit, vegetables, and whole grains. And because all that protein produces ketosis, which triggers bad breath, it's probably a good reason anyway not to hang out with Atkins dieters.

"Individuals need to understand that healthy carbs such as vegetables, fruits, beans, and whole grains (eaten in proper amounts) are essential components of a well-balanced diet," says Dr. Cedric Bryant, chief exercise physiologist for the American Council on Exercise. "The consumption of these healthy carbs has been linked to a reduced risk of heart disease, certain types of cancer and a number of other chronic ailments."

If you are exercising for several hours a week, you will need to consume more carbs for energy, but this is where you should tread carefully and not overdo it. Excess carbs are stored as fat. It makes no difference whether it's a box of low-fat pretzels or apple pie à la mode.

Napoleon once famously remarked that an army marches on its stomach. It's the same with cyclists and long-distance runners, who must learn to ride and run, respectively, on their bellies. Tour de France bike racers devour between 6,000 and 7,000 calories per day—breakfast, pre-race meals, dinner, and snacking and drinking fluids while in the saddle. Most of the calories during riding come from carbohydrates since they are the primary fuel source for energy. Bonking often happens when the brain is running low on glucose, or sugar, from the blood. It can lead to confusion, nausea, disorientation, and fatigue.

Six-time Hawaii Ironman champion Mark Allen was once hailed by *Outside* as "The Fittest Man in the World." In a column on nutrition for *Triathlete*, Allen, who is now retired from competition but offers online training programs, says that "any [activity] that lasts less than an hour-and-a-half will be affected very little by the calories you take in. Water can be a huge issue, but the calories you have stored up as glycogen [from carbohydrates] plus your pre-race meal should get you through with flying colors. Research shows that, in general, a person cannot absorb more than 500 calories per hour. The challenge in getting in those calories comes from what happens deep inside your digestive system." Above all, Allen believes in one word: *experiment*. Try different sports drinks and gels on your runs and rides. See which one agrees with your taste buds, digestive system, and how they replenish your energy reserves. Those sweet-tasting bars or drinks with high-fructose content might give you a quick energy boost, but that power surge will quickly taper off and leave you listless again; seek out products with low-glycemic ingredients that might give you less rapid but more long-lasting, sustained energy.

Fat

Let's now turn our chat to fat—an integral, if not overlooked, part of the athlete's diet. Fat plays an important role here—physiologically, hormonally, and nutritionally. The body's largest endocrine organ is fat tissue. The fat cell's main job is to store excess calories. The fat cell of an overweight person can expand to three times its normal size, and a swollen fat cell retards the body's production of insulin, which is the hormone that instructs the muscles to burn energy. The pancreas must work harder to produce more insulin, which in turn can lead to insulin resistance, artery damage, and inflammation because the fat cells are leaking fat and proteins into the blood system.

In 2006, the U.S. Food and Drug Administration required food manufacturers to list trans fats alongside saturated fats on product labels (think margarine, chips, cookies, fries). Some trans fats occur naturally in beef, lamb, and dairy products. But most are created when hydrogen is added to liquid vegetable oil to create solid margarine or shortening. Both trans fats and saturated fats, which are prevalent in meat, raise blood levels of bad cholesterol. But trans fats also reduce levels of good cholesterol, increasing the risk of heart disease even more. Trans fats also increase blood levels of triglycerides, the chemical form in which most fat exists in food as well as in the body.

Trans fats account for about 0.5 to 2 percent of daily calories for Europeans. That compares with an estimated 2.6 percent for Americans, according to the

U.S. Food and Drug Administration. Mediterranean countries are at the lowest end of the scale, reflecting their use of olive and other vegetable oils rather than spreads.

Until recently, fat had a Rodney Dangerfield reputation among athletes; it got no respect. This was unfortunate because good fats (oils and spreads of almonds, avocado, nuts, olives, or cold-water fish like salmon) help strengthen the immune system, ward off common infections, and stem inflammation. They also aid in the manufacture of hormones, such as testosterone and estrogen. Moreover, fat is the body's best source of energy. "Theoretically, even the skinniest athlete has enough fat stored to last for forty hours or more at a low intensity without refueling," writes Joe Friel in *The Cyclist Bible*, "but only enough carbohydrates for about three hours at most."

Friel also makes this high-five claim for fat: "After three decades of believing that very high-carbohydrate eating is best for performance, there is now compelling evidence, albeit in early stages, that increasing fat intake while decreasing and properly timing carbohydrate may be good for endurance athletes, especially in events lasting four hours or longer. Several studies reveal that eating a diet high in fat causes the body to preferentially use fat for fuel, and that eating a high-carbohydrate diet results in the body relying more heavily on limited stores of muscle glycogen for fuel."

Protein

Protein is a macronutrient made up of smaller parts called amino acids. While there are about twenty different amino acids, many of which the body can produce, there are eight that the body cannot. These eight must be found through foods, and are therefore essential. Animal proteins contain all eight of these essential amino acids in appropriate proportions, while the proteins found in plants often do not. But by mixing plant foods—for example, rice with beans—the amino acids in one protein can compensate for the comparative deficiencies of another.

While carbs and fat are necessary for endurance and energy, you need adequate amounts of protein in your diet because it serves these vital roles: muscle and tissue repair, growth, and maintenance. It is also a major component of cell structure and vital for enzymes, such as those necessary for the production of anti-inflammatory hormones. Protein can also be a source of energy when the body runs out of carbohydrates and fat for fuel.

But how much protein should you eat daily? The daily protein requirement for adults, established by the World Health Organization, is pegged at 0.75 grams per kilogram of body weight for Western diets, but this number tends to be higher for Americans (0.8 grams). One cautionary note: Excess protein is converted to fat and stored. An overabundance of protein may produce metabolic stress on liver and kidney function.

And what if you are a vegetarian like me? How can one avoid a protein deficit in his or her diet? *Go Ask Alice!*, a clearinghouse of nutritional and health information published by Columbia University, offers these tips:

Protein has certainly been the source of hot debate in the nutrition world as vegetarianism and veganism become more popular dietary and lifestyle choices for a growing number of people. There have been scores of arguments about protein in all its facets: how much you need, what kinds are most useful to the body, and how to prepare it. But what it comes down to is this: Everybody is different, has different needs, and digests foods uniquely, so the best non-meat sources of protein for one person might be the worst for someone else. Research has shown that we do best consuming between 40 and 65 grams of protein a day, those with very active lifestyles or who consume more calories consuming towards the higher end of the spectrum. Almost every food contains protein: nuts, seeds, beans, soy products (tofu, soy milk, tempeh), grains (wheat, oats, quinoa, rice), eggs, and dairy products all being excellent vegetarian sources.

Because muscle tissue is comprised of 15 to 20 percent protein, 70 to 75 percent water, and glycogen (carbohydrate), fat, vitamins, and minerals for the rest, it is important for those on the fitness rebound to eat more protein. With a protein deficit, you will lag behind in muscle and tissue repair, enzyme and hormone production, fluid balance, and red blood cell production.

"What is most important is that your elevated protein requirements are easily met by a well-planned sports diet," writes sports nutritionist expert Monique Ryan. "For athletes, consuming enough calories to meet their energy needs, this often translates into increased protein intake. When calories go up, the percentage from protein often remains constant, and the total grams of protein you consume increase. Average protein intake for most endurance athletes ranges from 70 to 200 grams daily depending on calorie intake."

ARE YOU A VEGETARIAN?
HOW TO AVOID THAT "PROTEIN DEFICIT"

Rising health fears are associated with mad cow disease, *E. coli*, salmonella, and listeria contamination of meat and poultry products. This concern, coupled with an increased revulsion at how cattle—a "food delivery system"—are penned, fed, drugged, and slaughtered, has led to vegetarianism gaining adherents. The "meat anxiety" is not solely felt in green meccas like Berkeley, Cambridge, Seattle, Madison, and Boulder. Fourteen million Americans call themselves vegetarians. But vegetarian athletes are especially at risk due to certain deficits in their diets. Strict vegans (who eschew any animal derivative in their food) won't do dairy.

Does a vegetarian diet leave some important nutrients out? Do vegetarians need a booster shot of supplements? Most experts agree that protein and minerals like zinc and iron, all found in important quantities in meat, are necessary for a healthy diet. Besides eliminating fat and cholesterol, a meatless diet removes protein, which is loaded with essential amino acids the body uses to repair its tissues. That replenishment is critical for athletes who are constantly stressing their muscles. There are many ways to make up the protein gap, depending on your type of vegetarianism:

- *Combining grains and legumes.* Vegetable sources of protein lack some of the amino acids the body needs for renewal, unless you eat grains (whole-grain wheat, quinoa, barley, or rice) with legumes (chickpeas, black beans, pinto beans, or lentils) every day.
- *And eat a lot.* For a 160-pound sedentary man to get his daily requirement of 8 grams of protein per kilogram of body weight, about 60 grams, he must consume 4.5 cups of pasta, 3 cups of broccoli, and 1.5 cups of tomato sauce. Athletes, who burn protein as a form of energy during exercise, need nearly double that—about 1.2 to 1.6 grams per kilogram of body weight, which adds up to about 80 to 110 protein grams for a 150-pound person.
- *Load up on soybeans.* This super-legume is prevalent in Asian countries with soybean-rich diets that include tofu, tempeh, and soy milk.

PUTTING IT ALL TOGETHER

So what is the optimal eating plan? Which one will satisfy your taste buds, keep your weight stabilized, provide you with energy throughout the day, and replenish muscles stressed from exercise? Judging by how most Americans shop, dine, or eat, we're doing almost everything wrong.

An eating lifestyle colloquially known as the Mediterranean diet might be the answer to our troubled relationship with food. "The Mediterranean diet is specific to a certain climate and culture," Walter Willet, chairman of the department of nutrition at the Harvard School of Public Health, told *Discover* magazine in 2009. "By paying attention to healthy ingredients rather than specific recipes, anyone can adapt this plan to his own tastes." The end result is better weight management, clearer arteries, and improved health. And the data supports his belief.

A recent study published in the *Journal of the American Medical Association* detailed sufficient evidence that the Mediterranean diet, combined with regular exercise (thirty minutes daily), is essential for longevity. For ten years, the study followed 2,300 active elderly Europeans, aged seventy to ninety, whose diet emphasized moderate red wine consumption, whole grains, fruits, vegetables, legumes, nuts, and olive oil and was low in saturated animal fats, trans fats, and highly processed grains. They died at a rate over 50 percent lower than those who didn't exercise and ate poorly.

The *Journal* also cited a study that looked at the Mediterranean diet's cardio-protective benefits, suggesting that it may inhibit inflammation in blood vessels, which is believed to be a major factor in heart disease and type 2 diabetes. According to a report on WebMD.com, "Patients at high risk for these diseases who followed the Mediterranean diet for two years showed more improvements in weight loss, blood pressure, cholesterol, and insulin resistance—conditions that promote heart disease—than a similar group placed on a conventional diet. Adherence to the Mediterranean diet was effective in reducing inflammatory blood markers, which have been linked to a high risk of heart disease."

The Mediterranean eating plan is largely based on the dietary traditions of the Greek island of Crete and southern Italy, where, until recently, rates of chronic disease were among the lowest in the world, and adult life expectancy was among the highest. The *New York Times* health blog offered this meaty morsel about the Mediterranean diet: "While the traditional diet included meat only about once a month or on special occasions, most health experts say adhering to Mediterranean eating doesn't have to mean giving up meat. It just means consuming smaller portions less often. If you are packing your diet with produce, nuts, legumes and whole grains, you won't have a lot of room left on your plate for big servings of meat anyway. In the traditional diet, someone wasn't eating a 12-ounce Porterhouse steak. They ate small bits of meat in a sauce. It was there to get flavor and taste from. Meat is delicious and they knew that."

Bottom line, the Mediterranean diet is largely based on plant foods and whole grains. And this leads us straight to food guru Michael Pollan's recommendation about how to rehabilitate the Western diet, which has been overtaken by nutritionism, fast-food addiction, packaged and processed foods, questionable meat-industry practices, and gargantuan agri-business. Pollan emphatically states at the outset of *In Defense of Food*, "Eat food. Not too much. Mostly plants." By basing your diet on those seven words—an easy enough regimen to follow—he argues that healthy eating is within everyone's reach. It is neither complicated nor confusing.

The Healthy Eating Pyramid, created by the faculty in the Department of Nutrition at the Harvard School of Public Health, supports Pollan's dietary fiat. Its website states that "eating a plant-based diet is healthiest. Choose plenty of vegetables, fruits, whole grains, and healthy fats, like olive and canola oil. Cut way back on American staples. Red meat, refined grains, potatoes, sugary drinks, and salty snacks are part of American culture, but they're also really unhealthy." In addition to eating better, Harvard's pyramid authors suggest that you "start with exercise. A healthy diet is built on the base of regular exercise, which keeps calories in balance and weight in check." That's good, sound common sense, and will keep you from straying off the return-to-fitness path.

A MOUTH-WATERING LOOK AT THE MODERN HISTORY OF DIETING

We live in a nation of excess—McMansions, SUVs, retail superstores, ballooning waist sizes. "Overeating is an act of heroism," says novelist, poet, and gourmand Jim Harrison. Seventeen years ago, 33 percent of U.S. citizens were overweight. Now that figure has expanded to 40 percent. Yet diet products and weight-loss programs total $33 billion a year. A real growth industry! Here then is a lip-smacking tour of the modern history of dieting. Have you

(continues)

ever tried any of these diets, or know someone who did? Not all eating plans are created equally—as you will see.

1830s. The Bland Diet. Presbyterian minister Sylvester Graham, following in the killjoy footsteps of Puritans, counseled that only by denying the flesh would one's spirits grow strong. Overeating caused sickness, sexual obsession, and social chaos. He advocated bland foods such as his very own "Graham Cracker" and avoiding meat, spices, and stimulants. A case of the bland leading the bland, his program crumbled when adherents became weak and starving.

1863. First low-carb diet. Obese British casket maker William Banting visited an ear, nose, and throat surgeon named Dr. William Harvey who advocated no starch, sugar, beer, and potatoes. Banting, who lost forty-five pounds on a diet of lean meat, fish, vegetables, dry toast, soft-boiled eggs, and a few glasses of wine a day, eventually wrote a self-published popular booklet called *Letter on Corpulence Addressed to the Public*, which stayed in print until 2007.

1909. Upton Sinclair's Fasting Clubs. As the pioneer crusading investigative journalist and author of *The Jungle*, which took on the Chicago meatpacking industry, Upton Sinclair also wrote that periodic fasting was a cure for obesity. A craze of fasting clubs resulted.

1910. The Mega-Bite Diet. Horace Fletcher, a San Francisco art dealer, became known as "The Great Masticator" for advocating chewing each bite at least thirty-two times and turning the food into liquid gruel. "Fletcherizing" supposedly led to weight loss and less desire for that other vice—alcohol.

1918. Counting Calories. Dr. Lulu Hunt Peters' *Diet and Health, with Key to the Calories* sold two million copies and was the first bestselling diet book. The formerly chunky physician said she lost seventy pounds by counting calories—her diet was 1,200 calories a day. Peters' book included a list of food portions that contained only a hundred calories, as well as suggested target weights. Written primarily for women, Peters warned against the use of diet drugs, which often contained arsenic and mercury.

1930s. The Hollywood Eighteen-Day or Grapefruit Diet. This was a daily starvation diet of 585 calories, with worship of grapefruit at its core. It was sponsored by the fledgling citrus industry, of course. But why this fruit? The diet was based on the unsupported claim that grapefruit contains a fat-burning enzyme.

1950. DuPont Diet. After DuPont hired Dr. Alfred Pennington to find out why traditional low-calorie diets were not working, he put company executives on a high-fat, high-protein, low-carbohydrate unrestricted-calorie diet. Pennington theorized that people can metabolize fat completely but not carbohydrates; hence people get fat because they can't fully break down carbohydrates and so most of them are converted to fat.

1952. Diet pills. In 1952, 3 billion ten-milligram Dexedrine tablets were sold. The market was truck drivers and college students trying to stay alert as well as housewives hoping to shed a few pounds. Long-term use of this artificial stimulant, also known as "uppers," led to heart damage, strokes, kidney failure, and psychosis.

1963. Weight Watchers. In 1961, Jean Nidetch went to a New York City Department of Public Health obesity clinic and lost weight on a special diet. Sensing the emotional pain behind the weight gain, she later turned her diet into a women's support group and then started marketing the overall concept. In 1964, Weight Watchers did $160,000 in sales; it is now a multinational corporation with revenues of $1 billion, and 25 million grads internationally.

1967. Stillman Diet. Dr. Irwin Stillman published *Dr. Stillman's Quick Weight Loss Diet*, which advocated eating lean meat, poultry, eggs, and low-fat cheese. The theory was that proteins took more energy to digest and thus you could eat as much as you wanted and be promised weight loss of seven to fifteen pounds the first week and five pounds a week thereafter. But with little carbs, excess protein triggered ketosis, resulting in bad breath, constipation, nausea, and weakness. Stillman died of a heart attack in 1975, but not before 20 million followed in his foul footsteps.

1971. Wild Foods. As a frequent guest on *The Tonight Show*, country bumpkin Euell Gibbons looked the look, talked the talk, and walked the walk as the father of modern wild foods. Before he became the bestselling author of *Stalking the Wild Asparagus*, as well as pitchman for Post Grape Nuts cereal, he had spent a lifetime doing odd jobs that included being a cowboy, hobo, carpenter, surveyor, boat builder, beachcomber, newspaperman, school teacher, farmer, and educator. Organic groups credited him with helping to launch the burgeoning back-to-nature movement. An unexpected heart attack at the age of sixty-four returned Gibbons back to nature in Beavertown, Pennsylvania.

(continues)

1972. Atkins Diet. In 1972, Dr. Robert Atkins published one of the most influential weight-loss books of all time, *Dr. Atkins' Diet Revolution*. He informed over 15 million readers to cut back on the carbs, while devouring as many protein-laden dishes and fatty foods as they could possibly stomach. Atkins claimed that the human body would burn its own fat if it had no carbohydrates to burn first. Not everyone agreed with this hypothesis, believing that this radical diet would not work beyond a few months, and that it could cause heart problems, blocked bowels, exhaustion, and bad breath. In other words, Atkins dieters make for lousy dates and roommates. Right before he died in 2003—the seventy-two-year-old slipped on some ice near his office, conked his head, and went into a coma—the *Journal of the American Medical Association* suggested that "people on [his diet] lost weight because they consumed fewer calories, not fewer carbohydrates."

1978. The Complete Scarsdale Diet. The late Dr. Herman Tarnower's highly regimented program demanded that followers give up alcohol, butter, and oil, and subsist on seven hundred calories a day of food with high levels of protein. If you wanted to snack, you had to stick with carrots and celery. His rigid ideas and lack of coauthor credit on his popular book drove jilted lover and former headmistress Jean Harris to gun him down. Biting a bullet was not part of the Scarsdale Diet. A manslaughter conviction landed Harris in prison, where she learned to survive on starchy inmate fare.

1976. Pritikin Program. Dr. Nathan Pritikin believed that a very low-fat diet could reverse heart disease. John Travolta (he was *Saturday Night Fever* thin then) and Barbra Streisand signed up and millions followed the Pritikin diet, which consists mainly of fresh and cooked fruits and vegetables, whole grains, breads and pasta, and small amounts of lean meat, fish, and poultry, all coupled with a daily regimen of aerobic exercise. Pritikin founded the world-renowned Pritikin Longevity Center in 1976, but died nine years later at age seventy due to complications resulting from experimental drug therapy used to treat his leukemia.

1981. The Beverly Hills Diet. Judy Mazel, at age thirty, said she heard voices telling her to pull off an L.A. freeway to get some cashews at a health food store, where she somehow arrived at the realization that enzymes produced by a combination of tropical fruits such as papayas and mangos would create total digestion. All that fruit meant loose bowel movements.

1983. Jenny Craig. When dieters sign up with Jenny Craig, they learn about portion control and eat specially prepared meals until they can't stand them much longer. No salt, caffeine, tea, or alcohol. Former JC spokesperson Kirstie Alley watched her weight soar when she stopped following the program; her main weakness, she admitted in interviews, was a fondness for chocolate treats and Chinese takeout. Alley then cannily parlayed her weight issues into her own reality television show.

1990s. Weight-Loss Surgery. Stomach stapling and gastric bypasses are meant for the morbidly obese and are now performed on 25,000 patients a year for $20,000 a pop. And yes, medical complications are common. And yes, the weight often comes back.

1991. The Zone Diet. Dr. Barry Sears, co-author of the bestselling book *The Zone,* focused on the weight-gaining effects of high carbohydrate diets. He advocated a balanced diet of 40 percent carbohydrates, 30 percent protein, and 30 percent fat. Too many high-glycemic carbohydrates can cause a rise in blood sugar and the release of large amounts of insulin. He also suggested the consumption of healthy monosaturated fats like olive oil.

1993. Life Choice: Eat More, Weigh Less. Californian Dr. Dean Ornish weighed in with a more spiritual content. The Life Choice Diet purported to heal emotional pain through meditation, yoga, regular exercise, and a low-fat vegetarian diet. The average daily amount of calories ranges between 1,200 and 1,350 calories. Eat fat, stay fat, was Ornish's key message; he felt that calories from fat cause one to become fat. Critics, however, believe that this plan is too low in fat (10 percent of the total calories) and that dietary fat is important to the body.

1993. Stop the Insanity! Susan Powter, high school dropout, mother of two, and former topless dancer, claimed a 133-pound weight loss with her high fiber and low-fat diet. Powter flaunted her lack of credentials, claiming that she was "just a housewife who figured it out," and her high-decibel infomercials urged plenty of exercise. Her real fuel seemed to be anger, and the biggest lure was the premise that you could eat all you wanted. Somehow, along the way, she went bankrupt, and late-night TV viewers were finally spared her sales pitches.

1995. Sugar Busters. Several New Orleans doctors locally published a thin weight-loss volume called *Sugar Busters.* It preached that sugar and

(continues)

refined carbohydrates are bad since they raise your insulin levels, which leads to increased body fat storage—pretty much the same message as the Zone Diet, but this was more like Dieting for Dunces. When Ballantine Books republished the book nationally in 2001, it raced to the top spot on the *New York Times* bestseller nonfiction list. Mind-candy for the masses indeed. An analysis of the menu plan by the American Dietetic Association pointed out that the daily caloric yield was approximately 1,200. It was not fewer carbohydrates that contributed to weight loss but rather the very low calorie intake.

1999. NutriSystem. After it emerged from bankruptcy, NutriSystem's business model changed from marketing a liquid protein diet drink to selling portion-controlled packaged meals through the Internet and infomercials. The "send you the food" diet plan was shrewdly calculated to bypass time-consuming shopping and cooking chores. The company uses celebrities like Marie Osmond and NFL Hall of Famer Dan Marino to pitch its message of convenience and weight loss. NutriSystem relies on low-glycemic foods and vegetables to keep your hunger at bay. The downside for long-term users can be a lack of variety and freshness in the dishes.

2000. Subway Diet. Supersized 425-pound Jared Fogle, then twenty, devised his own Subway fast-food diet: a six-inch turkey sub for lunch and a foot-long veggie sub for dinner. He combined the two daily subs with walking, and his pounds melted away faster than you can say "hold the cheese." Jared lost over 240 pounds and, to his own surprise, he ended up becoming the highly visible ad pitchman for the restaurant chain. After airing its first series of Jared television commercials, Subway sales spiked 18 percent the first year.

2002. Raw Foods. Raw foodies passionately believe in their cause—that foods heated above 115°F lose much of their nutritional value and are harmful to the body. Heating food above this temperature degrades or destroys certain valuable enzymes. A typical raw food diet is comprised of fruits, vegetables, nuts, seeds, sprouted grains, and legumes. Leslie Kenton's book *Raw Energy: Eat Your Way to Radiant Health* first popularized this diet in 1984, but a 2002 *New York Times* magazine profile of raw foodism put this austere eating plan on the national mealtime map. Detractors claim that only eating raw foods can lead to a nutritional shortfall and vitamin deficiencies.

2003. South Beach Diet. A super-strict eating regimen designed by cardiologist Dr. Arthur Agatston and dietician Marie Almon, the diet's original intent was the prevention of heart disease, but word quickly spread about its weight-losing efficacy. The diet replaces bad carbs and bad fats with good carbs and good fats. It's *sayonara* to heavily refined sugars and grains as a way to eliminate food cravings. Some critics feel that the diet, while healthy-heart promoting, is difficult and challenging to follow in the early stage and can cause dehydration, electrolyte imbalance, and bad breath.

2007. Eat-Clean Diet. Give Tosca Reno complete credit for taking control of her life. In 2000, the forty-year-old Canadian mother of three was trapped in a bad marriage, seventy pounds overweight, and sick and tired of being "a fat housewife." She dumped both hubby and the excess weight by regularly exercising and eating more frequent but smaller, healthier portions—five to six small meals every two to three hours. She avoided prepackaged, over-processed refined foods, white sugar and flour, saturated and trans fats, soft drinks, and alcohol. Instead, her meals were comprised solely of complex carbs (fresh fruits, vegetables, and whole grains) and lean proteins from nuts, legumes, soy and soy-based products, low-fat dairy, or fish. The nutritional goal was to curb her appetite and keep the blood sugar and metabolism steady throughout the day. Reno's diet and lifestyle makeover plan have been widely popularized with a series of bestselling *Eat-Clean Diet* books.

2008. Flat Belly Diet. Want to lose the bulge? Then you need to eat monounsaturated fatty acids (for example, olive oil)—and all without doing any exercise or giving up many of your favorite foods! This is the women-centric message of *The Flat Belly Diet!,* a bestseller co-authored by Liz Vaccariello, editor-in-chief of *Prevention* and Cynthia Sass, the magazine's nutrition director. With single meal plans of only four hundred calories, the goal is to eat every four hours to maintain energy levels and prevent hunger. The book contains a thirty-two-day diet plan that the authors claim can help dieters lose up to fifteen pounds and several inches of belly fat, but the science says otherwise: Diets targeting specific body parts don't work, and you will never keep the weight off without regular exercise.

2009. Hydroxycut. Widely known for its before and after photos of dieters, Hydroxycut is a line of herbal weight-loss products that supposedly increases your fat-burning metabolism and reduces hunger cravings. Its primary

(continues)

ingredients include substances derived from two Indian fruits, *Garcinia cambogia* and *Gymnema sylvestre,* as well as chromium polynicotinate, caffeine, and green tea. But in May 2009, the Food and Drug Administration warned consumers to stop using the Hydroxycut line of weight-loss products, citing reports of a death due to liver failure and other instances of serious health problems, including kidney failure and heart damage.

2010. Drive-Thru Diet. Following Subway's lead with Jared, Taco Bell launched a new national marketing campaign centered around a regular customer named Christine Dougherty, a twenty-seven-year-old business consultant from Pensacola, Florida, who says that she lost fifty-four pounds by choosing "fresco items" on the drive-thru menu. It took her two years of eating at Taco Bell five to eight times a week, while exercising more, to shed the weight. The caloric difference is actually quite minimal—a Crunchy Taco Supreme clocks in at two hundred calories, and the fresco version reduces that amount by only fifty calories. Dr. Stephen Sinatra, author of *The Fast Food Diet,* told the *New York Times,* "With fast food you get the good, the bad and the ugly. If you do the Fresco Burrito Supreme Chicken, it's got an enormous amount of sodium—1,410 milligrams—which is a disaster." The PepsiCo-owned, faux-Mexican food chain makes no specific claims about its fresco tacos' fat-reducing capabilities—and explicitly states on its website that the "Drive-Thru-Diet is not a weight-loss program." But will that disclaimer have any meaning to those looking for a quick-fix diet at any of Taco Bell's 5,600 restaurants? They'd be better off while getting out of their cars when ordering. Or driving right past, not thru.

ASK THE EXPERT

"YOU ARE WHAT YOU EAT": INTERVIEW WITH DR. PHIL MAFFETONE ON THE IMPORTANCE OF NUTRITION FOR GOOD HEALTH

Dr. Phil Maffetone cuts a popular swath in multisport circles. Named coach of the year by Triathlete *magazine, he pioneered the use of the heart-rate monitor for endurance athletes, developed a comprehensive approach to individualizing diets, and introduced the concept of fat-burning and aerobic function. He helped guide professional triathlete Mark Allen to a record six Hawaii Ironman triathlon championships. Several years ago, Maffetone took a radical career detour by deciding to become a songwriter and moved to Los Angeles where he also became the wellness and nutritional guru to music mogul and producer Rick Rubin. Named by MTV as "the most important producer of the last 20 years," Rubin, then forty-four, was responsible for resurrecting Johnny Cash's late-in-life second career, and in 2007 was appointed co-chairman of Columbia Records.*

Through his close relationship with Rubin, Maffetone was introduced to Johnny Cash when the music legend was gravely ill. "My association with Johnny began soon after the death of his wife June Carter Cash," says Maffetone. *"Johnny's health had been failing in recent years and was now worsening. He had asked me for help in restoring as much health as possible and bringing back life to a man who still had a mission. However, for me, the task would be quite difficult. This was not because he was so frail but because Johnny was regularly taking more than thirty prescriptions, and at the time of his death, that number had increased to more than forty. This was clearly a problem of over prescribing, and a problem common in many elderly.*

"When I first saw Johnny, at age seventy-one, he was relegated to invalid status. He had been sent to a wheelchair, given leg braces, and prescribed special shoes that cost thousands of dollars even though he couldn't walk. In addition to the obvious difficulty this posed on a man who had been extremely active, it was restricting him from regaining any part of his health, and as he said to me more than once, it was even embarrassing. Together, we devised a strategy to improve his diet, stimulate his physical and mental capacities, and set goals, one of which was to attend the MTV Music Awards and another to record another CD. This sounded just great to Johnny, who was still actively engrossed in his life's work.

"The first day of therapy with Johnny yielded a few unsteady but pain-free steps. I utilized what I call "manual biofeedback" and other techniques that I've employed during my twenty-five years of practicing complementary medicine. Within two more days, he was able to take upward of one hundred steps. More improvements came in the following weeks. Performing these exercises barefoot was part of my approach and something Johnny liked. As he was able to venture outdoors, he wore a comfortable seven-dollar pair of flat sandals, which replaced his expensive, embarrassing footgear.

"Other therapy included sitting outside, a place he previously would only go when he had to go to a hospital or dentist, for some healthy sunrays, riding a stationary bicycle, and eventually walking up and down steps. I also assigned him music therapy—to which he joyfully agreed—to help restore other lost function in his vision and writing. Among other things, this resulted in him writing the first song in a long time, and sadly, what would be his last. In addition to these physical activities, Johnny's body chemistry needed help. He was a diabetic, but by improving his diet—finding the foods that best matched his specific needs—his blood sugar became much improved. I worked with his home chef to develop an organic kitchen and focus on real,

healthy foods, including more fruits and vegetables and proteins, while reducing refined foods and sugars.

"My approach was to improve his body function with physical activity and proper diet, and let nature take its course. Johnny became very functional at the end of his life. And, despite the prescriptions, his condition had actually improved leading up to the time of his death. So why did Johnny pass on when his health was actually improving? Maybe he died because it was his time, or as he stated to me, it was time to go see June. Certainly this issue can be debated, something I have no intention of doing."

Maffetone's overall approach regarding health and fitness, whether it's for world-class endurance athletes or bedridden music legends, follows a few basic rules: Eliminate stress, practice proper nutrition, and learn to listen to your body. (See his website www.philmaffetone.com for more information.) For those just returning to fitness after years of inactivity, injury, or illness, the Maffetone Method embraces commonsense and holistic principles that too often get ignored by those seeking an instant solution. All throughout my own return to fitness, I emailed or spoke regularly with Phil. The following interview focused on the importance of good nutrition. As Phil told me often, "You are what you eat."

Question: What is your opinion of low-fat diets?

Phil Maffetone: One of the most popular and health-damaging diet plans is the low-fat diet. The basic idea is built on the fallacy that dietary fat only causes weight gain and is detrimental to health. Some people on low-fat diets avoid fat like the plague and often develop "fat phobia." Low-fat diets are also popular among calorie-counters because they are a seemingly easy way to reduce calories. There are several problems associated with low-fat diets. They can slow metabolism, and also increase hunger through reduced satiety. People on low-fat diets also tend to eat more carbohydrates.

But the worst problems associated with low-fat diets are essential-fatty-acid imbalances, hormonal problems, and disease. Women who have been on low-fat diets are especially vulnerable to hormonal imbalances.

Q: What happens within the body by eating too many carbs?

PM: The human body is not adapted to processing large amounts of refined carbohydrates. For 99.6 percent of our existence on Earth, humans consumed diets that averaged almost 30 percent protein with about 30 percent carbohydrates and the rest fat. In addition, early humans were very active physically. Only in the last 10,000 years has this changed. The Agricultural Revolution brought a dramatic increase in carbohydrate intake, and the Industrial Revolution brought highly refined carbohydrates to the table. The intake of carbohydrates by humans has never been so dramatically high as it has been in the last hundred years. This relatively short period of significant dietary change has contributed to many problems leading to heart disease, cancer, obesity, and other diseases. This explains why, for many people, eating carbohydrate foods can prevent a higher percentage of fats from being used for energy, lead to an increase in body-fat storage, greatly diminish human performance, and negatively affect health. Yet, in the last few decades the nutritional trend has been toward a more high-carbohydrate, low-protein, and low-fat diet. Many people have a strong emotional attachment to this belief, created mainly through advertising.

Part of this problem has to do with education and society. Before the USDA changed its food pyramid, its approach advocated eating the bulk of calories from carbohydrate foods such as bread, cereal, rice, and pasta, which form the base of the pyramid. From there the pyramid suggests you eat lesser amounts of vegetables and fruits, dairy products, meats, and eggs. Lastly, small amounts of fats and sweets make up the tip of the pyramid. The food pyramid turned out to be a misguided public-information program. Following this high-carbohydrate program is equivalent to eating two cups of sugar a day.

Specific problems with the current USDA pyramid include high-glycemic carbohydrate excess, imbalances of essential fatty acids, and low levels of other nutrients. The revised food pyramid suggests that most foods consumed should be bread, cereal, rice, and pasta—between six and eleven servings a day! Most people consume carbohydrates in their processed form as white bread, including rolls, bagels, crackers, processed cereals, white rice, and white-flour pasta. These high-glycemic products are among the most harmful foods; they rapidly raise blood sugar and insulin.

Additionally, certain dietary fats are essential for good health. These include omega-6 and omega-3 fats found in certain oils such as fish and flaxseed oil. However, the current food pyramid recommends that fats be used sparingly. Even worse is the food pyramid recommendation promoting the use of margarine, which is often made of hydrogenated and partially hydrogenated fat; its consumption can disrupt the balance of fats and promote ill health and disease.

Q: What kind of healthy, balanced diet would you recommend instead?

PM: Typically most people eat too much carbohydrate foods, especially refined carbohydrates. Most people also eat too much of the wrong kinds of fats and not enough of the right kinds. Many people do not get enough protein. Almost nobody eats sufficient amounts of vegetables. Worse yet, most people are deficient in the most important nutrient of all—water. While carbohydrates form the base layer of the USDA's food pyramid, these types of foods would be nearer to the middle of my pyramid. And what's more it would not include refined items such as white bread and pasta, or processed cereal. Instead, my slimmer carbohydrate layer would be made up of fruits, legumes, 100-percent whole grains. Proteins and healthy fats would share a layer in my pyramid. Many nutritional experts are now beginning to realize that many people, including those over age fifty, do not meet protein requirements.

And while many people eat too much fat from saturated and omega-6 vegetable-oil sources, most people are deficient in heart-healthy monounsaturated fats such as those obtained from extra virgin olive oil. In addition, omega-3 fats found in fish and flaxseed oil are essential and are basically devoid from the USDA pyramid. Today it is virtually impossible for people to obtain enough of these fats from a normal diet and so vitamin supplementation is often necessary.

Q: Should one be concerned by wheat's affect on good health?

PM: Absolutely! Over the centuries, wheat has become the staple of many diets. This is very unfortunate, as wheat is a common cause of intestinal problems, allergies, and sometimes disease. Wheat also can prevent absorption of various nutrients, induce weight gain, and trigger other health problems. Some people are more sensitive to the harmful effects of wheat than others. The most practical way to tell is to note how you feel after eating wheat or products made from it, such as pasta, bread, bagels, cereal, and most snack foods, such as cookies and pretzels. The most common symptom is intestinal bloating, but symptoms may also include belching, diarrhea, or other abdominal discomfort, as well as sleepiness or reduced mental focus.

Wheat can bind important minerals such as calcium, magnesium, iron, zinc, and copper from food and prevent their absorption. This grain can also reduce digestive enzymes, especially those from the pancreas, rendering key foods—including protein and fats—less digestible. With poor fat digestion, essential fatty acids may not be absorbed, leading to problems such as reduced skin quality, inflammation, and hormonal imbalance.

Eating wheat and then exercising can trigger allergic reactions in some people. These reactions range from mild problems, like skin rash or hives, to more severe problems including anaphylaxis and occasionally even death. If you're sensitive to wheat, reducing or eliminating it from your diet is the most effective way to correct the problem and reduce the unhealthy effects.

Q: Getting enough protein is problematic for many like myself who are vegetarians, or those who are rightly scared off by non-organic processed beef, poultry, or even farm-grown salmon. Can insufficient protein lead to poor muscle recovery?

PM: Once you've adjusted to the right amount of carbohydrates for your body, and added the proper balance of fats to your diet, proper protein intake is relatively easy to determine. For example, if you find that 45 percent of your diet is carbohydrate, and 30 percent is fat, the remaining 25 percent as protein would probably be the optimal amount for you. As convenient and oversimplified as that may sound, that's how it turns out for most people. Think of it as a puzzle; once you find the first two pieces, the third one falls neatly into place. Even moderately active adults need protein to rebuild muscle tissue on a daily basis. In other words, throughout your life, your body continually makes new cells for your muscles, organs, glands, and bones, all of which require protein as a main building block. Athletes or those who exercise require even higher protein intakes. In addition to growth and repair of muscles and other tissues, some protein is used for energy.

Protein is also necessary to make natural antibodies for the immune system. Those who lose muscle mass through reduced protein consumption have reduced immunity. And those who consume inadequate protein may not get enough of certain nutrients necessary for immune function. For example, the amino acid cysteine is contained in protein foods such as whey and can improve immune function. This amino acid is necessary for the body to make its most powerful antioxidant, glutathione. Presently, many experts in this field feel the RDA of 0.8 grams of protein per kilogram of body weight is too low, with some suggesting three to four times that amount. Using the RDA values as the guideline—the minimum requirements—a significant number of people are protein-deficient. This is typical of what I saw when I was in private practice.

Some say that excess protein is dangerous. I agree; eating more protein than the body can utilize can be unhealthy. But if your body requires more than a hundred grams a day, that's not excessive, it's what your body needs. Eating the amount of protein your body requires is not a high-protein diet—it's getting your requirements! But remember, as your protein intake increases, so does your need for water, which helps eliminate the byproducts of protein through the kidneys. That's why some say that protein is a stress on the kidneys; it most certainly is if you are dehydrated. Many people are frightened away from eating enough protein by unfounded concerns, or by concerns that can be addressed simply by drinking enough water. In general,

animal foods are the best sources of complete protein, containing essential and non-essential amino acids. Overall, the highest-rated protein food is eggs, followed by whey, beef, and fish.

Q: Tell me more about eggs.

PM: Eggs are not just incredible, but what I would call the perfect food all wrapped up in one single cell. Yes, that's right, an egg is an individual cell. In this single cell, an egg contains the most complete and highest protein rating of any food, containing all essential amino acids. Two eggs contain more than twelve grams of protein, just over half in the white and the rest in the yolk. In addition, eggs also contain many essential nutrients, including significant amounts of vitamins A, D, E, B1, B2, B6, folic acid, and especially vitamin B12. Eggs also contain important minerals including calcium, magnesium, potassium, zinc, and iron. Choline and biotin, also important for energy production and stress management, are contained in large amounts in eggs. Most of these nutrients are found in the yolk of the egg. The fat in egg yolks is also nearly a perfect balance, containing mostly monounsaturated fats, and about 36 percent saturated fat. And, egg yolks contain linoleic and linolenic acids— both essential fatty acids. Eggs have almost no carbohydrate (less than one gram), making them the perfect meal or snack for the millions who are carbohydrate intolerant. Ounce per ounce, eggs are also your best food buy with hardly any waste. People love the taste of eggs, but many are concerned about eating them because of cholesterol; but the cholesterol in eggs is not something to be feared, and adding more eggs to your diet can actually decrease your risk of cardiovascular disease. While eggs are one of nature's most perfect foods, they are only as healthy as the hens that lay them, since the nutritional make-up of eggs, especially the fat, is very dependent on what the chickens eat. For this reason you should avoid run-of-the-mill grocery-store eggs that have been produced in chicken factories. Unfortunately this includes most eggs on the market. The healthiest eggs are those that come from organic, free-range hens.

Q: How about fish as a healthy protein source?

PM: Fish are a good source of protein and some also contain significant quantities of essential fatty acids, especially omega-3 fats. However, just as with other protein foods, some fish are healthier choices over others. For instance, if you are eating farm-raised salmon or other fish, your catch of the day may include antibiotics, pesticides, steroids, hormones, and artificial pigments. In addition, pollution of waterways and oceans has increased the potential dangers of eating all fish and seafood. Farm-raised salmon—which make up 95 percent of the salmon on the market and the bulk of fish purchased by consumers—are raised in aquatic pens, the undersea equivalent to cattle feedlots and chicken and hog factories. Since these fish are raised in confined, crowded, and unsanitary conditions, the threat of disease and parasites is great. To combat disease and parasites, some fish farmers add antibiotics to salmon feed, and treat the salmon and their pens with pesticides. Some salmon are also treated with steroids to make the fish sterile, and growth hormones to speed them to market size and reduce production costs. In addition, since farm-raised salmon do not naturally eat crustaceans, which makes the flesh pink or orange, salmon growers often feed color additive to pigment the flesh. If you choose to eat fish, it is best to buy wild-caught fish. In general, avoid seafood that includes the so-called bottom feeders, those fish and other sea species that eat from the ocean's floor, where the potential for consuming toxic material is highest. This is especially true for those species that feed close to shore. Flounder, sole, catfish, and crab are some examples of foods to avoid eating regularly. Oysters, clams, mussels, and scallops are also sources of potential pollutants. Clams are perhaps the worst seafood to eat, especially when raw.

Q: What are some tips for healthy cooking?

PM: How you cook your food can be just as important as how you select it, since even the healthiest ingredients can be destroyed through improper kitchen practices. The biggest problems are overcooking, using too-high heat, and overheating certain types of oils. The worst method for cooking anything is deep-fat or high-heat frying, especially using vegetable oils. While many healthy foods may be lightly sautéed in butter or olive oil, deep-frying overheats the oil and can be deadly. In addition, the high heat may destroy other nutrients in the food itself. Meats, fish, and poultry can be grilled, roasted, or cooked in their own juices with sea salt. Less oil or butter is needed for pan-cooking meats because they often contain sufficient fats. Additionally, most people overcook meats and destroy some of the valuable nutrients. It's also important to not use too-high heat for too long. For instance, when grilling a steak, remember to turn it every minute or so to prevent the excess formation of chemicals that can be harmful to your health. This goes for vegetables as well—if using high heat, remember to turn them often. Vegetables can be steamed, stir-fried in olive oil, roasted, baked, or grilled. Cook vegetables minimally to avoid destroying vitamins and phytonutrients—they also taste better when not overcooked. If boiling or steaming, use as little water as possible to avoid leaching of nutrients. Eggs can be soft-or hard-boiled, or cooked sunny-side up, over-easy, poached, or lightly scrambled. Use low heat to avoid "tough" or rubbery eggs.

If using oils for cooking, it's important to remember that all oils contain varying ratios of monounsaturated, saturated, and polyunsaturated fats. Monounsaturated and saturated fats are not sensitive to heat, but polyunsaturated oils are very prone to oxidizing when exposed to heat. This oxidation produces free radicals, which are related to many health problems. Butter is one of the safest oils for cooking, as it contains a low amount of polyunsaturated fat, only 4 percent. Olive oil can also be used for cooking but its polyunsaturated content is a little higher at 9 percent. This is still much better than, for instance, peanut oil, which contains 33 percent polyunsaturated, or worse yet, safflower oil at 77 percent. As strange as it may sound, another fat you may consider is lard, which contrary to popular belief may be a healthier choice for cooking than butter.

Q: How rigorous should one be in terms of counting calories, especially when one is trying to lose weight while exercising more often?

PM: The calorie-counting theory is based on the idea that the calories in the food you eat, minus the calories you burn for energy, equal the weight you lose or gain. The idea is that balancing energy intake and output results in stable weight. If you eat fewer calories than you burn, you lose weight. But if you take in more than you use, you gain. The problem with this theory is that it does not work as simply as it sounds for most people. The reason is that everyone has a different metabolism, so food is utilized differently. In addition to the number of calories taken in, the amount of carbohydrates, fats, and proteins eaten also significantly affects how the body burns energy. So to use only the total calories as a guide may be misleading. Calorie counting does not consider where those calories come from, the quality of food, or the balance of macronutrients. Calorie counting almost always results in eating less food. When you eat less food, especially less fat, which contains the most calories, one of the significant results can be that your metabolism slows down and you can eventually store more fat, despite your initial (short-term) weight loss. That's why so many people eventually gain more weight and fat after being on a calorie-restricted diet. The best way to speed up metabolism is to eat the amount of good-quality food you need each day. Other factors that increase the metabolism are dietary fats and aerobic exercise.

Q: You mentioned earlier the importance of water in one's diet. Can you elaborate?

PM: About 60 percent of the body is made up of water, with different areas accounting for various percentages. For example, about 80 percent of your blood, heart, lungs, and kidneys is water; your muscles, brain, intestines, and spleen are about 75 percent. Even areas like your bones, which are 22 percent water, and fat stores, 10 percent water, require a specific level that, if not maintained, results in poor function. Therefore, pure, clean water is the most essential of all nutrients. You can live for weeks without consuming food. But go more than a couple days without water and your very survival will be at risk. Proper intake of water is so vital to optimal function that a deficiency of less than 1 percent can begin producing signs and symptoms of dysfunction. Slightly more dehydration can produce significant health problems. The key to maintaining proper hydration is to drink plenty of water throughout the day. Water is the key ingredient in maintaining chemical balance in your body. This includes transporting nutrients to the cells, maintaining the function of blood, and eliminating wastes from the lungs, skin, and colon. Water also plays a major role in hormone regulation and balancing acid-base levels. One of the most significant functions of water is to regulate the balance of potassium (on the inside of the cell) and sodium (outside the cell). This balance is most important in nerve and muscle cells, producing nervous-system function and muscle contraction. More importantly, water is like your car's radiator, cooling the reactions that create heat in your body. For example, muscle contraction, digestion, and the processing of nutrients produce large amounts of heat, which must be cooled by water. If this regulation did not occur effectively, your temperature would rise to a level that would destroy your enzymes and other protein-based substances, and you would die. The water literally absorbs the excess heat and carries it to the skin, where it is dissipated through evaporation and other means.

Thirst is how most people remember to drink water. But this is a problem, since the brain's thirst center does not send a message until you are almost 2 percent dehydrated. By then, you already have problems associated with dehydration. The kidneys, however, respond to dehydration much sooner than the brain. In this case, if your urine output is diminished, you're beginning to dehydrate. What is meant by diminished? If you're not urinating at least six to eight times each day, you may be dehydrated. In addition, the color of your urine also tells how well you're hydrated. Your urine should be clear. If your urine is yellow, it probably means you need more water.

Here are some general everyday guidelines to preventing dehydration: Drink water throughout the day, with smaller amounts every couple hours rather than two or three large doses a day; avoid carbonated water as your main source because the carbonation

may cause intestinal distress; remember that the average person may need about three quarts of water each day; and avoid chlorinated and fluoridated water. In addition, get used to drinking water as your main source of liquid. While it's true you obtain some of your water needs through food and other beverages, most should come from plain water, consumed between meals. Certain drinks such as coffee, tea, soda, and alcohol can actually increase your need for water. So don't count these beverages as part of your water intake.

Q: What is your recommendation for taking vitamin supplements?

PM: We should be concerned about taking synthetic vitamins and other unnatural nutrients, because published research in the last few years concludes two important things: First, synthetic and other unnatural nutrients are mostly ineffective in preventing disease. Second, these chemicals may be dangerous to your health—some have been shown to increase the risk of death! This research should not be confused with the health-promoting roles of the natural versions of these nutrients found in natural foods. Decades of research and thousands of studies demonstrate the effectiveness of these natural food nutrients in successfully preventing and treating disease.

Q: Finally, for those trying to get or stay fit, what else do you suggest they eat?

PM: The necessary nutrients for a person coming back to a healthy lifestyle. It starts with the best diet. Supplements that may be most important include EPA from fish oil. This will help control recovery from workouts because it regulates the inflammatory and anti-inflammatory system. For many people, a protein supplement may also be important if the diet does not supply that: Egg powder and whey powder are the best protein powders, and useful in shakes. And stay hydrated!

⑪

ALL ABOUT BODY FAT

Before You Step on the Scale . . .

Why are the final ten pounds so difficult to lose? After six months of faithfully adhering to a consistent exercise program—running, biking, strength training—I was proud of my newly reformed body. Muscles had returned from hibernation. Chest, arms, legs. All good. The only region still requiring improvement was the gut. Sure, it had shrunk considerably. Instead of being able to grab Pillsbury Doughboy fistfuls of flab, all I could comfortably squeeze was a several-inch layer of fat.

I had lost weight—perhaps ten or fifteen pounds, though I refused to step on a scale because that's one daily obsession I could live without. Because muscles are denser and weigh more than fat, the results would have been imprecise. Yet wouldn't it have been grand to have eliminated the belly excess, to take it out into the execution yard and kill it once and for all? Fat chance! As long as my brain and taste buds strongly requested comforting carbs and sweets—bagels, fruit juice, brownies, cookies—the belly would forever balk at entering witness protection. If I wanted to acquire a slim breadbasket, I needed to ease up on bread and baked treats. Until that happened, a persistent layer of tummy lard would protrude, like Elvis's jutting lower lip.

To learn more about why most men like myself have trouble losing the extra baggage around their midsection, I did a Google search and came across "7 Things You Didn't Know About Fat," on the Canadian website Askmen.com. Topping the list was this eye-opener: "When you consume more calories than you burn off, fat cells in the body swell to as much as six times their minimum size. Everyone has fat cells; they begin to form and take shape before birth. Around the age of 16, the body's fat cells are mature, and then lifestyle and genes play a role in gaining or losing weight as you age."

But are love handles really such a bad thing? In her book, *Rethinking Thin, New York Times,* health and science reporter Gina Kolata, who spent two years researching America's fixation with dieting, eventually concluded that it's not a lack of willpower that keeps us above our idealized target weight.

> Scientists know that animals and people have a range of weights that they can comfortably sustain. Each person's range is different but any weight much above or below a person's range is almost impossible to maintain. No matter what the diet and no matter how hard they try, most people will not be able to lose a lot of weight and keep it off. They can lose a lot of weight and keep it off briefly, they can lose some weight and keep it off for a longer time, they can learn to control their eating, and they can learn the joy of regular exercise. . . . Those who do the best tend to be those who learn to gauge portions and calories and to keep the house as free as possible of food they cannot resist. The effort, the *lifelong* effort, can be rewarding. But true thinness is likely to elude them.

Kolata's right. True thinness was never encoded in my DNA. For appetite suppression, however, I kept the cupboards and fridge free of high-caloric temptations like Ben and Jerry's, gourmet potato chips, and Pepperidge Farm cookies. Plus, if I happened to eat a lot one day, I would back off the next. Following a strenuous workout, my appetite, stoked by a revved-up metabolism, usually kicked into high gear and this feeling would last for twenty-four or forty-eight hours. These periods generated some concern—eating when not hungry.

Is it futile to fight the battle of the bulge? My own history proved that this war could be successfully waged. But I was twenty-five years old and training twelve to fifteen hours a week for the Hawaii Ironman. Belly went bye-bye. But that kind of workout intensity seemed impractical and undesirable in my early fifties. Yet I discovered, much to my satisfaction, that through regular exercise and carefully monitoring what I ate (at least 75 percent of the time), the paunch had downsized.

WHAT IS YOUR BODY SHAPE?

When someone says, "I am out of shape" or "I want to get in shape," what do they really mean by these two common phrases? And what is their baseline or starting point, and how is it measured? Fitness is subjective and resists easy categorization; the term has multiple meanings for different sports. Sumo wrestlers and pixie gymnasts train several hours every day—and both are fit.

Fitness variables include stress, diet, injury frequency, activity, mental outlook, and of course, genetics. You rarely see pro cyclists over six feet tall in the Tour de France because they often get pulverized in the mountains by the smaller, lighter riders who have a higher strength-to-weight ratio. (Tour champions Miguel Indurain and Eddy Merckx were notable exceptions.) Or look at the small-boned, rail-thin Kenyans, Moroccans, and Ethiopians who dominate long-distance running. On the other hand, sports like football and basketball reward athletes who won a different kind of chromosomal lottery jackpot.

Success as an athlete obviously derives from a combination of natural ability, training, and body build. But is there a possible link between body shape and personality? Why do we equate fat with jolly, and mean with thin? (Or at least Hollywood and novelists do.)

In the 1950s and '60s, Columbia University psychology professor W. H. Sheldon conducted studies to prove that body shape could predict intelligence and personality. Sheldon divided the human structure into three types: (skinny) ectomorphs, (muscular) mesomorphs, and (pudgy) endomorphs. He assigned personality traits to each body type: endomorphs were relatively happy, easygoing, and lazy; ectomorphs were brainy, nervous, insecure, and high-strung; mesomorphs exuded strength, vitality, and self-confidence. He based this typology on an interesting pool of subjects. He was able to convince college administrators at Ivy League and Seven Sisters colleges to require entering freshman to remove their clothes for anonymous "nude posture" photographs.

Critics attacked Sheldon's methodology as pseudo-science with disturbing hints of Nazi-era "master-race" eugenics. But while his behaviorist theories eventually became discredited by other researchers, his taxonomic labels somehow survived and entered our vocabulary to describe body shapes and the sports they typically attract.

An endomorph has these somatic characteristics: pear-shaped body, wide hips and shoulders, and plenty of fat on the body, upper arms, and thighs. He or she usually has short arms and legs, as well as a large amount of mass on a shorter than normal frame. Sports of pure strength, like weightlifting, are well-suited to endomorphs. Their extra body weight can make it difficult to perform sustained weight-bearing aerobic activities such as running or cycling. They typically gain weight and muscle mass easily and rapidly lose conditioning if training stops. If you are endomorphic and your lighter cycling pals are always beating you on hill climbs, don't despair. Challenge them to arm-wrestling afterward.

A mesomorph has a wedge-shaped body, wide broad shoulders, muscled arms and legs, narrow hips, and has a minimum amount of fat. A mesomorphic individual excels in strength, agility, and speed sports like sprinting, tennis, and basketball. It's the ideal body type for most jocks. They can gain muscle and strength easily, which makes them superb athletes in any sport. Their physiology favorably responds to cardiovascular and resistance training.

An ectomorph has narrow shoulders and hips, small chest and abdomen, thin arms and legs, and little body fat. This individual typically dominates endurance sports like long-distance running, in part, because the smaller body surface area is better suited to managing body temperature. And there's less weight to move. You also see a lot of ectomorphs in pro cycling: powerfully chiseled legs and a scrawny upper body, since excess muscularity means extra weight on the bike. If you are an ectomoph, you might want to go to the gym to work on your upper body, but don't expect to grow massive muscles overnight.

Your body shape won't predict how fit you can become, but it will help you know why certain types excel in specific sports. When Frank Shorter (five feet, ten inches) won the Olympic gold medal in the marathon in 1972, he weighed just 135 pounds with an alarmingly low body fat of 2.2 percent. In his running heyday, Bill Rodgers, an inch shorter and seven pounds lighter, was unstoppable and never gained weight despite a crazy diet—he ate cold pizza topped with mayonnaise for breakfast. At the time, it was thought that a runner could never be too thin. That is still true at the world-class level. For elite runners, excess weight means slower times. But for the rest of the running population, a few extra pounds are perfectly okay. Your goals are much different from those of professional athletes and elite competitors who have been training hard for years. Don't let your own body type or size discourage you from doing what you enjoy.

WEIGHTY MATTERS: MEASURING BODY FAT

The Body Mass Index, or BMI, has long been considered the standard for measuring the amount of fat in a person's body. The Body Mass Index is defined as the individual's body weight (in pounds) divided by the square root of the height. For example, if you are five-ten and 185 pounds, your BMI is approximately 23. Generally, a BMI of 25 or above indicates a person is overweight; 30 or above indicates obesity. A person with a higher BMI is considered to be at greater risk for heart disease, diabetes, and other weight-related problems.

BMI Categories:

- Underweight = <18.5
- Normal weight = 18.5–24.9
- Overweight = 25–29.9
- Obesity = BMI of 30 or greater

. . .

The U.S. National Health and Nutrition Examination Survey of 1994 indicated that 59 percent of American men and 49 percent of women have BMIs over 25. Extreme or morbid obesity—a BMI of 40 or more—was found in 2 percent of the men and 4 percent of the women. There are differing medical opinions regarding the threshold for being underweight in females, with the range between 18.5 to 20 percent. Below these numbers and the person can be suffering from a severe eating disorder like anorexia.

In 1998, the National Institutes of Health brought U.S. definitions more into line with World Health Organization guidelines, lowering the overweight cut-off from BMI 27.8 to BMI 25. This had the effect of redefining approximately 30 million Americans, previously "technically healthy" to "technically overweight." It also recommended lowering the overweight threshold for South East Asian body types to around BMI 23.

The BMI was created in the mid-1800s by the Belgian social scientist Adolphe Quetelet, who was investigating "social physics," or methods of comparing different populations. But according to new research, the BMI may not be as accurate as originally conceived. A research group from Michigan State University and Saginaw Valley State University measured the BMI of more than four hundred college students—some of whom were athletes and some not—and found that in most cases the student's BMI did not accurately reflect his or her percentage of body fat. While BMI can be calculated quickly and without expensive lab equipment, BMI categories fail to take into account factors such as frame size and muscle mass. Also, BMI is often used as an imprecise substitute for percent body fat.

"The overlying issue is the same criteria for BMI are used across the board," said Joshua Ode, a PhD student in the MSU Department of Kinesiology and an assistant professor of kinesiology at Saginaw Valley. "Whether you're an athlete or a 75-year-old man, all the same cut points are used. A previous study of NFL football players found that a large percentage of them—around 60 percent—were considered obese. But when you look at an athlete like that, you see that in many cases he is not obese. Many athletes have huge BMIs because of muscle mass, but in many cases are not fat."

The U.S. Army stopped using the BMI because of too many overweight recruits—27.1 percent of all eighteen-year-olds who applied to join the military in 2006 were overweight. So the Army changed its fat policy to make it more lenient. New recruits are now measured based upon a statistical table that lists an appropriate weight for any given height. This table is more forgiving than the definition of "overweight" employed by the Centers for Disease Control and Prevention. To measure body-fat percentage, the Army conducts a series of measurements involving height and the circumferences of the abdomen, neck, and—for women—hips. Once a soldier makes weight, he or she is then required to take a physical-fitness test.

Some researchers think that waist size is a better indicator than BMI in determining one's overall health. *New York Times* health correspondent Tara Parker-Pope reported that "many studies of both men and women now suggest that it is not how much you weigh but where you carry your weight that matters most to your health. In the March 2008 issue of the *Journal of Clinical Epidemiology,* a study showed that body mass index is the 'poorest' indicator of cardiovascular health, and that waist size is a much better way to determine, for both sexes, who is at a higher risk for hypertension, [type 2] diabetes and elevated cholesterol."

What is the optimum waist size? According to Parker-Pope, "Studies suggest that health risks begin to increase when a woman's waist reaches 31.5 inches and her risk jumps substantially once her waist expands to 35 inches or more. For men, risk starts to climb at 37 inches, but it becomes a bigger worry once their waists reach or exceed 40 inches."

The *International Journal of Obesity* also reported that waist-to-height ratio, especially for younger people, might be a better indicator of overall health risks. "Put simply," the *Journal* wrote, "your waist should be less than half your height."

According to a survey conducted by the National Center for Health Statistics, the average waist size for a white American male was 39 inches. For a white American woman, the average waist size was 36.5 inches. But as obesity continues to trend upward, these figures will increase as well. Perhaps America should take its health cues from Japan where waist size is taken seriously. In 2008, government officials were concerned that the average adult was gaining weight due to less exercise and an adoption of the fattening Western diet. So they instituted a nationwide slimming campaign of measuring waistlines. The state-prescribed limit for male waistlines is 33.5 inches and for female waistlines it's 35.4 inches. Companies and local governments are legally required to measure the waistlines of anyone between the ages of forty and seventy-four as part of their annual medical checkups. Those who fail to make the weight limit are required to undergo mandatory health education and nutritional counseling. By trimming widening waistlines, Japan hopes to reduce health-care costs and lower the risk of diabetes and heart attacks. The downside, say critics, is that many Japanese go on harmful crash diets and take drugs to slough off weight right before testing.

For those who want to measure their body fat with scientific precision, there are home-based products that offer body composition analysis. The Bioelectrical Impedance Analysis (BIA), for example, uses a small electronic pulse that passes through muscle and fat at different rates. However, its measurements may be thrown off by how hydrated you are and how much you've eaten. Users are encouraged to establish a baseline measurement and repeat testing under consistent conditions over time to detect changes.

Skin-fold calipers are also used to determine body-fat percentages but are not recommended unless performed by a trained tester. While calipers have a 98 percent accuracy, in the hands of someone who doesn't know the correct placement on the body and the right amount of skin-fold to capture, this method of fat measurement is fairly worthless.

The most accurate body fat test is underwater or hydrostatic weighing. After first being weighed on dry land, the subject is seated in a chair, asked to expel all air in the lungs, and is then submerged in a tank with a weighted belt and nose clip. The individual must remain motionless while the underwater weight is recorded. Because fat is buoyant, body density and body fat percentage can be calculated by using a mathematical formula based on the Archimedes principle of water displacement. This test is time-consuming and usually only available at university research institutions.

But if science, skin-fold calipers, BMI, or the bathroom scale aren't your thing, you can always reach down and see how much of your belly you can grab. It's what I often did.

IS THERE AN IDEAL BODY FAT PERCENTAGE?

The ideal weight and optimal fat-to-lean ratio varies considerably for men and women and by age. The average adult body fat is 15 to 18 percent for men and 22 to 25 percent for women. The minimum percent of body fat considered safe for good health is 5 percent for males and 12 percent for females. Athletes tend to be at the low end due to their increased lean weight, or muscle mass. Women athletes with low body fat can experience low energy, weak bones, and menstrual disorders.

Body Fat Percentage for the Average Population

Age	Up to 30	30–50	50+
Females	14–21%	15–23%	16–25%
Males	9–15%	11–17%	12–19%

Average Body Fat Percentage of Athletes

Sport	Male	Female
Runners	5–10%	10–16%
Elite marathon runners	3–5%	9–12%
Baseball	12–15%	12–18%
Basketball	6–12%	20–27%
Shot putters	16–20%	20–28%
Bodybuilding	5–8%	10–15%
Skiing (cross-country)	7–12%	16–22%
Cycling	5–15%	15–20%
Swimming	9–12%	14–24%
Triathlon	5–12%	10–15%
Volleyball	11–14%	16–25%

Athletes who reduce their body fat by extreme measures—fasting or vomiting—are at great health risk because this can lead to decreased performance, injury, and illness. Nutrient deficiencies and electrolyte imbalances from low food intake can contribute to stress fractures, disease, inflammation, and dehydration. In fact, there is a dietary correlation between world-class athleticism and illness. As part of its 2004 Athens Olympics coverage, the *New York Times* reported that while athletes normally have very little body fat, sickness was "foremost in the athletes' minds." According to Professor Peter Fricker, the medical director of the Australian Olympic team in Athens, "There's no doubt that athletes are playing hard enough to suppress immune defenses. The normal population in Australia expects to get between three and four upper respiratory infections each year. But if you look at groups of elite athletes, about 15 percent of those athletes can have six or seven or more, up to even 11 or 12. They seem to get more vulnerable as they train harder."

If you had 0 percent body fat, you'd be dead. If you have 1 or 2 percent, you probably wouldn't even have sufficient energy to turn this page. Fat is a primary source of fuel for the body. Fat stores also serve an important function in hormone metabolism and tissue protection. Bodybuilders, for example, like aiming for a body fat percentage between 2 percent and 4 percent during competition, and to arrive at this dangerously low level, they often become severely dehydrated, have little pep, and risk damaging their joints and organs, which require an adequate amount of protective fat.

In his memoir, *Muscle: Confession of an Unlikely Bodybuilder*, Southern Californian bodybuilder Sam Fussell described the starvation diet that he put himself through one week prior to a top amateur championship. *Muscle* reads more like a dark, cautionary tale about why you shouldn't abuse your body in pursuit of "perfection." The health consequences are far too grim. With his body fat hovering around 8 percent, Fussell felt that his abdominal section looked bloated. "I wasn't really shredded, so with six days to go, I needed to lose at least 10 pounds of fat." To acquire the "shrink-wrapped" look, he lowered his daily food intake to just over six hundred calories, reducing his carbs by 90 percent. He dined on two egg whites for breakfast, 3.5 ounces of boiled chicken and one broccoli stalk for lunch, 3.5 ounces of halibut and ½ cup of spinach for a second lunch, and 3.5 ounces of halibut for dinner.

By mid-week, he had so little energy that he was forced to stop training altogether. All he could manage to do was rest indoors and "lay exhaustively on the sofa," while shivering underneath several layers of clothes and a winter parka. "I was freezing all the time. My diet had seen to that. I no longer had enough body fat to protect me from the outside world. It was 70 degrees Fahrenheit outside; to me, it felt like 40." Too weak to even practice posing moves, he used a chair as a walker to move about the room, "pausing every few feet to suck in great gasps of air."

While Fussell ultimately achieved the shredded look for the competition—"with no fat, my abdominal section was utterly 'sliced'"—he could hardly wait for the contest to end so he could increase his caloric intake and indulge in regular fare like oatmeal for breakfast. He also looked forward to another luxury—toothpaste. "I hadn't used my Crest for the last six weeks. It was off-limits. The sodium content was simply too high."

Just as too little body fat can lead to severe physiological complications, too much body fat is also harmful. "Fat cells behave differently in different parts of the body," says Askmen.com. "Belly fat increases the likelihood of bad cholesterol (LDL), triggers extra fat in the bloodstream, and raises blood pressure and blood sugar levels." It gets worse! "Fat cells within the abdomen are metabolically more active than fat cells located in other areas of the body. They release more fatty acids, which can lead to diabetes, coronary artery disease, stroke, and certain cancers. Abdominal fat cells may also affect the healthy functioning of the liver."

For men with over 25 percent fat and women over 32 percent fat, there is a dramatic correlation with illness and disease. "Overweight" athletes place an extra burden on their joints, bones, and heart by carting around excess pounds. Try this experiment: Get a ten-pound bag of flour or rice and put it inside your fanny pack and go for a short run. Notice how uncomfortable running now seems. Add another ten-pound bag. You're running with twenty extra pounds. It takes a lot more effort to go the same distance or speed.

One way to run faster is to turn that fat into muscle. David Costill, an exercise physiologist at the Ball State University Human Performance Lab, compared two runners whose body fat differed by 8 percent. Running at the same intensity, he found that the leaner person could run up to thirty seconds faster per mile than his heavier counterpart.

This is, obviously, food for thought, especially among those who are performance-minded. Serious cyclists and triathletes are obsessive about small weight differences in equipment, buying costly components only if it means saving a few ounces or grams in weight; but they can opt for a cheaper, simpler alternative by dropping a few pounds.

To summarize, a single, optimal, narrow range of body fat percentage simply does not exist across the board for athletes. More importantly, some people might feel and perform better at a higher or lower body fat percentage than others in their same age category.

FIT VS. FAT?

We tend to think that all thin people are "fit." But these beanpoles might never go to the gym or run a 10K, and could actually have chronic health issues. Conversely, when we hear or read about the thousands of mildly overweight men and women running in 10Ks and marathons, we think to ourselves, "They can't all be fit!" But they are!

In a recent study based on national health data collected from 5,440 adults, a surprising number of overweight people were found to be metabolically healthy, while large numbers of slim people had some of the same health problems often associated with obesity. The study, appearing in the *Archives of Internal Medicine*, tracked height, weight, blood pressure, "good" cholesterol, triglycerides, and blood sugar. About 24 percent of the thin adults showed unhealthy levels for at least two of these risk factors. *It's healthier to be fit and fat than be thin and inactive.* As the study's author, Mary Fran Sowers, a University of Michigan obesity researcher, told the Associated Press, "The results show that stereotypes about body size can be misleading, and that even less voluptuous people can have risk factors commonly associated with obesity."

"If you want to know who's going to die, know their fitness level," says Dr. Steven Blair, professor of exercise science, epidemiology, and biostatistics at the University of South Carolina. His research provided empirical evidence that "obese individuals who are fit have a death rate one half that of normal-weight people who are not fit."

Even the President's Council on Physical Fitness and Sports agrees with this assessment. In 2000, the Council reported, "Active obese individuals actually have lower morbidity and mortality than normal weight individuals who are sedentary . . . the health risks of obesity are largely controlled if a person is physically active and physically fit."

WHY SOME OF US CAN'T LOSE WEIGHT

Having a normal amount of body fat is good for you. You can still have washboard abs with body fat between 7 and 12 percent. But if you are constantly concerned about your body fat percentage, it makes better sense instead to fixate on something else, such as eating the right kind of foods or getting regular exercise. In fact, recent studies found that certain aspects of one's body composition are genetic, especially how and where you store fat, and can be one of the reasons why dieting doesn't often work for many people.

Researchers at the Karolinska Institute in Sweden found that no amount of dieting will alter the number of fat-hoarding cells in our bodies. According to their findings, published in the science journal *Nature*, the number of fat cells is predetermined during adolescence and stays the same later in life. By testing patients who lost huge amounts of weight, they found little change in fat cell numbers. Lead researcher Dr. Kirsty Spalding said, "It explains why it's so difficult to lose weight and to keep it off—those fat cells aren't going anywhere, and they're crying out for more."

Fad diets, with little or no exercise, can cause a person to lose as much muscle tissue as fat. Once you leave the diet, you will most likely return to your pre-diet weight but you will now have more fat and less lean muscle. And with a higher percentage of body fat, you have a lower metabolism—and that means you are burning fewer calories throughout the day. It's one of the reasons why daily regular exercise for up to an hour is beneficial because it trains your metabolism to burn more fat during the other twenty-three hours of the day. Dieting *without* exercise will not keep the weight off.

THE NATIONAL WEIGHT CONTROL REGISTRY

Yet all is not lost for chronic dieters with fluctuating weight issues. Obesity experts have long maintained that it didn't matter what kind of diet people followed to lose weight initially, but preventing its unwanted return was another matter. To break this maddening cycle, a solution exists for the overweight and it has nothing to do with diet pills or costly surgery. And it's free. Just sign up and join the National Weight Control Registry, which was founded in 1994 by Rena Wing, PhD, from Brown Medical School, and James O. Hill, PhD, from the University of Colorado. The Registry tracks over 5,000 individuals who have lost significant amounts of weight and kept it off for long periods of time. To be eligible for inclusion in the Registry, you need to have shed a minimum of thirty pounds and not gained it back for at least three years. According to the website, "detailed questionnaires and annual follow-up surveys are used to examine the behavioral and psychological characteristics of weight maintainers, as well as the strategies [people] use to maintain their weight losses."

Eighty percent of the Registry's volunteers are women and 20 percent are men. The average woman is forty-five years of age and weighs 145 pounds, while the average man is forty-nine years of age and weighs 190 pounds. Registry members have lost an average of sixty-six pounds and kept it off for 5.5 years.

So what is the secret of their success? According to the Registry's data, 45 percent of participants lost the weight on their own and the other 55 percent lost weight with the help of some type of diet program. But two numbers stand out: 98 percent of Registry participants report that they modified their food intake, such as eating reduced portion sizes, and 94 percent increased their physical activity, with the most frequently reported form of activity listed as walking. It's working out that makes a significant impact on weight-loss results: 90 percent exercise, on average, about one hour per day. Surprisingly, most volunteers don't adhere to a low-carb diet since it is difficult to sustain for long periods. But keeping track of calories is something they almost all do. If a Registry member backslides and has several days of overeating, he or she will typically eat less in the days that follow. These mini-weight swings are much more manageable than experiencing a large weight gain that is then followed by yet another crash diet—which perpetuates the cycle.

WHAT ABOUT THOSE INFOMERCIAL WEIGHT-LOSS SHORTCUTS?

There is simply no free lunch when it comes to body-toning weight loss. Gastric bypass surgery is expensive and risky. The same with liposuction since it can cause lethal blood clots to form inside your body. But how about those ab-sculpting electric gizmos constantly being promoted on late-night infomercials? Do they actually work as advertised?

These portable padded devices fit snugly around your waist, then a switch is thrown and an electrical current supposedly zaps the fat right away within minutes. The company pitchmen and pitchwomen proudly claim that you won't have to break a sweat or do any crunches and sit-ups. Nothing is required but to sit back and watch more television. As one brand promised, "You will lose up to four inches in thirty days, guaranteed!"

Since the FDA maintains that ab belts are "medical devices," they are required to be "safe and effective" before they can be sold to the public. Yet few companies do. As Jim Brown, editor of the *Georgia Tech Sports Medicine and Performance Newsletter* and a health education PhD, explained in an interview with Slate.com, electric stimulation can "help you make the kind of tiny improvements that matter when your muscle, because of some injury, is so weak that you'd have to start out with baby steps." But, he says, "If there's nothing wrong with you—other than that you're lazy—in order get a real benefit, you'd have to put so much current through your body that you'd get fried."

Another ab-belt study by the University of Wisconsin, La Crosse, concluded that "test subjects using the belts experienced no significant changes in weight, body-fat percentage, strength or overall experience. Not only was electric muscle stimulation ineffective, but it was also painful."

THE ULTIMATE BODY TRANSFORMATION

By changing our bodies with good nutrition and regular exercise, each of us has the power to become shape-shifters, not unlike an action hero undergoing a metamorphosis from ordinary to superhuman. Consider the extreme body makeover of former chowhound extraordinaire Joe Decker who, in 2000, was named "the world's fittest man" by *Guinness World Records.* To earn this prestigious honor, the personal trainer from Washington, D.C., went on a twenty-four-hour exercise binge in which he biked a hundred miles, ran ten miles, hiked ten miles, power walked five miles, kayaked six miles, swam two miles, NordicTracked ten miles, rowed ten miles, then cranked out 3,000 ab crunches, 1,100 push-ups, 1,100 jumping jacks, 1,000 leg lifts, and weight lifted 278,540 pounds.

It wasn't always this way with Joe. He used to be fat, not fit. He grew up on a farm in central Illinois. After suffering a leg injury in high school football, he abandoned sports and took up extreme eating. When he signed up to join the U.S. Army, he not only failed the mandatory physical fitness test but was put in a special "fat boy" group that limited what he could eat. The army whipped him into shape. He left the service after three years to attend college and then later became a bartender in New Orleans, where his eating habits really went south. He describes this gluttonous, backsliding period in his workout and training book, *The World's Fittest You*: "I became the best partier in New Orleans. They called me the 'Mess' because I had no self-control or discipline. I'd get off work, have a few drinks, then start partying for three straight days. During these partying binges, I hardly ate. I'd sleep for a day or so and then eat nothing but pizza, hamburgers, and French fries. Emotionally, I had become dependent on overeating [and] bingeing on alcohol. A typical dinner for me was thirty or forty chicken wings at Hooters, washed down with a few pitchers of beer."

Decker eventually realized that his "lifestyle was killing [his] body from the inside out." So he decided to make drastic changes in his diet and behavior. He substituted water for booze, and low-fat home cooking replaced greasy fried foods. He began working out at home with an old weight set from Walmart, pull-up bar, and some worn-out running shoes. He started walking, then gradually built his way up to slow jogging. A milestone was finishing a 5K. But Decker didn't stop there. He entered longer races, moving up to a marathon and then a fifty-miler. His next race was a 135-mile slog through Death Valley in the summer. Hooked on ultrarunning, he competed in a number of hundred-mile running races in North America. His *Guinness* feat was literally a fitting exclamation mark to his remarkable transition from obese party animal to heavily muscled endurance athlete. "I was ready for a change," writes Decker, who maintains that everyone has this capability, "no matter what your shape, size, or fitness level."

Decker is correct. We all have the potential to change. Consider the well-known example of Oprah. The media juggernaut has bounced from fat to fit to fat over the years. Looking at her current plus-size physique, it's hard to believe that she once ran a 4:29:20 marathon in 1994. Her televised confession in 2009 that she was unable to control her eating was a brave, gutsy thing to do. By publicly disclosing her embarrassment regarding her weight gain, she said that she wanted to do something about it, enjoining all of America to get healthy and fit. Despite the best intentions of a personal trainer and private chef, Oprah admitted to feeling like a diet failure. But she is simply the most highly visible example of someone who has battled lifelong weight concerns. Perhaps there are deep-rooted psychological issues affecting her eating, but for all her wealth, Oprah is like so many of us who have an uneasy, complex relationship regarding diet and regular exercise. But don't beat yourself up if you temporarily slip up and start eating poorly or engage in little or no physical activity for a few days or weeks. It's never too late to reverse course. Just don't wait too long before taking positive action. Otherwise, you will be surprised how fast the years race by, like calendar pages flipping forward in a 1940s movie. Like it did with me for a decade.

As I made my own return to fitness, I experienced positive, gradual changes to my body shape. Yet I considered myself a work in progress, and this provided further motivation to continue regularly working out. My quest lacked an expiration date. Instead, it was an open-ended promise to take better care of my body—and that all those years of apathy and neglect were like a bad dream.

Regardless of your own body shape, or your efforts to modify it through dieting, the most important thing is to stay active. "If the height/weight charts say you are five pounds too heavy, or even 50 pounds or more too heavy, it is of little or no consequence health-wise—as long as you are physically fit," says exercise physiologist Dr. Steven Blair. "On the other hand, if you are a couch potato, being thin provides absolutely no assurance of good health, and does nothing to increase your chances of living a long life."

So keep moving.

FAT TO FIT: DAVE LOW BECAME HAWAII'S "FITTEST CEO OF THE YEAR" BY LOSING SEVENTY-FIVE POUNDS AND TAKING UP RUNNING AND TRIATHLON

As a Wall Street and San Francisco financial trader and consultant, Dave Low, forty-six, dealt with business stress by overeating. He swelled up to 225 pounds, which made the five-nine Low look like a human bowling ball made of fat. Today, Low is a slimmed-down, svelte 150 pounds, who loves competing in triathlons and marathons, and is the managing director of a boutique investment firm in Honolulu. In 2007, he won Hawaii's "Fittest CEO" competition and appeared as a swimsuit model for Triathlete *magazine. The following year, he clocked a respectable 11:53 at the Hawaii Ironman Triathlon. Yet within two months of that race, he packed on another twenty pounds and stopped exercising. "After the Ironman, I took a trip around the world with my then-girlfriend, says Low, "and that meant giving up training for eating." Now single, Low worked himself back into triathlon shape. Here's the story behind his yo-yoing physical transformations—one that is marked by an ongoing duel pitting self-esteem issues against incredible self-discipline.*

I love to eat. My favorite foods are pizza, chips, chocolate, Chinese, beer, fast food burgers, and *all-I-can-eat* buffets. Coupled with an extreme personality disorder that is probably Obsessive Compulsive Disorder, my level of fitness and weight over the years looks like the volatile stock chart of a publicly traded company. My weight has fluctuated all over the scale, from 150 to 225 pounds. It has also reflected my relationships with women and stress from work. If I were comfortable in love or work, I would let my body go in terms of fitness and diet, and my weight would balloon up. But if things went wrong with my personal life or if I were stressed at work, I would then fall into a deep depression causing me to lose my appetite. I'd start working out again and the pounds would fall off. However, as I have gotten older and realized how unhealthy this weight volatility is, I decided that I wanted to have better control of my level of fitness and weight. I was determined to remain around 150 pounds. It is simply too hard emotionally and physically to start the cycle all over again.

As a kid, I was a mediocre athlete. In high school, I was a running back in football, wrestled at 145 pounds, and played ice hockey and baseball. Pound for pound, the wrestling coach said that I was the strongest on the team. In college, my very active social life made my fitness plummet. Though I dabbled in collegiate intramurals, it was only sporadic. Ultimate Frisbee was one of my activities, and it would normally be a great cardio workout, except that our team would take extensive breaks and just hang out to drink beer.

After I started working as a financial consultant at Lehman Brothers on Wall Street, it became stressful dealing with coworkers and management all day long. There were also highly demanding and wealthy clients. When I moved out to San Francisco in 1989 to work at Bear Stearns, I did a lot of windsurfing in the San Francisco Bay to vent some of the stress, but being a seasonal sport, I would balloon up during the non-windy period from October to April.

In 2001, after cashing out and witnessing the market implosion, I retired to Maui and invested in real estate. I got fat and lazy, and then went back up to 225 pounds. It was easy to do when lunch or dinner often consisted of a twelve-piece bucket meal from KFC, or three Big Macs, two large fries, and six-piece Chicken McNuggets, or two medium plain pizzas.

I knew that people were making fun of me behind my back. No one likes being called a "fat slob." I got motivated to lose weight and get in shape.

From my days as a high school and college wrestler, I knew how to restrict food intake for rapid weight loss. So while my body adjusted to eating less food, don't think I stopped craving a pepperoni pizza or two pints of Häagen-Dazs.

(continues)

I also knew that with a heavy cardio regimen, the weight knew plummet if I started running. But I had always hated running. So like a Wall Street analyst, I started doing research. I bought a bunch of running books and subscribed to fitness magazines in order to learn about training and healthy lifestyle strategies. Setting goals in everything I do was important in order to achieve financial success. Regaining my high school physique became my new job.

My first "run" was a slow jog/walk down the hill from my house and back up. It was about a quarter mile. It was painful. With every sluggish step and with sweat soaking my XXL T-shirt, I could feel my flab jiggle and undulate like Jell-O. The next day, my legs were sore, but I managed to eke out a half-mile.

It became a challenge to exceed the previous week's mileage, seeing how far I could push my body. The first week, it was five miles. Second week, eight miles. Third week, ten miles. I started running in the pineapple fields of Haleakala.

I loved seeing how the excess weight melted off and I noticed the results in the mirror. These results fueled my passion to get cut even more and start eating healthier foods—salads, brown rice, vegetables, avocados, skinless chicken, fish (salmon, ahi), fruit (bananas, mangos, papaya), and nuts (cashews, macadamias, almonds).

With every pound burned off, I regained pride in myself and eventually lost the self-loathing. As my waistline decreased, my positive energy, outlook, and focus increased. In three months, I lost about seventy-five pounds.

Five months after I had started running, I entered my first marathon and finished Honolulu in 3:17! I later ran in the world's hardest ultra—the infamous thirty-eight-mile Run to the Sun that goes from sea level all the way up to the summit of 10,000-foot Mount Haleakala. I placed fourteenth overall with a 7:17.

I then moved to Honolulu and, sadly, the self-destructive cycle of weight gain repeated itself because I got complacent and lazy. I started overeating. I was burned-out on running. I got fat again and went up to 215 pounds. So in 2005, I bought my first expensive bike—a Cervelo Soloist. I joined a local triathlon group to train for my first triathlon with distances of 660 meter swim, 30 K bike, and 4.5 mile run. I placed fifth in my age group. I was hooked by the sport! Swimming and cycling enhanced my training so I wouldn't get bored with running. I began to work out with weights three times a week.

It was great to be crowned "Hawaii's Fittest CEO." The competition was sponsored by 24 Hour Fitness, Pfizer, *Hawaii Business* magazine, and ESPN. The test included: life cycle (heart rate measured for endurance); shark skill (pro football test measuring dexterity); maximum push-ups in one minute (upper-body strength); and plank pose (core strength) for maximum time. Out of thousands of CEOs, the field was narrowed to the twenty-two finalists, and then I won. I beat guys much younger than me.

Yet I know that my love of food will always be a problem. I've learned to live with it. There's always the risk of reverting back to obesity. It's like being a recovered alcoholic or ex–drug addict. The addiction to food is overpowering to someone like myself. That's why I continue to work out ten or more hours per week.

Going from fat-to-fit more than once has made me aware that I can never let down my guard when it comes to diet and regular exercise. I know that I am an extreme example of this constant struggle experienced by so many others.

⑫

THE CLIMB BACK TO FITNESS WAS LIKE RUNNING UP A MOUNTAIN

Making it to the top of Mount Tam had been my fitness goal since Day One—6.5 uphill miles, immediately followed by 6.5 downhill miles and back home. A half-marathon actually, with 2,000 feet of elevation gain. This *idée fixe* provided the impetus and motivation to run in the cold and rain, or even at night with a flashlight. But when at the beginning you can only jog for two lung-sapping, leg-weakening minutes, the notion of eventually running uphill for that duration seemed insane and utterly ludicrous. It'd be like venturing off into the Alaska wilderness armed with a small hatchet, several books, and a ratty sleeping bag. We know how that tragic story ended for the young idealistic man.

Yet I needed a larger-than-life target to measure my fitness return, something grand, intimidating, and emotionally resonant. The Ultimate Fitness Report Card. Because getting back in shape *was* like running up a mountain. I was just fortunate to have one right in my own backyard.

Mount Tam was both the metaphor and real-life challenge of my athletic journey. At the peak's visitors area, there's a drinking fountain. Only after my lips tasted its cold water could I be granted the honor and privilege of genuine success.

I knew what had to be done. But was I up to the physical challenge? What if I failed to complete the run to the summit? What then? Would I feel like such a failure that I would stop working out and retreat into my former slothful ways? This solo Tam run was going to be one of the most important races of my life.

LESSONS LEARNED

Quite often during runs and bike rides, I would reflect upon what this struggle to become fit really meant. Not in terms of time spent working out or ground covered. But deeper, existential, life-defining concerns—because I still had difficulty confronting the painful truth that for years I had let myself slide backward and downward into a deep hole of inactivity precipitated by my own derelict choosing. Even in my current fit state, I wanted to further beat myself up for allowing this to happen—but then, to my satisfaction, these negative thoughts would soon disappear on their own accord. It's as if harmful self-criticism had nowhere to go so long as I stayed physically active.

Anyway, here are several lessons I learned along the way that shaped my odyssey, and hopefully, they will help you define yours as well.

It Always Takes Longer Than Expected, So Be Patient and Think Long Term. Since it took a decade to become unspeakably unfit, it made no sense to expect quick results. Eliminate the several false starts and temporary setbacks, my return-to-fitness campaign required six solid months of regularly working out, averaging between five and seven hours a week.

Don't Dwell in the Past. I continually felt the urge to compare my current training with long-ago Ironman triathlon workouts. Instead it was imperative to stay focused in the present, even reminding myself out loud: "You are twice the age. Now shut up and be grateful that you ran and biked five times this week!"

Even a Small Amount of Regular Exercise Makes a Big Difference. Just five minutes of basic calisthenics—push-ups, sit-ups, squats, lunges—only three times a week is better than going completely slack. Do the math: Five minutes multiplied by three equals fifteen minutes; do this every week for a year, we're now up to 780 minutes, or thirteen hours of exercise that can burn up to 6,500 calories, or just under two pounds of fat. A decade of this minimalist regimen will keep you twenty pounds lighter, while maintaining some muscle tone. Yet I went nearly 4,000 days without working out. So even during my rest or easy days, I made sure that I did some exercise, even if it were only a ten- or fifteen-minute walk, Here's another example: Go for a one-mile walk just three times a week. In one year, you will have traveled 156 miles. Now continue this same walking regimen for seven years. Total ground covered will be 1,092 miles, which is the actual distance from New York City to Miami. But what if someone said to you, "Hey, I want you to walk from New York to Florida"? You'd consider the ambulatory request nonsensical.

Listen to Your Body. A heart-rate monitor was an indispensable biofeed-back tool in terms of helping me incrementally build an aerobic base without stepping into the tar pit of overtraining—and risk possible injury. I also main-tained a training log whose filled-in cells offered concrete, empirical evidence of athletic progress. Both the monitor and diary reined in an impulsive ten-dency to overdo things, thereby ensuring a "look-how-tough-I-am!" zeal was continually kept in check.

Progress from Small Achievable Goals to Successively Larger Ones. It had been humiliating to be so woefully out of shape. Not being able to jog more than two hundred yards, or do more than one chin-up, or thirty push-ups had a demoralizing effect. Yet as my running increased from five minutes to ten, then fifteen, then for a half hour after several months of steady effort, or when I made it up to five chin-ups, I embraced these minor accomplishments with quiet pride. Then imagine the jubilation I felt when one morning I cranked out 130 consecutive push-ups and twenty-five chin-ups (both personal records), or on another occasion ran a hilly eight miles to begin the day. It also felt nice to have my resting heart rate drop from 72 to 59.

Redemption. I got a second chance with my return-to-fitness body as it successfully bounced back from all the prior abuse, bouts of illness, and lengthy inattention. I forgot how resilient and forgiving the body can become through better nutrition and regular exercise. The human body, in most cases, is able to right the wrongs that were cruelly waged against it.

(continues)

> **Workouts Actually Get Easier Over Time!** Surprise, Surprise.
> **Looking Ahead.** With my fitness and conditioning base in place, I could now confidently look ahead to many years of health-affirming exercise. It was liberating to start dreaming again—dreaming about pursuing new endorphin-inspired adventures that would inevitably lead to other tributaries of athletic desire—all determined on my own terms.

February 12, 2010. A Friday. I had marked this date on my workout calendar eight weeks earlier as the big day. For the previous two months, I had gone on two-hour runs at least once a week. I then tapered the final week by running only fifteen minutes on two separate days. The enforced slowdown left me feeling antsy.

After a breakfast of coffee, glass of orange juice, and buttered bagel, I was ready. It was around nine thirty in the morning and raining hard when I began the run, but I hoped that the weather would improve at the higher elevations. I wore black Lycra tights, rain pants, adventure racing floppy hat, fleece jersey, yellow rain jacket, and my dependable, minimalist, thin-soled Nike Frees without insoles. Stashed inside my fanny pack were a small plastic water bottle, six GU energy gels (Chocolate Outrage), and some cash if I needed to take a cab home. I decided not to wear a heart-rate monitor because this run was solely between Tam and me. *Mano a* mountain.

Since I was starting from my cottage, and not at the bottom of Railroad Grade, I had a 500-foot elevation head start from sea level, but this advantage was offset by this: The first half-mile straight up Summit Avenue marked the steepest part of the entire run. Think San Francisco's most vertical streets, but set among redwoods, oak, and eucalypti.

I went at a slow, consistent pace, with shortened leg stride and relaxed breathing and heart rate. Summit ended at Fern Canyon Road, and there was another half-mile of paved road before the fire road trail began. I had run this section many times before. So the familiarity helped calm my jittery nerves as I began to have serious doubts about this run. I already wanted to quit! I did my best to tamp down the anxiety, and soldiered onward, or rather upward into the soup.

The rain had lessened into a thick mist. The trail was muddy and slick, requiring extra care where I placed my feet. Clouds socked in the entire mountain. Visibility was limited to several hundred yards. I could barely see past whichever switchback I was on. It felt like I was running through an endlessly serpentine tunnel, following a wet brown ribbon, with green vegetation lining both sides, and everything else swallowed up in a dull chiaroscuro of grays and whites. No sweeping views of the Bay Area in this walled-off environment.

There was a degree of monotony in what I was doing. One sodden shoe in front of the other. Each step taking me infinitesimally closer to the peak that indifferently loomed somewhere high above in the distance and hidden in the clouds. At least, I wasn't able to look up and see how far I needed to go. These rain clouds had a silver lining.

The mountain was desolate. I only saw one cyclist and two hikers. But all the rain had brought Tam musically to life. Small creeks thundered with rushing water, creating a mighty celebratory roar as the white frothy tumult fought past rocks and fallen tree branches. Here was nature showing off all her resplendent glory. I felt magically blessed and inspired each time I passed one of these forceful, splashing streams cutting down the mountain's heavily forested flanks.

I reached West Point Inn in fairly good shape. It too was deserted. Little more than two miles remained, all a steady uphill grind. My legs were starting to feel tired and a general fatigue had settled in, so I squeezed a GU into my mouth—and repeated this every thirty minutes. These hundred-calorie serial injections staved off a bonk. My running pace stayed consistent, moderate, relaxed, aerobic. I began to overheat, but right after I took a ninety-second clothing break and stuffed my jacket into the pack, the rain picked up. Without stopping, I put the jacket back on.

I was both surprised and pleased to realize how easy this run was turning out. I had expected an epic death run in the mud and rain, along with pain, and mind-bending suffering for the last half. How very wrong this portent proved to be. All my training had been adequate preparation for this challenge.

Railroad Grade ended at Ridgecrest Boulevard. With less than a half-mile remaining before reaching East Peak's visitors center, I resisted the urge to run faster and go anaerobic, because I needed to conserve energy for the descent. Which also meant that I knew I would make it to the top. Victory hovered tantalizing close.

But awaiting me at the summit was something that I never envisioned during all those months of training, when I used to frequently fantasize about what it would feel like to arrive here after a ten-year absence.

There was nothing. Just a claustrophobic carapace of dense clouds and rain-slicked asphalt. Visibility was at best a hundred yards. The summit lookout observation hut was hidden inside the misty maw. The snack bar was shuttered closed. The large parking lot was empty. There was nobody. I was all alone. And instead of soaring high with triumphant exaltation, I felt the finish to be anticlimactic. Maybe even disappointing.

Of the hardy, privileged few who successfully climb a mountain like Everest, the overwhelming desire is to rejoice in the moment as long as possible. But Everest adventurers must not linger at the top, because it's life threatening at that altitude and they must reach their last base camp before dark or risk probable death.

Mount Tam is just over 2,500 feet—nowhere close to being classified a "death zone." Yet I felt like I was marooned in a numb zone—an emotionally blank state. I was puzzled by this odd, void-like sensation. After two and a half hours of running, I certainly didn't feel like I was standing on top of the world.

Even the drinking fountain came as a letdown; its water gave off an unpleasant metallic tang. I fed a wet dollar bill into the Coke vending machine—it was the only thing alive up here—and guzzled down half the can, then tossed it into a recycling bin, and decided to head back downhill. Total elapsed time on the cold, lonely windswept summit: five minutes.

It was only after several downhill miles, with my quads taking the percussive brunt of the long, punishing descent, that my mood began to brighten and lift, and when the exact nature of what I had just accomplished gradually began to emerge. It struck me that I had been looking at everything the wrong way. Of course there wasn't some cinematic ending once I made it to the peak. That kind of finale would have been false and delusional, a fiction commonly made palpable by Hollywood's insistence on manufactured drama and artifice.

The real mountain, all along—and present even when I had been unfit all those years—had been a seemingly unmovable mental barrier. While my training had successfully enabled me to make it to the top of Tam, this physical feat simply marked the new beginning of a return to fitness. In the future, there will be other mountains—figuratively and literally—that will demand running up. The true test is whether I will continue to build upon what I had already achieved. Honestly, I don't know yet. But I have no intention of ever getting out of shape again.

RECOMMENDED READING

Bingham, John. *The Courage to Start: A Guide to Running for Your Life.* (Fireside, 1999).

Cheever, Ben. *Strides: Running Through History with an Unlikely Athlete.* (Rodale, 2007).

Crowley, Chris and Henry S. Lodge, MD. *Younger Next Year: Live Strong, Fit, and Sexy—Until You're 80 and Beyond.* (Workman, 2007).

Friel, Joe. *The Cyclist's Training Bible.* (VeloPress, 2003).

Galloway, Jeff. *Marathon:You Can Do It!* (Shelter Publications, 2010).

Karnazes, Dean. *Ultramarathon Man: Confessions of an All-Night Runner.* (Tarcher, 2005).

Kolata, Gina. *Ultimate Fitness: The Quest for Truth about Health and Fitness.* (Farrar, Straus and Giroux, 2003).

Kolata, Gina. *Rethinking Thin: The New Science of Weight Loss—and the Myths and Realities of Dieting.* (Farrar, Straus and Giroux, 2007).

Maffetone, Philip. *In Fitness and In Health, 5th Edition.* (BookSurge, 2009).

Maffetone, Philip. *The Big Book of Endurance Training and Racing.* (Skyhorse, 2010.

McDougall, Christopher. *Born to Run: A Hidden Tribe, Superathletes, and the Greatest Race the World Has Never Seen.* (Knopf, 2009).

Murakami, Haruki. *What I Talk About When I Talk About Running.* (Vintage International, 2009).

Pollan, Michael. *In Defense of Food: An Eater's Manifesto.* (Penguin, 2009).

Solomon, Andrew. *The Noonday Demon: An Atlas of Depression.* (Scribner, 2001).

Wallack, Roy. *Run for Life: The Breakthrough Plan for Fast Times, Fewer Injuries, and Spectacular Lifelong Fitness.* (Skyhorse, 2009).

INDEX